Practical
Radiotherapy

Practical Radiotherapy

Physics and Equipment

Third Edition

Edited by

PAM CHERRY MSC TDCR

Senior Lecturer, School of Health Sciences,
Division of Midwifery & Radiography,
City, University of London, London, UK

ANGELA M. DUXBURY MSC FCR TDCR

Emeritus Professor of Therapeutic Radiography,
Sheffield Hallam University, Sheffield, UK

WILEY Blackwell

Registered Office(s)
John Wiley & Sons, Inc., 111 River Street, Hoboken, NJ 07030, USA
John Wiley & Sons Ltd, The Atrium, Southern Gate, Chichester, West Sussex, PO19 8SQ, UK

Editorial Office
9600 Garsington Road, Oxford, OX4 2DQ, UK

For details of our global editorial offices, customer services, and more information about Wiley products visit us at www.wiley.com.

Wiley also publishes its books in a variety of electronic formats and by print-on-demand. Some content that appears in standard print versions of this book may not be available in other formats.

Library of Congress Cataloging-in-Publication Data
Names: Cherry, Pam, editor. | Duxbury, Angela, editor.
Title: Practical radiotherapy : physics and equipment / edited by Pam Cherry, Professor Angela M. Duxbury.
Description: 3rd edition. | Hoboken, NJ : Wiley-Blackwell, 2020. | Includes bibliographical references and index.
Identifiers: LCCN 2019024040 | ISBN 9781119512622 (paperback) | ISBN 9781119512721 (adobe pdf) | ISBN 9781119512745 (epub)
Subjects: | MESH: Radiotherapy–methods | Radiotherapy–instrumentation | Health Physics | Radiation, Ionizing
Classification: LCC RM849 | NLM WN 250 | DDC 615.8/42–dc23
LC record available at https://lccn.loc.gov/2019024040

Cover Design: Wiley
Cover Image: © Mark_Kostich/Shutterstock

Set in 10/12pt STIX Two Text by SPi Global, Pondicherry, India
Printed and bound in Singapore by Markono Print Media Pte Ltd

10 9 8 7 6 5 4 3 2 1

Contents

LIST OF CONTRIBUTORS   vii
FOREWORD   ix
PREFACE   xi
ACKNOWLEDGEMENT OF PREVIOUS CONTRIBUTORS   xiii

1   Introduction to Radiotherapy Practice   1
    Angela M. Duxbury and Anne J. Jessop

2   Mathematical Skills Relevant for Radiotherapy Physics,
    Atomic Structure, and Radioactivity   7
    Erica Chivers

3   X-ray Production   23
    Dora Meikle and Gareth Hill

4   Radiation Detection and Measurement   35
    Jan Chianese and Fiona Chamberlain

5   X-ray Interactions with Matter   47
    Kathryn Cooke

6   Principles of Imaging Modalities   59
    Caroline Wright, Katheryn Churcher, and Jonathan McConnell

7   Principles of Treatment Accuracy and Reproducibility   111
    Nick White and Helen P. White

8   Radiotherapy Beam Production   145
    David Flinton

9   Principles and Practice of Treatment Planning   195
    Pete Bridge

10 Image-guided Radiotherapy and Treatment Verification   221
    Cath Holborn and Ros Perry

11 Quality Management in Radiotherapy   241
    Renee Steel

12 Radiation Protection   255
    Pete Bridge

13 The Use of Radionuclides in Molecular Imaging and
    Molecular Radiotherapy   267
    Paul Shepherd OBE and Terri Gilleece

14 Brachytherapy Physics and Equipment   289
    Gemma Burke

INDEX   305

List of Contributors

Pete Bridge PhD MSc BSc Hons BSc SFHEA
Senior Lecturer in Radiotherapy, School of Health Sciences, Liverpool University, Liverpool, England, UK

Gemma Burke MSc PgC, BSc Hons FHEA
Senior Lecturer, Faculty of Health and Wellbeing, Sheffield Hallam University, Sheffield, England, UK

Fiona Chamberlain MA MIPEM RSci PgCert (HE) FHEA
Senior Lecturer, Faculty of Health and Social Care, University of West of England, Bristol, England, UK

Jan Chianese MSc TDCR
Head of Radiotherapy, Faculty of Health and Social Care, University of West of England, Bristol, England, UK

Erica Chivers MA MSc HDCR(T) CertISM PgCert
Lecturer in Radiotherapy, School of Health Care Sciences, Cardiff University, Cardiff, Wales, UK

Katheryn Churcher MSc BSc
Advanced Radiation Therapist, Adem Crosby Centre, Sunshine Coast University Hospital, Birtinya, Australia

Kathryn Cooke MSc DCR(T)
Former Senior Lecturer in Radiotherapy, Faculty of Health and Wellbeing, Sheffield Hallam University, Sheffield, England, UK

Angela M. Duxbury FCR MSc TDCR
Emeritus Professor of Therapeutic Radiography, Faculty of Health and Wellbeing, Sheffield Hallam University, Sheffield, England, UK

David Flinton EdD MSc BSc Hons DCR(T) SFHEA
Associate Dean Education (Quality and Student Experience), School of Health Sciences, City, University of London, London, England, UK

Terri Gilleece MSc DCR(T) PgD(NucMed) PgCHEP FHEA
Lecturer in Radiotherapy, School of Health Sciences, Ulster University, Belfast, Northern Ireland, UK

Gareth Hill MSc BSc Hons FHEA
Head of Therapeutic Radiography, Radiotherapy Department, Ninewells Hospital, NHS Tayside, Dundee, Scotland, UK

Cath Holborn MSc PgCert BSc Hons
Senior Lecturer, Faculty of Health and Wellbeing, Sheffield Hallam University, Sheffield, England, UK

Anne J. Jessop MSc BA Hons DCR(T)
Former Senior Lecturer, Faculty of Health and Wellbeing, Sheffield Hallam University, Sheffield, England, UK

Jonathan McConnell FCR PhD MSc PgCLTHE PgCRII BSc DCR (R) CoR Accred
Consultant Reporting Radiographer, Queen Elizabeth University Hospital, Glasgow, Scotland, UK

Dora Meikle MSc BSc
Former Lecturer in Therapeutic Radiography, Queen Margaret University, Edinburgh, Scotland, UK

Ros Perry PDip BSc
Professional Lead Radiotherapy Treatment, Radiotherapy Centre, Ipswich Hospital, Ipswich, England, UK

Paul Shepherd OBE MSc DCR(T)
Head of Radiotherapy, School of Health
Sciences, Ulster University, Belfast,
Northern Ireland, UK

Renee Steel PGDip, BHSc(RT)
Radiotherapy Quality Manager,
Cancer Centre, Guy's and St Thomas' NHS
Foundation Trust, London,
England, UK

**Helen P. White Med PgDip(ClinOnc)
BSc Hons FHEA**
Head of Department –Radiography
(Therapeutic, Diagnostic and Ultrasound),
Division of Radiography, Birmingham City
University, Birmingham, England, UK

**Nick White MSc BSc Hons BSc
Hons BA SFHEA**
Senior Lecturer in Radiotherapy, Department
of Radiography, Birmingham City University,
Birmingham, England, UK

**Caroline Wright PhD MSc PGCE BSc
(Hons) DCR(T)**
Associate Professor-Radiation Therapy,
Department of Medical Imaging and
Radiation Sciences, Monash University,
Melbourne, Australia

Foreword

The field of radiotherapy is a very rapidly changing and developing one. When I first started in the field in the early 1980s I was counseled on more than one occasion to the effect that radiotherapy was a dying trade and I would be best advised to find a different specialism within medical physics. In practice the opposite has proved to be the case. The last few decades have seen incredible developments in treatment delivery and imaging and the process shows no sign of running out of steam anytime soon. Online image-guided radiotherapy with IMRT (intensity-modulated radiotherapy) or VMAT (volumetric arc radiotherapy) is now in routine clinical use in every department; a situation which would have been unthinkable only 10 years ago. There are also some very exciting developments just over the horizon including the MR (magnetic resonance)-LinAc and proton beam therapy.

With this background a new edition of this book is very timely and the editors and authors have taken the opportunity to bring the text right up to date. The new edition builds upon its predecessors with the first eight chapters providing an introduction to the basic scientific principles of radiotherapy. These are followed by chapters on modern treatment planning, image-guided radiotherapy, and verification. There are also chapters on the role of quality management in radiotherapy and the principles of radiation protection. The final two chapters cover the fields of molecular radiotherapy and brachytherapy.

As with the previous editions the book is primarily intended as a comprehensive resource for student therapy radiographers but it will serve as a very useful introductory text for medical physicists, oncologists, nurses, and other radiotherapy professionals.

Andrew Poynter, CPhys, FIPEM

Preface

The primary aim of the first edition of this book in 1998 was to produce a much needed 'reader friendly' up-to-date text on all aspects of radiotherapy physics and equipment, as many find this a challenging subject. This theme continued into the second edition, published in 2009. Radiotherapy is a fast-changing, dynamic profession driven by continual advances in technology and so in the last 10 years much has changed. We have sought feedback from academic and clinical staff as well as students, and in keeping with the previous editions, each chapter in this book has been updated and written by contributors in both academic and specialist clinical fields.

As with the previous editions, this book is written primarily for the undergraduate therapeutic radiographer but it is hoped that it will be a useful reference book for medical physicists, nurses, and clinical oncologists alike. Whilst comprehensive in its own right, the book is also intended to complement other texts currently on the market in order to provide a complete and up-to-date understanding of radiotherapy physics and equipment.

Pam Cherry and Angela M. Duxbury
London and Sheffield 2019

Acknowledgement of Previous Contributors

The editors and authors of chapters would like to recognize the following authors who have contributed to chapter content that has been published in the previous edition.

Dr Christopher M. Bragg, Dr John Conway, Dr Elaine Ryan, David Duncan, Dr Tony Flynn, Elizabeth Miles, Alan Needham, and Dr Bruce Thomadsen.

CHAPTER 1

Introduction to Radiotherapy Practice

Angela M. Duxbury and Anne J. Jessop

Aim

The aim of this chapter is to provide a brief introduction and overview of the principles of current radiotherapy practice and to act as a guide for the other chapters presented in this text.

1.1 Introduction

Venturing into the field of radiotherapy physics is one of the most interesting and exciting aspects of radiotherapy practice. The rapid developments in computer and technological innovation continue to impact on changing and advancing practice.

1.2 What Is Radiotherapy?

Radiotherapy is a speciality that uses high-energy ionising radiations to treat cancer and some benign conditions. In 2015, there were 359 960 new cases and 163 444 deaths recorded from cancer in the UK. Over 50% of cancer patients survive for 10 years or more and 27% of cancer patients will receive radiotherapy [1].

The intention of radiotherapy can be curative, known as radical treatment, or it can be given to reduce the symptoms of cancer, known as palliative treatment. It can be used as a treatment modality on its own and/or combined with cytotoxic (cell toxic) chemotherapy and/or surgery.

Radiotherapy delivered from outside the body is known as external beam radiotherapy, using X-rays (photons) or electrons from a linear accelerator machine or protons produced by a cyclotron (see Chapter 8). It can also be delivered from within the body as internal radiotherapy, by placing sealed radioactive sources directly into tissue or cavities, known as brachytherapy (see Chapter 14), or by administering a fluid/capsule of radioactive material, an unsealed radionuclide, into the body (see Chapter 13).

Once a patient has been referred for radiotherapy, the aim of the treatment process is to undertake detailed imaging to visualise the tumour (see Chapter 6) followed by complex treatment planning (see Chapter 9) to ensure that accurate treatment delivery is achieved (see Chapters 7 and 10) in order to

Practical Radiotherapy: Physics and Equipment, Third Edition. Edited by Pam Cherry and Angela M. Duxbury.
© 2020 John Wiley & Sons Ltd. Published 2020 by John Wiley & Sons Ltd.

deliver a radiation dose that can destroy the tumour whilst minimising the dose to the surrounding healthy organs.

Radiation absorbed dose (see Chapter 4) is measured in Grays (Gy) and the therapeutic radiation dose administered varies depending upon: the curative intent of therapy; the radio sensitivity of the tumour; the volume of tissue to be treated; and the site of the tumour. To enhance the effectiveness of treatment and to allow normal tissue time to recover from the radiation injury, treatment is given in fractions over a specific period of time, for example, 45 Gy in 15 fractions over 21 days.

A combination of skill, accuracy, and complex technology are dedicated to delivering safe and effective radiotherapy in order to achieve the two competing goals – high tumour control and few treatment complications. Treatment failure to meet the treatment intent can result in the patient's clinical outcome being seriously affected in both the short and the long term. Many things can go wrong in this multi-step/person/department process and error prevention and quality management (see Chapter 11) is essential to minimise catastrophic consequences for the patient [2].

1.3 Working with Ionising Radiations

The nature of ionising radiations means that they cannot be detected by the human senses therefore, in order to be able to detect and accurately measure the amount of radiation being delivered several different methods of radiation detection and measurements have been developed (see Chapter 4).

Working with ionising radiations is safe providing a raft of measures are adopted and followed. Safe working practices are a legal requirement and follow the Ionising Radiation Legislation, the Ionising Radiation (Medical Exposure) Regulations (IR[ME]R) 2017 (IR[ME]R NI 2018) [3] (see Chapter 12).

1.4 How Radiotherapy Works

There are several interaction processes that occur when ionising radiation interacts with matter. These depend on the nature and energy of the primary radiation beam and the structure of the medium through which the radiation beam passes. For X-ray energies utilised in radiotherapy, these interaction processes are described in Chapter 5.

High-energy radiation used for radiotherapy treatment can be lethal to both normal and abnormal tissue; this is due to either direct or indirect actions occurring when the radiation is delivered to the target volume within the patient.

Direct action occurs when the cells within the normal tissue or tumour are in the mitosis phase of the cell cycle and the DNA strands are exposed as part of the cell division. The X-rays strike the DNA chain and cause either a single or double strand break; the result of a double strand break is cell death, however there is a possibility that following a single strand break cells can go on to have further cell divisions.

Indirect action occurs when the radiation ionises the water molecules within the cells and is not directly linked with the cell cycle. When the water molecule is ionised this leaves a H_2 element and an O element to restabilise and both these ions seek a partner to join with; some will become a water molecule again (H_2O) with no resultant effect. Other ions will combine as H_2O_2 (hydrogen peroxide), which is toxic to the cells' internal environment, with the resultant effect that cell death will occur.

Both of these actions are based on the probability that radiation will come into contact with either the cell during mitosis, or water molecules along their path through the patient. As the radiation cannot discriminate between normal and tumour cells there is the likelihood that normal tissue will be affected, along with the tumour, as it is impossible to clearly define the tumour boundary. As a result of any tissue damage, cells in the vicinity will be stimulated to move into the mitosis phase of the cell cycle to repair the damage; this is true for both normal and tumour cells. With all of the tumour cells being included within the treatment volume during a course of radical treatment, the aim is to deliver a tumouricidal dose of radiation to the tumour whilst sparing as much normal tissue as possible; this is known as tumour control probability (TCP) and normal tissue complication probability (NTCP).

1.5 Radiotherapy Beam Production

Most commonly used radiotherapy beams are electronically produced using a linear accelerator; a machine consisting of a discrete number of components that function together to accelerate electrons before they strike the target to then produce high-energy photons (X-rays). These X-rays are then directed towards the patient and subsequently the tumour through a series of collimation systems. Electron beams are produced using the same principles of accelerating electrons, however the target is removed from the exit window and the electron beam is then used to treat the patient (see Chapter 8).

Proton beams are produced using either a cyclotron or a synchrotron to accelerate the particles by magnetically pulling them through a circular path until the protons reach their maximum speed. The advantage of using a proton beam is that the Bragg Peak depth can be manipulated to more closely match the tumour shape by modulating the beam as it emerges from the head of the machine (see Chapter 8).

Kilovoltage machines were historically the main provider of external beam radiotherapy, until the introduction of Cobalt-60 units, and subsequently linear accelerators; both of which have the capability to improve the delivery of dose at depth. However, kilovoltage machines (see Chapter 8) still have an important role within radiotherapy when treating superficial tumours, especially smaller lesions or lesions close to the eye.

1.6 Treatment Delivery and Planning

Radiotherapy can be delivered in different ways using a linear accelerator to deliver high energy X-rays (photons) or electrons; the majority of patients prescribed radiotherapy will receive their treatment by external photon beams. Treatment can be given with a curative intent, known as radical treatment, or to relieve symptoms, known as palliative treatment.

When delivering radical treatment the radiation dose is higher than for palliative treatment, for example, 60 Gy, and may be delivered using multiple static fields or more commonly by single or multiple radiation beams that sweep in uninterrupted arc(s) around the patient, called volumetric arc therapy (VMAT) incorporating intensity-modulated beams known as intensity-modulated radiotherapy (IMRT) designed to deliver a lethal dose across the tumour or tumour site, whilst sparing the surrounding normal tissue (see Chapter 9). Radiotherapy delivered using a linear accelerator for palliative treatments can be given by using a single field or parallel opposed fields, although IMRT/VMAT are increasingly being used for palliative treatments due to the reduced side effects of treatment. Palliative treatment usually delivers a lower dose of radiation, for example, 30 Gy.

In using IMRT/VMAT delivery the treatment planner has the ability to sculpt the doses to the shape of the target thereby optimising the radiation delivery to irregular shaped volumes. It is possible to produce concave distributions of dose in radiation treatment volumes. IMRT/VMAT has the advantage of (i) greater sparing of normal structures like salivary glands, mandible, pharyngeal constrictors, oesophagus, optic nerves, brain stem, and spinal cord; (ii) delivery of a simultaneous integrated boost; and (iii) eliminating the need for multiple field matching. VMAT is an advanced form of IMRT which delivers IMRT-like distributions in a single rotation of the gantry, varying the gantry speed and dose rate during delivery, in contrast to standard IMRT, which uses fixed gantry position with either step and shoot or dynamic multileaf collimator shaping of the beam (see Chapters 8 and 9). Planning studies using VMAT as the mode of delivering radiotherapy demonstrate shorter planning and treatment times, fewer monitor units for treatment delivery, better dose homogeneity, and normal tissue sparing.

1.7 Treatment Accuracy and Patient Immobilisation

The first step in the radiotherapy treatment process is the accurate localisation of the tumour in reference to external landmarks. Firstly the patient must be CT (computed tomography) scanned (see Chapter 6) in the position in which they are going to be treated, for example supine with their arms elevated to remove them out of the treatment fields. The patient must be immobilised with the aim to ensure the patient is in the same position for each treatment fraction (see Chapters 7 and 10). This is required in order to deliver the planned radiation doses accurately.

Typically, a patient is CT scanned one to two weeks before they start radiotherapy and multiple tattoos may be applied to the patient's skin so that the patient's external anatomy can be aligned accurately with the treatment plan when they come back for their radiotherapy treatment. If external tattoos are to be solely relied upon for accuracy we must assume that the patient's external anatomy is constant and that the target inside the patient remains in the same position every day in relation to the external anatomy.

The patient's CT images are then loaded into a treatment planning system (TPS) which has software that is specially designed to model the energy absorption of multiple beams traversing through the body. The treatment planner selects the target volumes to be treated and the volumes or organs that are to receive as low a dose as possible (known as organs at risk) and the TPS calculates and produces a map of dose distributions, known as a treatment plan. This plan is used as a reference plan to ensure accurate and safe treatment is delivered for each treatment (see Chapter 9).

Image-guided radiotherapy (IGRT) is any imaging at the pretreatment and treatment delivery stage that leads to an action that can improve or verify the accuracy of the radiotherapy treatment (see Chapter 7). IGRT encompasses a wide range of techniques ranging from simple visual field alignment cheques, through to the more complex volumetric imaging that allows direct visualisation of the radiotherapy target volume and surrounding anatomy. The complexity of the imaging required depends on the anatomical site to be treated (see Chapters 6 and 7).

Techniques can be adopted that will assist accurate dose delivery, for example, Deep Inspiration Breath Hold (DIBH) can be used for patients with left-sided breast tumours. This can decrease the radiation dose delivered to the heart and can lower the incidence of ischaemic heart disease. This technique involves the patient inspiring to a specified threshold and then holding that level of inspiration during every radiation therapy field delivered (see Chapter 10).

1.8 Technology and Techniques

Recent technological advances allow for radiotherapy to be delivered in different modalities, such as intraoperative radiotherapy (IORT) during surgical procedures (see Chapter 8). IORT is defined as the application of therapeutic levels of radiation to a target area, such as a tumour, whilst the area is exposed during surgery. The treatment can be applied using low-energy (kV) X-rays, or with electrons. These techniques are most commonly used in the treatment of breast cancer, but can be used for other tumours, e.g. cancer of the cervix.

Proton therapy is a well-established, effective form of radiation treatment that uses a high-energy beam of protons rather than high-energy X-rays to deliver a dose of radiotherapy for patients with cancer. It works best on some very rare cancers including tumours affecting the base of skull or the spine. Proton beam treatment can be a more effective form of therapy because it directs the all-important radiation treatment to precisely where it is needed with minimal damage to surrounding tissue. The treatment is therefore particularly suitable for treating childhood cancers.

Stereotactic body radiotherapy (SBRT) or stereotactic ablative radiotherapy (SABR) is a way of giving relatively high doses of radiotherapy to a very small tumour. SBRT is delivered using a linear accelerator and delivers radiotherapy from many different positions around the body; the beams are designed to meet at the tumour. The tumour receives a high dose of radiation and the tissues surrounding it receive a relatively lower dose. This lowers the risk of side effects and increases the TCP.

1.9 Current Radiotherapy Practice

The underpinning physics principles, details of the equipment, and all aspects of practice that embrace safe and effective radiotherapy treatment are detailed throughout the chapters in this book.

References

1. Cancer Research UK. Cancer statistics for the UK [cited 4 December 2018]: Available from https://www.cancerresearchuk.org/health-professional/cancer-statistics-for-the-uk#heading-Four.
2. The Royal College of Radiologists, Society and College of Radiographers, Institute of Physics and Engineering in Medicine, National Patient Safety Agency, British Institute of Radiology. Towards Safer Radiotherapy [Internet]. London: The Royal College of Radiologists; 2018 [cited 3 May 2018]. Available from: www.rcr.ac.uk/system/files/publication/field_publication_files/Towards_saferRT_final.pdf.
3. European Union Directive of Euratom. The Ionising Radiations (Medical Exposure) Regulations 2017 [Internet]. Legislation.gov.uk. 2017 [cited 4 February 2018]. Available from: www.legislation.gov.uk/uksi/2017/1322/contents/made.

Further Reading

Symonds, R.P., Mills, J.A., and Duxbury, A.M. (2019). *Walter and Miller's Textbook of Radiotherapy, Radiation Physics, Therapy and Oncology*, 8e. Edinburgh: Churchill Livingstone, Elsevier.

CHAPTER 2

Mathematical Skills Relevant for Radiotherapy Physics, Atomic Structure, and Radioactivity

Erica Chivers

Aim

The aim of this chapter is to provide a review of the mathematics and basic physics that will help in the understanding of radiotherapy physics.

2.1 Mathematical Skills Relevant for Radiotherapy Physics

This section introduces relevant mathematical skills and relates them to radiotherapy practice using radiotherapy examples.

2.1.1 Fractions

A fraction is one number divided by another. The top number, a, is the numerator and the bottom number, b, is the denominator:

$$x = \frac{a}{b}$$

Radiotherapy is usually given as a total (overall) dose that is split into a number of fractions. A total dose of 45 gray (Gy) may be given in 15 fractions of equal weight. The dose per fraction may be calculated as

$$\text{Dose per fraction} = \frac{45}{15} = 3 \text{ gray (Gy)}$$

2.1.2 Clinical Application

When using radioactive sources for imaging or treatment purposes, the radioactive source

---

Practical Radiotherapy: Physics and Equipment, Third Edition. Edited by Pam Cherry and Angela M. Duxbury.
© 2020 John Wiley & Sons Ltd. Published 2020 by John Wiley & Sons Ltd.

will undergo decay (where it changes into its daughter product) over a period of time. This may be considered in terms of a reduction in its whole amount, i.e. its fractional reduction.

After a specific period of time (its half-life, t½) one half of the original number of radioactive atoms will remain.

We start off with the complete (i.e. 1) radioactive substance.

- After the 1st half-life, ½ of the amount of the radioactive substance remains.
- After the 2nd half-life, ¼ of the amount of the radioactive substance remains.
- After the 3rd half-life, 1/8 of the amount of the radioactive substance remains.
- After the 4th half-life, 1/16 of the amount of the radioactive substance remains.

i.e. $\boxed{\dfrac{1}{2^n}}$ where n = half-lives elapsed

2.1.3 Ratios

A ratio is another way of expressing a fraction but is more useful when trying to compare two quantities. A ratio is expressed as $m:n$ (the ratio of m to n).

To divide a quantity A into a ratio $m:n$ to find $p:q$:

$$p = \frac{A}{(m+n)} \times m$$

$$q = \frac{A}{(m+n)} \times n$$

2.1.3.1 EXAMPLE

Question: a treatment regimen with a total dose of 50 Gy is to be given in two phases. The ratio of the dose in each phase is 3:1. What dose must be given for each phase?

Answer:

(p = phase 1 dose: q = phase 2 dose)

$$\text{Phase 1 dose} = \frac{50}{3+1} \times 3 = 37.5 \text{ Gy}$$

$$\text{Phase 2 dose} = \frac{50}{3+1} \times 1 = 12.5 \text{ Gy}$$

The ratio of the phase 1 to phase 2 dose is 37.5 : 12.5.

Sanity check! $\dfrac{37.5}{12.5} = \dfrac{3}{1} = \dfrac{m}{n}$

2.1.4 Proportionality

If two quantities are linearly proportional, then they have a constant scaling or multiplication factor, k. When $a \, \alpha \, b$ then $a = kb$, where k is a constant of proportionality.

2.1.4.1 EXAMPLE

Question: a treatment machine delivers a dose of 0.75 Gy in 15 seconds. How long will it take to deliver a dose of 2 Gy?

Answer:

$$k = 15 / 0.75 = 20 \left(s / Gy \right)$$

$$t = k \times 2 = 40 \, s$$

2 Gy will be delivered in 40 seconds.

2.1.5 Percentages

Percentages are often used to indicate the amount by which a value has changed or by how much a value should be changed. Per cent means 'per 100' or 1/100. Therefore 50% = 50/100 or one half.

To change a fraction (a/b) to a percentage (x):

$$x = \left(\frac{a}{b} \times \frac{100}{1} \right)\%$$

2.1.5.1   EXAMPLE

Question: a CT (computed tomography) plan shows a 95% coverage of the prostate on 21 slices out of 30. What percentage of the prostate volume is covered by the 95% isodose?

Answer: $x = \left(\dfrac{21}{30} \times \dfrac{100}{1} \right)\% = 70\%$

2.1.5.2   EXAMPLE

Question: the spinal cord is covered by the 90% isodose in a plan. If the patient is given 1.75 Gy, what dose will the spinal cord receive?

Answer: $z = \left(\dfrac{90}{100} \times \dfrac{1.75}{1} \right) = 1.575\,\text{Gy}$

To work out x% of y:

$$x\% = \frac{x}{100} \times \frac{y}{1}$$

2.1.5.3   EXAMPLE

Question: a field size (FS) of 14 cm needs to be increased by 12% in order to allow for organ motion. What is the correct enlarged FS?

Answer: $z = (12/100 \times 14) + 14 = 15.68\,\text{cm}$

To find z, an increase of y by x%:

$$z = \left(\frac{x}{100} \times y \right) + y$$

2.1.6 Clinical Application

Similarly, using a clinical example of brachytherapy, the percentage reduction in radioactive substance is shown by the following example.

We start off with the complete (i.e. 100%) radioactive substance.

- After the 1st half-life, 50% of the amount of the radioactive substance remains.
- After the 2nd half-life, 25% of the amount of the radioactive substance remains.
- After the 3rd half-life, 12.5% of the amount of the radioactive substance remains.
- After the 4th half-life, 6.25% of the amount of the radioactive substance remains.

2.1.7 Significant Figures

A radiotherapy total dose of 40 Gy in 15 fractions may be recorded as 2.67 Gy per fraction or 2.666 666 Gy per fraction. The information from both sources is correct but is given to a different degree of accuracy.

2.666 666 might be more accurate, but when we round to three significant figures, it is 2.67.

The first non-zero digit, reading from left to right in a number, is the first significant figure, and the second significant figure is the second non-zero digit.

'Rounding' to a significant figure is often used.

2.1.7.1   EXAMPLE

2.666 666 rounded to 1 significant figure is 3.

2.666 666 rounded to 2 significant figures is 2.7.

2.1.8 Standard Form

A number in standard form has a number between 1 and 10 multiplied by 10 raised to a power. A very large or very small number may need to be expressed in standard form, or scientific notation. The power is easy to work out by counting the number of times that you shift the significant figure.

2.1.8.1 EXAMPLES

Question: find 0.0895 in standard form.

Answer: move the decimal place twice to the right so the power = 8.95×10^{-2}

Question: find 800 000 in standard form.

Answer: move the decimal place five places to the left so the power = 8.0×10^{5}

Question: find 47 000 000 000 in standard form.

Answer: move the decimal point a total of 10 places to the left so the power = 4.7×10^{10}

2.1.9 Logarithms

A log is just a way of expressing a number as the 'power' of another number (the 'base').

For the general equation:

$$y = b^x \qquad \log_b y = x$$

If b is given the value 10, then $y = 10^x$. Now, if x is given the values 1, 2, 3, etc.:

y	10^x	x
10	10^1	1
100	10^2	2
1000	10^3	3
10 000	10^4	4
100 000	10^5	5

This is a 'log' table to the 'base' 10. Therefore:

- $\log_{10} 10 = 1$
- $\log_{10} 100 = 2$
- $\log_{10} 1000 = 3$.

The value for y gets very large, but when it is expressed as a logarithm it stays small.

When data covers a large range of values, it may be useful to use a logarithmic scale to present the data. This enables the wide range of values to be presented in a manageable manner. In a semi-log graph the y-axis is logarithmic, which means the separation on the graph is proportional to the logarithm of numbers. The x-axis has a linear scale, which means it is evenly spaced.

A semi-logarithmic scale may be used when one set of data covers a large range of variables and one set covers a smaller range. In radiobiology, this is seen when presenting a cell survival curve. This visually displays the relationship between the fraction of irradiated cells retaining their reproductive integrity and the absorbed dose of radiation. Conventionally, the surviving fraction of cells is depicted on a logarithmic scale and is plotted on the y-axis against radiation dose on the x-axis.

2.1.9.1 Exponentials

A special logarithmic case is 'e', where a constant change in x results in the same fractional change in y. The example, $y = e^x$ can also be expressed as $\log_e y = x$ or as $\ln y = x$. A log to base e is a 'natural logarithm' (ln) and 'e' has the value 2.718. Log e is log to the base e (2.781) instead of 10.

If e^x is plotted against x, an exponential curve is obtained. This type of curve describes many naturally occurring events such as radioactive decay.

Radioactive decay is exponential because the number of atomic nuclei decaying into a daughter product, at a given moment, is proportional to the number of radioactive nuclei that actually exist at that moment. Exponential decrease starts fast and get slower – therefore, depending on $t\frac{1}{2}$, radioactive materials decay into a stable (and therefore safe) material over a very long period of time, and so storage of radioactive materials is a long-term concern.

2.1.10 Similar Triangles

If one triangle is an enlargement of another, they are similar triangles. The triangles must have the same corresponding angles. Figure 2.1 shows two similar triangles.

In radiotherapy, similar triangles are used in three ways: field size (FS); inverse square law (ISL); and magnification.

2.1.11 Field Size

To find the FS variation with the source to skin distance (SSD).

In Figure 2.2 the ratio $SSD_1 : SSD_2$ is equal to the ratio $FS_1 : FS_2$, therefore:

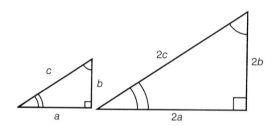

FIGURE 2.1 Two similar triangles.

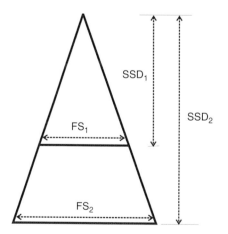

FIGURE 2.2 Similar triangles to illustrate how field size (FS) changes with source to skin distance (SSD).

$$\left(\frac{SSD_2}{SSD_1}\right) = \left(\frac{FS_2}{FS_1}\right)$$

Provided that any three of these variables are known, it is possible to calculate the fourth, unknown value.

2.1.11.1 EXAMPLE

Question: at an SSD of 100 cm, the field length is 12 cm. What is the field length if the SSD is increased to 150 cm?

Answer:

$$\left(\frac{SSD_2}{SSD_1}\right) = \left(\frac{FS_2}{FS_1}\right)$$

$$FS_2 = FS_1 \left(\frac{SSD_2}{SSD_1}\right) = 12 \times \left(\frac{150}{100}\right) = 18\,cm$$

2.1.12 The Inverse Square Law

It is a geometrical consideration that any point source which spreads its influence equally in all directions, without limit to its range, will obey the ISL. Point sources of ionising radiation (and other electromagnetic radiations), sound, and gravitational forces all obey the ISL. This relationship considers similar triangles in three dimensions. In Figure 2.3 the top of the object is a point source of X-rays. All photons travel in straight lines. Photons in the shaded area 'A' have come from the point source, are at a distance 'd' from it and are travelling directly away from it. Photons in the shaded area 'B' are further away from the point source at a distance '2d', but the number of photons in area B is the same as in area A. Therefore, the number of photons per unit area, or the intensity, is less in B than in A. The decrease in intensity can be derived using similar triangles.

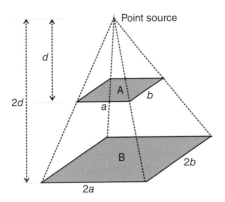

FIGURE 2.3 A diagram of the inverse square law (ISL).

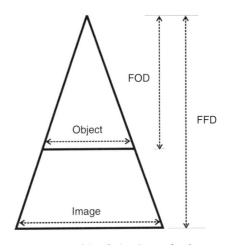

FIGURE 2.4 An object being imaged using a point source.

In Figure 2.3, if the distance from the source is doubled, then all sides of the triangles will double. Therefore:

$$\text{Area A} = a \times b = ab$$

$$\text{Area B} = 2a \times 2b = 4ab$$

Therefore, the area is four times greater but the number of photons is the same and:

$$I = \frac{I_0}{4}$$

where I is the intensity and I_0 is the initial intensity of the beam.

$$I = I_0 \times \left(\frac{a \times b}{4 \times a \times b}\right)$$

If the distance is increased from d to $10d$:

$$\text{Area A} = a \times b = ab$$

$$\text{Area B} = 10a \times 10b = 100ab$$

$$I = I_0 \times a \times b$$

$$100 \times a \times b$$

When the distance from the source increases, I always decreases by:

$$I = I_0 \times \left(\frac{d_1}{d_2}\right)^2$$

or it can be said that I is inversely proportional to d^2.

$$I \propto \left(\frac{1}{d}\right)^2$$

As the ISL is geometric in its origin, all photons must be travelling from the same point and in a straight line. Therefore, there must be a point source and no scatter (change of direction).

2.1.13 Magnification

Figure 2.4 shows an object being imaged onto an imaging device using a point source (a single identified point of origin). The magnification (M) is defined as

$$M = \frac{\text{size of image}(I)}{\text{size of object}(O)}$$

Where FFD is the focus to film distance and FOD is the focus to object distance, similar triangles can be used to work out dimensions, if three quantities are known.

$$M = \frac{I}{O} = \frac{\text{FFD}}{\text{FOD}}$$

2.2 Basic Physics Relevant to Radiotherapy

2.2.1 Units of Measurement

It is often necessary to present the results of measurements or calculations in a numerical fashion. The number used to do this requires two parts: a pure number and the unit in which the quantity has been measured or calculated, e.g. 50 Gy, where the unit is the 'gray' and the pure number is 50. There are, however, some basic units on which all measurements are based and a number of derived units that are based on combinations of the basic units. SI Units (from Système International d'unités) is the modern form of the metric system and is widely used.

2.2.1.1 Basic Units

All measurements used in science are based on three basic units of measurement (Table 2.1). These are the basic units of measurement because they are independent of each other and cannot be converted from one to another.

2.2.1.2 Derived Units

Any physical quantities other than mass, length, or time are measured in derived units. A derived unit is a SI unit of measurement comprised of a combination of base units, for example the SI unit of force is the derived unit Newton or N.

2.2.1.3 Prefixes

As discussed, it is easier to present very large or small numbers in standard form. A way of

TABLE 2.2 Common prefixes.

pico	p	10^{-12}	kilo	k	10^{3}
nano	n	10^{-9}	mega	M	10^{6}
micro	μ	10^{-6}	giga	G	10^{9}
milli	m	10^{-3}	tera	T	10^{12}
centi	c	10^{-2}			

simplifying this further is by the use of universal prefixes. Table 2.2 shows common prefixes.

For example, $0.000\,007\,\text{m} = 7 \times 10^{-6} = 7\,\mu\text{m}$
$3000\,\text{m} = 3 \times 10^{3} = 3\,\text{km}$
$400\,\text{cGy} = 4 \times 10^{2} = 4\,\text{gray (Gy)}$

2.2.2 Energy

Energy is defined as the ability to do work. Two special forms of energy must be considered: potential and kinetic.

Potential energy (PE) is the energy a body possesses by virtue of its position relative to other objects. PE is therefore 'stored' energy such as that in a battery or coiled spring. A body's PE is equal to the amount of work that has been performed to put it in its particular position, i.e. the force applied multiplied by the distance moved. For a body of mass m above the ground by a distance h and under the effect of gravity, g, its PE = mg h.

Kinetic energy (KE) is the energy that a body possesses by virtue of its motion. A body's KE is that energy that would have to be applied to the body to bring it completely to rest. Electrons, when released from their bound state within an atom, are able to move throughout material when they possess KE.

2.3 Heat and Temperature

Heat and temperature are related to each other but are different concepts. Heat is energy and temperature is a measure of energy. This relationship is seen in Table 2.3.

TABLE 2.1 Basic units of measurement.

Unit	Symbol	SI unit
Mass	m	kilogramme (kg)
Length	l	metre (m)
Time	t	second (s)

TABLE 2.3 Heat and temperature.

	Heat	Temperature
	The amount of energy in a body	The measure of intensity of heat
Measures	Total kinetic and potential energy contained by molecules in an object	Average kinetic energy of molecules in a substance.
Property	Flows from hotter object to cooler object.	Rises when heated and falls when cooled.
Unit of measurement	Joules	Kelvin. Celsius
Measurement device	Calorimeter	Thermometer

2.3.1 Heat

The atoms and molecules of any material are in constant motion. The type of motion varies depending on the form of the material. Within a solid, particles vibrate about a fixed position, whereas in liquids and gases motion is much more random as the particles have much greater freedom of movement. All materials therefore possess KE due to this motion. Heat is the form of KE possessed by a material resulting from the motion of its particles and, as heat is a form of energy, the SI unit for it is the joule.

2.3.2 Temperature

Temperature is a measure of the level of KE of the atoms and molecules of a material. As the speed of vibrations increases within a body, the measured temperature increases, as more vibration means higher energy. The temperature determines the direction of heat flow when one object is brought into thermal contact within another. Heat will flow from a region of higher to lower temperature.

Temperature can be expressed in several units of measurement.

2.3.3 Heat Transfer

Heat energy can be transferred from one body to another by the processes of conduction, convection, and radiation.

2.3.3.1 Conduction

This process applies principally to solids or objects that are in direct contact with each other. Transfer of heat is by collision of particles in one body with those in the other body. If the temperature of one end of a body is increased, this heat will flow along the body due to the collisions of neighbouring particles. The flow of heat in a body will be affected by a number of physical factors:

heat flow $\propto$ cross-sectional area (A);

heat flow $\propto$ length (l);

heat flow $\propto$ temperature difference ($T_1 - T_2$).

Heat flow is also dependent on the material itself, in particular its thermal conductivity (k).

Metals are examples of good heat conductors.

2.3.3.2 Convection

Convection is the main process by which heat is transferred in a fluid (liquids and gases). Heat energy is moved around by circulation of the heated fluid. As a fluid is heated it becomes less dense and will therefore rise. As it rises, it is replaced by cooler fluid, which is then heated and rises, so the process continues creating convection currents in the fluid by virtue of this movement.

2.3.3.3 Radiation

This is the only form of heat transfer that can take place in a vacuum. As particles in a body vibrate, they emit energy in the form of electromagnetic waves. Heat radiation occurs in the electromagnetic spectrum just beyond the red part of the visible spectrum (infrared). One of the properties of electromagnetic radiation is that it can travel in a vacuum. Therefore, it is possible to transfer heat across a vacuum. It is by this process that heat from the sun is felt, because it has to pass through a vacuum before it reaches the earth.

Applications to radiotherapy of these processes of heat transfer can be seen in the cooling of the target/anode of a stationary anode X-ray tube. Heat builds up in the tungsten/rhenium target when it is bombarded by electrons, and is transferred by conduction to the copper anode. From the copper anode, the heat is transferred to the surrounding oil and from there by convection to the surrounding housing. Heat is conducted through the housing and then transferred by convection to the air. Additionally, electromagnetic radiation (infrared range) travels through the vacuum of the X-ray tube from the target. When this radiation reaches the metal ceramic envelope, it interacts with the envelope's atoms imparting energy. This causes the envelope to heat up. From here, heat is transferred by conduction to the oil surrounding the metal envelope.

2.4 Electricity, Magnetism, and Electromagnetic Radiation

Electricity and magnetism are important to the understanding of radiation. The movement of charges in an electric field and the combination of electric and magnetic fields in the form of electromagnetic waves underpin X-ray production and interactions.

2.4.1 Electric Fields

Separate but similar charges repel each other and unlike charges attract each other. As two electrons are both negatively charged, they repel each other.

An electric field can be created across two electrodes with the application of a potential difference. In a device such as an X-ray tube, the cathode is negative, and in a device which provides energy (such as battery in use), the cathode is positive (electrons flow into it and charge flows out).

2.4.2 Current

Current is the motion of electrons from one electrode to another through a conductor. Current is defined as the net charge (Q) flowing through an area A per unit time (t).

The unit of current is the ampere (A), which is equal to Coulombs per second (C/s). This is shortened to 'amp'. Currents in radiotherapy X-ray tubes are of the magnitude of milliamps (mA).

2.4.3 Voltage

The force that drives current around a circuit is the potential difference. This is measured in volts. An electron moving through a potential difference experiences a net change in energy, measured in electron volts. This effect is analogous to a mass falling through a given height difference in a gravitational field. One electron volt (eV) is the energy required by an electron to move through a potential difference of 1 V.

2.4.4 Resistance

The voltage of a circuit divided by its current is known as the resistance of the circuit. This is given as:

$$R(\Omega) = \frac{V(V)}{I(A)}$$

This is Ohm's law. The unit of resistance is the ohm (Ω), which is equal to 1 V per ampere (*V/A*).

2.4.5 Magnetism

A magnetic field produced by a magnet has a north and a south pole. As with electric charges, opposite poles attract and like poles repel; however, unlike electric charges the opposite charges in a magnet cannot be isolated, but always come in pairs. The magnetic field lines produced by a magnet run from north to south.

2.4.6 Electromagnetic Induction

When a magnet is moved through a coil of wire, a current is induced in the coil. The opposite is also true: a current passing through a coil generates a magnetic field through the centre of the coil. This is known as electromagnetic induction.

2.4.7 Electromagnetic Waves

Electromagnetic waves all travel in a vacuum with a velocity equal to the speed of light (*c*) where $c = 3 \times 10^8$ m s^{-1}. All waves have a wavelength, λ, the distance travelled in one cycle, and a frequency, v, the number of cycles per second, measured in hertz (Hz). Figure 2.5 shows the wavelength, frequency, and amplitude of a wave. The wave in this example has a frequency of 3 Hz.

The phenomenon of electromagnetic induction tells us that electric and magnetic fields that vary with time are not independent – one affects the other. When a magnetic field moves with time it induces an electric field perpendicular to it (see Figure 2.6), and the same is true of the inverse situation when a time-varying electric field induces a magnetic field. Electromagnetic waves are so called because they are waves of energy transmitted by oscillating interdependent electric and magnetic fields. As an electromagnetic wave is energy radiating away from an oscillating source it is also called electromagnetic radiation.

Radio waves, microwaves, ultraviolet light, infrared light, visible light, X-rays, and

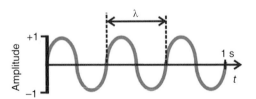

FIGURE 2.5 The wavelength, frequency, and amplitude of a wave.

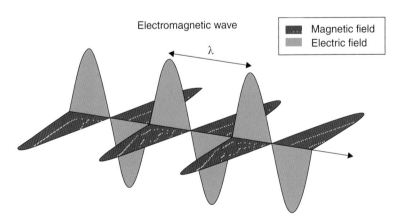

FIGURE 2.6 Electromagnetic wave showing direction of wave. Source: image courtesy of Nick Strobel at www.astronomynotes.com.

gamma rays are all types of electromagnetic radiation, but have different wavelengths. Electromagnetic radiation can be considered to behave as both a wave and a particle because it demonstrates both wave and particle-like properties.

2.4.7.1 Wave-like Properties

Electromagnetic radiation is usually thought of as being a wave. How is it known that it behaves like a wave? If visible light is considered, it can be demonstrated that visible light can undergo reflection, refraction, diffraction, interference – all of which are properties of waves. Experimental work with mass spectrometers has also demonstrated the diffraction of X-rays.

2.4.7.2 Particle-like Properties

Some phenomena associated with electromagnetic radiation, such as the photoelectric effect and Compton scattering, cannot be explained by the wave theory. To explain these phenomena, electromagnetic radiation must be considered to behave as particles or packets of energy rather than as waves.

2.4.8 Wave–Particle Duality

The wave- and particle-like properties of electromagnetic radiation can be related. From the wave-like properties, it is known that the wave can be described by the following relationship:

$$E = v\lambda$$

If particle-like properties are considered, it can be shown that the energy carried by the particles or photons is given by:

$$E = hv$$

Key: E is the energy of the photon, expressed in joules

h is known as Planck's constant and is equal to 6.62×10^{-34} J

v is the frequency expressed in cycles per second (s^{-1})

λ is the photon's wavelength

c is a universal physics constant noted as the speed of light in a vacuum, 3×10^8 m s^{-1}

These two equations can be combined because it is known that $v = c/\lambda$ and we can therefore substitute for v in the equation $E = hv$ which results in the relationship:

$$E = \frac{hc}{\lambda}$$

It is also known that $h = 6.62 \times 10^{-34}$ J and $c = 3 \times 10^8$ m s^{-1} and, if energy is converted to electron volts, where $1\,eV = 1.602 \times 10^{-19}$ J, then the relationship simplifies to:

$$E = 1.24 \times 10^{-6} / \lambda$$

where E is expressed in electron volts (eV) and λ is expressed in metres (m). From this relationship it can be seen that, as the energy increases, the wavelength will decrease.

2.5 The Electromagnetic Spectrum

The electromagnetic spectrum includes radiation from the longest wavelength radio waves to the shortest wavelength X- and gamma rays. All forms of electromagnetic radiation have an associated frequency and energy. The greater the energy, the larger the frequency and the shorter the wavelength. Given the relationship between wavelength and frequency – the higher the frequency, the shorter the wavelength – it follows that short wavelengths are more energetic than long wavelengths. Photon energy is inversely proportional to its wavelength.

It should be noted that there may be a degree of overlap between the different types of electromagnetic radiation and that there

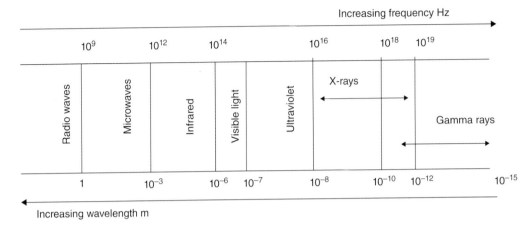

FIGURE 2.7 Electromagnetic spectrum.

are therefore no distinct boundaries between them. Of particular relevance in radiotherapy, there is an overlap between X-rays and gamma rays. Both of these electromagnetic radiations have a short wavelength and therefore a high energy – they are distinguished from each other in that gamma rays result from nuclear conversions and X-rays are produced as a result of electron rearrangement within an atom or when electrons strike a target.

Figure 2.7 shows the electromagnetic spectrum.

All electromagnetic radiation types share some common properties:

- They are composed of transverse electric and magnetic waves.
- They travel at the speed of light in a vacuum.
- In free space they travel in straight lines.
- In free space they obey the ISL.

These properties are relevant in radiotherapy as they influence X-ray production, radiotherapy treatment, and radiation protection.

2.6 Atomic Structure

All matter such as solids, liquids, and gases, is composed of atoms. The atom is the basic component of an element and elements are the individual entities from which all matter is composed. Although originally believed to be the smallest discrete particle (the word atom derives from the Greek for indivisible), an atom consists of a central nucleus, which is positively charged and electrons orbiting this nucleus, which are negatively charged.

2.6.1 Atomic Particles

Particles are classified by their mass as leptons or hadrons. Leptons are lightweight particles and include electrons. Leptons are elementary particles and cannot be further divided.

Hadrons are heavy particles and can be further divided. Neutrons and protons are hadrons and are composed of particles called quarks. Combinations of quarks yield neutrons, protons, and other hadrons. Up quarks and down quarks are generally stable and the most common. Protons consist of two up quarks and one down quark. Neutrons consist of one up quark and two down quarks. Up quarks have an electrical charge of $+\frac{2}{3}$. Down quarks have an electrical charge of $-\frac{1}{3}$. Therefore, protons have a positive charge and neutrons have no charge. In radioactive decay, protons or neutrons may change into each other.

E.g. β- decay involves a down quark changing into an up quark (a neutron becomes a proton and an electron). β + decay involves an up quark changing into a down quark (a proton becomes a neutron and a positron).

2.6.2 Nucleus

Protons (p) are positively charged with a charge of 1.602×10^{-19} C whereas neutrons (n) have no charge, thus giving the nucleus its overall positive charge. The electrons (e) orbiting the nucleus are negatively charged and their charge is equal in magnitude to that of the proton, i.e. -1.602×10^{-19} C. The number of electrons orbiting the atom is equal to the number of protons in the nucleus and the overall charge of the atom is therefore balanced, i.e. there is a zero net charge.

The mass of a proton is the same as that of a neutron and is 1.67261×10^{-27} kg as they are both composed of quarks whilst the mass of an electron is much less, 9.109×10^{-31} kg, which is approximately 1/1840 of the mass of the proton or neutron.

2.6.3 Mass Numbers and Atomic Numbers

For an element X, with mass number A and atomic number Z, its chemical symbol is written as:

$$_{Z}^{A}X$$

A is equal to the number of nucleons, i.e. the total number of protons and neutrons in the nucleus, whereas Z denotes the total number of protons in the nucleus. As the number of protons and electrons is equal, the atomic number also indicates the number of electrons outside the nucleus. For example, an atom of carbon would be written as:

$$_{6}^{12}C$$

where the mass number 12 indicates that the total number of protons and neutrons in the nucleus is 12 and the atomic number 6 indicates that there are 6 protons (and 6 electrons). As the mass number indicates that there are a total of 12 nucleons, and from the atomic number it is known that there are 6 protons, it can be calculated that there are also 6 neutrons.

2.6.4 Electron Orbits

Within the atom, the electrons orbiting the nucleus may be regarded as arranged in shells, each being identified by a letter K, L, M, etc. starting from the shell closest to the nucleus. Each shell has a limit to the number of electrons that it can contain, and the inner shells are always occupied first. The K-shell can accept up to 2 electrons, the L-shell up to 8, the M-shell up to 18, etc. For example, carbon with its atomic number of 6 has 2 electrons in the K-shell and the remaining 4 electrons in the L-shell. A diagram of a carbon atom is illustrated in Figure 2.8.

The electron configuration of the atom determines its chemical properties. Neon ($Z = 10$), for example, is chemically inert because both the K- and L-shells are full. Fluorine ($Z = 9$), however, has one electron missing from its outer shell and is chemically reactive. Another example, argon ($Z = 18$), suggests the presence of subshells. It is chemically inert but has only eight electrons in its M-shell, suggesting that atoms are also stable when subshells are full.

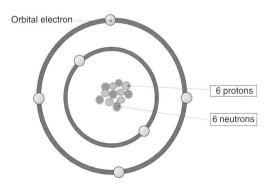

FIGURE 2.8   Representation of the particles in a carbon atom.

TABLE 2.4 **Classifications of nuclides.**

	Atomic number	**Mass number**	**Examples and radioactive emission (where appropriate)**
Isotope	Same for all	Different for all	$^{59}_{27}$Co stable
			$^{60}_{27}$Co (beta particles and gamma rays)
			$^{57}_{27}$Co (electron capture)
Isomer	Same for all	Same for all	^{99}Tc stable
			^{99m}Tc (gamma rays)
Isobar	Different for all	Same for all	^{60}Co
			^{60}Ni

2.6.5 Atomic Energy Levels

Electron orbits around a nucleus also have an energy associated with them. This is known as the atomic energy and is dependent on the force of attraction between the nucleus and the orbiting electrons. Electrons thus experience a binding energy within the shell or energy level. The binding energy associated with the K-shell is greater than for shells further away from the nucleus because the force of attraction on the K-shell electrons will be greater. The binding energies of the electrons go down as the shell number increases.

It is the binding energy that must be overcome if an electron is to be removed from its shell (ionisation). The potential energy associated with shells further from the nucleus will be greater than for those shells close to the nucleus.

2.7 Classification of Nuclides

Atoms of the same element can exist with different mass numbers but the same atomic number, i.e. the number of neutrons present in the nucleus is different, but the number of protons remains the same. Such elements are known as isotopes.

The important point to remember about isotopes is that, as the number of protons and therefore the number of electrons is unchanged, the chemical properties of the element are unchanged. When the imbalance in the number of protons and neutrons becomes too great, the atom and therefore the isotope may become radioactive and the isotope is called a radioisotope. Table 2.4 shows the classifications of nuclides and that they exist in different forms.

2.8 Radioactivity

Radioactivity may be defined as the spontaneous emission of particles, electromagnetic radiation, or both as a result of unstable nuclei. Nuclear binding energy is the energy required to split a nucleus of an atom into its component nucleons.

The initial nucleus is referred to as the 'parent'. The decay of a parent nucleus gives rise to a 'daughter' product. The daughter product itself may also be unstable and so undergoes further radioactive decay. The term 'radioactive family' describes multiple radioactive decay processes until a stable nucleus is reached.

Radioactive decay is identified in three main types – alpha, beta, and gamma after the first three letters of the Greek alphabet. It is relevant to note that other decay processes also take place.

2.8.1 Alpha Decay

A nucleus may be unstable as a result of too many protons or neutrons so that the nuclear binding energy is unable to bind the nucleus together. An alpha particle is made up of two protons and two neutrons bound together – their mass number is 4 and they have a positive electrical charge. Alpha decay occurs most often in large nuclei that have too many protons in comparison to the number of neutrons (nuclei larger than lead may decay in this manner). Alpha radiation reduces the ratio of protons to neutrons in the parent nucleus, bringing it to a more stable configuration. The alpha particle, once released, is repelled away from the parent nucleus and travels with its own KE at approximately 5% of the speed of light.

The original atom transforms or 'decays' into a different atomic nucleus, with a mass number that is reduced by four and an atomic number that is reduced by two. For example, uranium-238 will decay to thorium-234.

Alpha particles have a relatively large mass, electric charge of $+2\,e$, and relatively low velocity, and so they are very likely to interact with other atoms and lose their energy. Their forward motion can be stopped by a few centimetres of air. Alpha particles have relatively few uses in radiotherapy but recent developments include the use of radium-223. This is an alpha emitter that mimics calcium and is delivered and taken up by the bone cells. The alpha particles are emitted internal to the patient. This internal form of radiotherapy leads to longer survival for patients with bone metastases from prostate cancer.

2.8.2 Beta Decay

Beta decay itself comes in two forms: β^- and β^+.

β^- emission occurs by the transformation of one of the nucleus's neutrons into a proton, an electron (may be referred to as a negatron), and an antineutrino. This occurs when a nucleus has an excess of neutrons. The net charge of this particle is $-1\,e$ and it has negligible mass. It is able to penetrate a few millimetres within tissue. Strontium-89 (Metastron) and samarium-153 (Quadramet) are β^--emitters that are taken up like calcium into bone. This internal treatment is useful in the treatment of metastatic disease in the bone.

β^+ decay is a similar process, but involves a proton changing into a neutron, a positron, and a neutrino. This occurs when a nucleus has an excess of protons. The proton inside a radionuclide nucleus is converted into a neutron whilst releasing a positron and a neutrino (ν_e). A positron is regarded as a 'positive electron'.

The emission of positrons is utilised in positron emission tomography (PET). Since positrons are antimatter, they exist for a fraction of a second. As soon as they collide with an electron, they destroy each other and produce energy in the form of two gamma rays – annihilation energy. These gamma rays have a specific energy of 0.51 MeV each and travel at 180° to each other. These gamma rays are detected using a specific imaging device and are the basis of PET scanning and PET-CT (see Chapter 6).

2.8.3 Gamma Decay

After a nucleus undergoes alpha or beta decay, it is often left in an excited state with excess energy. An atomic nucleus loses this excess energy by emitting electromagnetic radiation in the gamma ray region. The gamma ray γ is a photon of high energy and short wavelength.

Gamma rays are used for radionuclide imaging and radiotherapy (see Chapter 13).

2.8.4 Half-lives and Probability

It isn't possible to work out when any particular atom will decay, but it is possible to make predictions based on the statistical behaviour of large numbers of atoms.

The half-life of a radioactive isotope is the time after which, on average, half of the original material will have decayed. Half-lives for various radioisotopes can range from a few microseconds (polonium-215) to billions of years (uranium-238)

'background radiation'. This arises from cosmic rays, radon gas and its decay products, and radioactive materials in the ground.

2.9 Background Radiation

There is a natural level of radiation all around us, which comes from several sources. Many radioisotopes occur naturally and result in there being a certain amount of radiation in our environment all the time – the

Further Reading

Graham, D.T., Cloke, P., and Vosper, M. (2011). *Principles of Radiological Physics*, 6e. Edinburgh: Churchill Livingstone.

Symonds, R.P., Mills, J.A., and Duxbury, A.M. (2019). *Walter and Miller's Textbook of Radiotherapy, Radiation Physics, Therapy and Oncology*, 8e. Edinburgh: Churchill Livingstone, Elsevier.

CHAPTER 3

X-ray Production

Dora Meikle and Gareth Hill

Aim

The aim of this chapter is to provide an overview of the design and mechanisms adopted to generate X-rays. This will enable an understanding of X-ray production within a range of equipment utilised in a radiotherapy department. Developing an awareness of how X-rays are generated within differing tube targets will allow the reader to relate X-ray production to the output spectrum of different imaging equipment used in radiotherapy practice.

3.1 Introduction

The essential elements of X-ray production have not changed over the last 100 years, since Wilhelm Conrad Roentgen discovered rays (X-rays) that could pass through matter. The application of X-rays within modern medicine has dramatically changed, although the same basic components used by Roentgen to produce X-rays are still required today. Modern X-ray tubes require an electron source, the cathode, and a target which the electrons can be directed towards, the anode. They also require a current capable of liberating the electrons from a tungsten filament,

set within the cathode, along with a high voltage across the tube to ensure the electrons will flow towards the anode at the required speed to produce X-rays, commonly referred to as photons.

X-rays or photons are a form of electromagnetic radiation. They cannot be detected by the human senses and are not affected by electric or magnetic fields (see Chapter 2). Within the field of therapeutic radiography and the treatment of malignant disease, X-rays within the diagnostic kilovoltage (kV) range have two purposes. The first is to treat superficial disease such as skin cancers, due to the location of this disease and the depth to which kV X-rays can travel within tissue; for a 60 kV beam the maximum dose is deposited at the skin surface and the 90% dose level will be approximately 2 mm deep, and for a 220 kV beam, the 90% dose level depth will be up to 10 mm. Most cancers are located in central positions within the body, therefore higher energy photons, produced by a linear accelerator (LinAc), are required to treat a tumour at depth (see Chapter 5 for X-ray interaction with matter).

The second purpose for using kV X-rays is to allow detailed imaging to be gathered whilst planning a patient's treatment, prior to the delivery of the radiation treatment. Photons have the ability to ionise other substances; this means photons cause the atoms

Practical Radiotherapy: Physics and Equipment, Third Edition. Edited by Pam Cherry and Angela M. Duxbury.
© 2020 John Wiley & Sons Ltd. Published 2020 by John Wiley & Sons Ltd.

they interact with to eject electrons from their electron shell, which explains the photons' imaging properties. This was the principle first adopted by conventional simulators and X-ray fluoroscopy within radiotherapy practice. Nowadays, more advanced technologies such CT (computed tomography) simulation and onboard imaging (OBI) found on modern LinAcs, utilise the basic concepts of kV X-ray production to enable the capture of images with better detailed definition and superior image resolution throughout the patient's pathway. The ability to generate a varied X-ray beam is key when balancing the quality of an image and dose received by a patient.

3.2 The X-ray Tube

The electrical production of X-rays is only possible under certain conditions such as having a source of electrons, an appropriate target material, a high voltage, and a vacuum. X-rays are produced when electrons with kinetic energy impact upon a high-density target. Each component part of the X-ray tube has been designed with the desire to produce electrons, supply them with energy, and enable an efficient as possible interaction with a target. A high voltage measured

in kilovolts (kV) is applied across the tube by a generator, which is a separate component from the X-ray tube. This high voltage will create a potential difference between the negative cathode and positive anode. The aim is to provide a small area on the target, where X-rays are emitted (the focal spot), as a high-intensity beam. This has to be traded off with the large amount of heat produced in the anode as a by-product. The components of the tube are enclosed in a glass, evacuated envelope and protective housing as indicated in Figure 3.1. The protective housing contains oil to help remove heat from the X-ray tube. A more durable design of X-ray tube is more commonly used for helical CT simulation due to the continuous rotating of the gantry when acquiring data. This section will examine the components of a typical X-ray tube and provide some information on the functions of each part to develop the reader's understanding of the X-ray tube.

3.2.1 Cathode

The cathode is the negatively charged electrode, where electrons are produced and released to be accelerated across the X-ray tube. The cathode contains two parts: a filament and a focusing cup. The primary

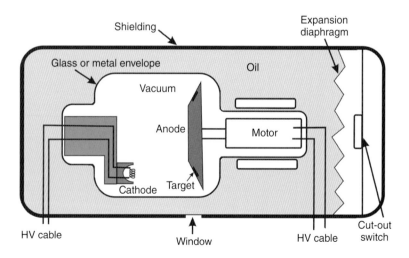

FIGURE 3.1 A diagram of components of a rotating-anode X-ray tube.

function of the cathode is to produce electrons and focus these electrons towards the anode.

3.2.2 Filament

The filament is a coil of tungsten wire, which is about 2 mm in diameter. It is tightly coiled, similar to the heating element in a bar heater, in order to increase the surface area of the metal. A high current is passed through this coil, which heats the metal to such an extent that the outer electrons of the tungsten atoms are boiled off and ejected from the surface of the coil. This phenomenon is known as thermionic emission. Tungsten is a good material for this purpose because it has a high melting point (3380 °C) and high thermal conductivity. This means that it can heat and cool quickly, allowing it to be heated rapidly for thermionic emission, and it can withstand high temperatures without becoming damaged. The rate at which the electrons are emitted by the cathode is directly related to the tube current which is measured in milliamps (mA).

X-ray tubes have dual filaments which permit the selection of a large or small source of electrons. The length and width of the filament control the ability of the X-ray tube to produce fine imaging detail. This is related to the focal spot size found on the rotating anode of the X-ray tube. An example of a small focal spot would be 0.6 mm, and large, 1.0 mm. The selection of a small or large focal spot is associated with the small and large filaments, found within the focusing cup.

3.2.3 Focusing Cup

When electrons are produced by the filament they spread out, because their negative charges electrostatically repel each other. This would result in some electrons not reaching the target, which would reduce the efficiency of the tube. To stop this from happening, a focusing cup is used, which is a negatively charged block of nickel that shapes the electrons coming from the filament into a focused beam, and hence produces a small focal spot on the target.

3.2.4 Anode

The anode is the positively charged electrode within the X-ray tube, which receives electrons from the opposing cathode. It consists of a high-density metal target, embedded in a copper disc. The electrons from the cathode hit the target area of the anode and interact (see Chapter 5). Tungsten is usually chosen as a target material because it has a high density, which increases the number of interactions per projectile electron. It also has a high melting point, allowing the target to become very hot without becoming damaged. Tungsten has a high thermal conductivity that allows the heat generated in the target to be quickly dissipated to the surrounding copper, which acts as a heat dissipater for the anode. Most tubes have a rotating anode, driven by a motor that operates by electromagnetic induction. Rotating the anode increases the efficiency of removing heat from the target area during the production of X-rays, which makes it possible to produce a higher-intensity beam without damaging the area of the anode struck by the projectile electrons. Key aspects of the anode include the target and the line focus principle.

3.2.5 Target

The area where the electrons from the cathode strike the anode is called the target or focal spot. This is the point at which X-ray photons are produced and begin to follow a divergent path. When the electrons hit the anode they interact, transferring their kinetic energy to the target atoms. These interactions take place in a very small depth of penetration into the target (0.25–0.5 mm). They result in either the conversion of kinetic energy into thermal energy, in the form of heat, or electromagnetic energy in the form of X-rays. The X-ray photons are emitted from the anode target at a 90° angle from the incoming electron pathway. Hence why the targets used in production of kV X-rays are known as reflective targets, as the electron beam does not pass through the target. Divergence of X-ray photons follow the same pathway as divergent sun rays; as the sun rays get closer to earth, they fan out more from their source which is millions of miles away. Like sun rays, X-rays diverge more the greater the distance they are from their focal spot or source.

3.2.6 Line Focus Principle

The smaller the focal spot, the greater the detail seen within the kV image produced by an OBI. However, with a small focal spot the amount of heat transferred to the target by the electrons becomes concentrated in a small area. If the heat from the target cannot be dissipated fast enough the target may become damaged and crack, causing the tube to fail. A good solution to this issue of creating more heat and still maintaining image detail is to angle the target as shown in Figure 3.2. The actual focal spot size is the area of the target that interacts with the electron beam. The angle of the anode means that the X-ray beam exiting the tube is much smaller than this area. This is called the line focus principle, illustrated in Figure 3.2. The angle marked θ is known as the target angle. Most X-ray tubes have a target angle from 7 to 20°.

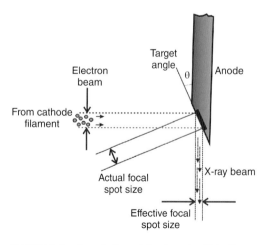

FIGURE 3.2 Angulation of the target within the rotating anode (taking advantage of the line focus principle), allows a larger geometric area to be heated whilst a small focal spot is maintained, ensuring greater resolution of the produced image.

3.2.7 Envelope

The cathode and anode are housed inside a glass or metal envelope. The envelope is sealed, and maintained at vacuum pressure. This is necessary so that the electrons can travel from the cathode to the anode without losing any energy during unwanted interactions with air molecules. The envelope was traditionally made of glass, because this is an easy material to mould and it is resistant to high temperatures. More modern tubes have housing made from metal, reducing the buildup of tungsten deposits on the glass envelope. These deposits on the inside of the glass envelope can reduce tube life and cause arcing.

3.2.8 Protective Housing

The envelope is in turn contained inside sturdy housing, which has several purposes. It provides protection and support for the components of the X-ray tube. There is a low attenuation window where the radiation beam exits towards the patient. The housing is filled with oil, which is used to dissipate heat from the anode. The oil expands as it heats up, and if this expansion becomes too great a cutoff switch is activated to prevent the tube from overheating. The housing is also coated in lead to provide shielding, and prevent radiation leakage in any direction during exposure except via the window. Finally, filters and collimators can be attached to this housing; this is commonly undertaken in superficial radiotherapy when treating skin cancers.

3.2.9 Extension of X-ray Tube Life

There are several practical steps that a therapeutic radiographer can undertake to extend the life of an X-ray tube. The manufacturer's warmup procedure on a CT simulator should always be followed to prevent excessive heat load on a cold anode. Many systems have a digital display of the heat capacity of the tube after a series of exposures; this is usually measured in percent. This tool is useful when monitoring the heat units created, which is the capacity of the anode and tube housing to store thermal energy. Utilising low mA values during an exposure decreases filament evaporation, which has a positive effect on the life expectancy of a tube. Multiple exposures near the tube limit are not advisable, as this can cause unnecessary heat stress on the anode which can cause serious damage.

3.3 X-ray Production

X-rays are one of the many forms of electromagnetic energy organised by wavelength on the electromagnetic spectrum (EMS); therefore X-rays will follow the same physical sciences rules as other forms of energy such as radio waves, microwaves, and visible light. All energies on the EMS share certain properties, listed as follows:

- all travel at the speed of light $(3 \times 10^{10} \, \text{cm s}^{-1})$;
- take the form of a wave, each with a differing rise and fall pattern expressed as wavelength and frequency (wavelength is the distance between crests of waves, frequency is number of completed cycles per second);
- consist of photons, which are bundles of pure energy which have no mass and no electric charge.

To understand the varying behaviours observed between the different forms of electromagnetic radiation, it is important to comprehend the relationship that exists between photon wavelength and frequency. An example of this would be to consider microwave television signals which can transmit sound and image information across a distance, but cannot readily pass through matter. You cannot see the television image if there is an object between the eye of the observer and the source, the television. In contrast to this, X-rays can penetrate matter and

alter atomic structure through ionisation (the ejection of orbital electrons). As the velocity (speed) of all forms of electromagnetic radiation is the same, the differing properties of each type of energy (consider the example just discussed microwaves and X-rays) can only be attributed to variations in their wavelength and frequency.

X-rays are located at the high end of the EMS as they possess short wavelengths. The relationship between wavelength and frequency is inversely proportional (i.e. as wavelength decreases, frequency increases). Quantum theory also states that frequency and energy are directly proportional. Despite the constant velocities of different electromagnetic radiations, they may have varying energies due to their wavelengths and frequencies. Radio waves have a long wavelength and lower frequency therefore are found at the low end of the EMS, whereas X-rays and gamma rays have short wavelengths and high frequency so are located at the high end of the spectrum. However both radio waves and X-rays have the same velocity.

X-rays are the classic form of artificially produced electromagnetic radiation. The X-ray tube is designed to accelerate a large number of electrons in a focused manner from the cathode to the anode, such that when the electrons arrive at the anode, they have acquired kinetic energy. This kinetic energy is then either converted to thermal energy (heat) or electromagnetic energy (X-rays). There is no equivalent energy to X-rays within nature; this type of energy is purely a human-made phenomenon. Within X-ray production there are several processes utilised to produce the end product, X-rays, which will now be discussed.

3.3.1 Thermionic Emission

In simple terms, X-rays are produced when electrons removed from the cathode are directed across the vacuumed tube at extremely high speeds to interact with the anode. The cathode electrons are released from the tungsten filament atoms in a process called thermionic emission, which refers to heat and the release of ions. The process of liberating electrons through heat application is similar to that observed in a light bulb. An electrical current (mA) is applied to the filament in the bulb which, because of its resistance, begins to glow. Whilst the current increases, the filament reaches a white-hot state necessary for the outer shell electrons to leave their orbits; this is known as incandescence. The resulting electrons which leave their orbits are called thermions. Thermionic emission will begin when the filament circuit receives energy via the tube current.

3.3.2 Potential Difference

The electron cloud, otherwise known as space charge, produced from the filament will stay in close vicinity of the cathode unless encouraged to move. As the exposure switch is depressed, the motivation force to move the electrons is released in the form of high voltage (typically 70–120 kVp). This high voltage creates a high potential difference between the negative cathode and positive anode. This in turn causes the negatively charged electrons to be strongly repelled from the cathode and drawn at high velocity to the positively attracting force of the anode. kVp is the voltage that determines the kinetic energy of the accelerated electrons within a X-ray tube. The potential difference may not be constant, therefore it is usual to quote the 'peak' (maximum) value. The kVp setting also determines the maximum energy of the X-ray photon emitted. Therefore a 50 kVp potential difference gives a maximum photon energy of 50 kV, however the average energy of that X-ray photon beam would be a half to a third of this value.

3.3.3 Target Interaction

X-rays are produced when the kinetic energy of the accelerated electron interacts with the atom of the target anode. When considering interactions that will occur at the anode target, it is important the reader has a basic understanding of atomic structure and electron orbits (see Chapter 2). Here is a quick revision: an atom consists of a nucleus and surrounding electron orbits. An incoming electron can interact with any of these orbiting electrons causing excitation, where the incoming electron transfers enough energy to raise the orbiting electron to a higher orbit, or ionisation, in which the incoming electron completely removes the electron from the atom.

As discussed earlier, when considering the X-ray tube, the anode (or target) is composed of a material with a high atomic number and high melting point, called tungsten. A high atomic number means that there are a greater proportion of electrons in the outer electron orbits of the tungsten atoms which create the anode target. The outer electron orbits within the tungsten atoms are less tightly bound to the nucleus of the tungsten atom; therefore projectile (incoming) electrons interact with outer shell electrons of the target tungsten atoms but do not transfer enough energy to remove (ionise) them and only raise them to a higher energy level. These outer electrons immediately drop back down to their normal energy state with the emission of heat. This happens frequently, making the X-ray tube very inefficient, because this energy has effectively been wasted. The probability of X-rays being emitted from the target is only around 1%. The remaining 99% of emissions result in the kinetic energy of the electron beam being converted into heat. Most of the kinetic energy of the electron beam hitting the target is converted into heat. However the fact that tungsten has a high melting point minimises the potential damage to the anode target due to the intense heat produced by the electron interactions. There are two interactive processes between incoming accelerated electrons and the atoms of the anode target which are crucial to understand when considering X-ray production within a X-ray tube: these are bremsstrahlung and characteristic radiation.

3.3.3.1 Bremsstrahlung

The principle interaction in X-ray production results in the output of X-ray photons known as bremsstrahlung, which comes from the German for 'braking' (*brems*) and 'radiation' (*strahlung*). The closer a projectile electron gets to the nucleus of a target atom the more it is influenced by the electrostatic field of the nucleus. As it passes close to the nucleus it is slowed down and it changes course, leaving in a different direction with reduced kinetic energy. This loss of kinetic energy appears as an X-ray, as shown in Figure 3.3. The electron may lose all or any intermediate amount of its kinetic energy, resulting in X-rays being emitted with a spread of energies, ranging from 0 to the maximum energy of the electron beam, which is the kilovolt setting on the console. A low-energy bremsstrahlung X-ray is produced when the incoming electron is only slightly influenced by the nucleus, producing a low-energy X-ray photon and then continuing with reduced energy. A high-energy bremsstrahlung X-ray is produced when the electron loses all its energy. The more pronounced the degree of deceleration the more energy is released. The intensity (*I*) with which bremsstrahlung radiation is produced increases with the atomic number (*Z*) of the target and the energy of the electrons (*E*):

$$I \propto ZE^2 \qquad (3.1)$$

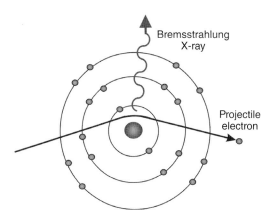

FIGURE 3.3 An incoming electron changing direction, due to the atomic nucleus, and giving off a low-energy bremsstrahlung X-ray.

Equation 3.1 also illustrates why heavy metal targets, such as tungsten, are used, because the efficiency of bremsstrahlung production is directly proportional to the atomic number of the target material. Bremsstrahlung accounts for approximately 75–80% of the X-ray tube's output.

3.3.3.2 Characteristic Radiation

The second interactive process which has a lesser contribution to X-ray production is characteristic radiation. Characteristic radiation is created by the direct interaction of projectile electrons from the cathode with inner shell electrons of the target material, tungsten. Ionisation results in an electron being ejected from the atom and leaving a hole in its place. If this hole is in an inner shell, this is a very unnatural state for the target atom to be in and the hole is very quickly filled by one of the outer electrons. The electron that moves from an outer to an inner shell has excess energy, which is emitted as an X-ray photon. This X-ray has an energy equal to the difference between the binding energies (BEs) of the electrons involved. Figure 3.4a shows an atom being ionised by an incoming projectile electron with high energy. The target electron has been ejected and has left a space in the K-shell. In Figure 3.4b an electron from the M-shell has moved into the vacancy, emitting a characteristic X-ray photon with an energy of 66.7 keV. For this interaction to occur in a tungsten atom, the energy of the emitted X-ray is calculated as 69.5 keV (BE of K-shell) − 2.8 keV (BE of M-shell) = 66.7 keV.

As demonstrated here, the energy of the characteristic X-ray is dependent on the binding energy of the target atom's electrons. BEs decrease the further away the electron orbits are from the nucleus. Outer-shell electrons have an extremely low binding energy and are easily ejected from the orbit. Ionisation events in the O or P shell of the tungsten atom do not produce significant characteristic X-rays as the energy output is extremely low. The resultant X-ray energies can be calculated if an M, N, O, or P electron fills this space, but all are called K X-rays because they result

(a)

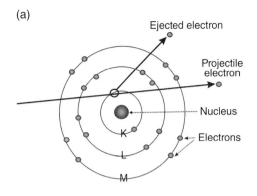

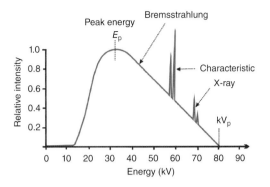

FIGURE 3.5 An X-ray emission spectrum for a tungsten target tube, with an operating voltage of 80 kV and a current of 400 mA.

(b)

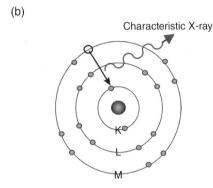

FIGURE 3.4 (a) An atom being ionised when a K-shell electron is ejected by an energetic projectile electron. (b) The vacancy in the K-shell, resulting from ionisation of the atom, is filled by an M-shell electron. A characteristic X-ray is given off.

from an ionisation of the K-shell. In the above example, the M-shell electron would also be replaced by an electron from an outer orbit and so on, producing a cascade of replacements with each one emitting a photon of energy equal to the difference in the BEs. This emission spectrum of the material is known as characteristic radiation because it is characteristic of the target element. It is a line spectrum of these discrete energy X-rays. The next area to consider in relation to X-ray production is the emission spectra of an X-ray tube and how this relates to each interaction process within the target.

3.3.4 The X-ray Spectrum

As described in Section 3.3.3, either characteristic X-rays, which have discrete photon energies, or bremsstrahlung X-rays,

which can have any photon energy up to the maximum kinetic energy of the electron hitting the target, can be produced. This X-ray spectrum can be represented graphically as a plot of the frequency with which X-rays are emitted as a function of their energy. Figure 3.5 shows the characteristic X-ray line spectrum superimposed on top of the continuous spectrum for the bremsstrahlung X-rays. The characteristic line spectrum is so called because the lines represent high intensities of single energy X-rays. Only the K X-rays are shown because these are the only characteristic emission from tungsten with sufficient energy to be of value when utilising kV energy radiation.

The general shape of the X-ray spectrum is the same for all X-ray machines. The maximum energy of the X-ray photons is equal to the voltage across the tube, which is set by the operator. This setting is actually the peak kilovoltage (kVp). The low-energy radiation is decreased in intensity as a result of the self-absorption of the anode itself. The average energy of the X-ray beam is about one-third of the maximum X-ray energy and its total intensity is given by the area under the curve. The maximum energy of the X-ray photons is inversely proportional to the wavelength (λ) Eq. (3.2):

$$\lambda(m) = \frac{1.24 \times 10^{-10}\left(\text{keV} \cdot m\right)}{\text{kV}_{\text{p}}\left(\text{keV}\right)} \qquad (3.2)$$

For example, the minimum wavelength associated with the X-rays emitted from a unit operated at 100 kVp is 0.0124 nm.

3.4 X-ray Output Intensity

The X-rays produced at the target are given off in all directions. Most are absorbed by the target itself or the surrounding shielding. The small amount of X-rays that leave the tube through the window is called the exit beam; these are the useful X-rays. A measure of the amount of these X-rays is the output intensity, which is the number of photons in the useful beam. The intensity of the beam is determined by the number of X-rays produced at the target. This firstly is affected by the number of electrons arriving at the target, i.e. the tube current (mA). Secondly, the velocity of the cathode stream which is determined by the potential difference (kVp) influences the energy available within the electrons for conversion into X-ray photons. Finally, if there is anything in the pathway of the exiting beam, this may cause X-rays to be absorbed. When any of these factors are altered, the output intensity of the useful beam changes.

High-energy X-ray photons pass through matter more readily than low-energy photons. This ability is referred to as penetration and is critical to the production of a useful radiographic image. A radiation beam of high energy penetrates human body tissues with greater ease than a low-voltage X-ray beam; this is the key concept in diagnostic and therapeutic radiography. Intensity is defined as the X-ray energy passing through unit area per unit time and is measured in roentgens or expressed as air kerma in Grays. The intensity of the X-ray tube is equal to the tube efficiency multiplied by the tube power, Eqs. (3.3)–(3.5).

$$\text{Tube power} \propto \left(\text{W} \right) \\ = \text{voltage} \left(\text{KV}_p \right) \times \text{current} \left(\text{mA} \right) \quad (3.3)$$

$$\text{Efficient} \propto \text{voltage} \left(\text{kV}_p \right) \quad (3.4)$$

therefore

$$\text{Intensity} \left(I \right) \propto \left(\text{kV}_p \right)^2 \times \text{mA} \quad (3.5)$$

3.5 Beam Quality

It is difficult to quote an energy for the spectrum that comes from an X-ray tube, due to the fact that it is polyenergetic. This means it has a spread of energies between zero and the maximum kilovoltage (kVp) of the tube, with the shape of a bremsstrahlung spectrum. As a polyenergetic beam travels through material, lower-energy photons are attenuated more than higher-energy ones. This means that the spread of energies present in the beam will determine how far it will travel in a material, or how penetrating it is. The greater the velocity of the cathode electron stream, the greater the resultant energy of the X-ray photons produced by target interactions. Therefore increasing voltage (kVp) increases photon energy. This energy is commonly termed beam quality.

3.5.1 Half-value Layer

This is a way to measure beam quality. The output of a well-collimated X-ray beam is measured and thin aluminium foils, usually of 1-mm thickness, are placed into the beam pathway until the intensity is half its original value. The thickness of aluminium producing this 50% reduction is called the half-value layer of the beam (HVL). The HVL is found by plotting the series of readings on a graph and is quoted as millimetres of Al. The HVL is measured at 80 kVp for a standard X-ray tube. It gives a measure of the penetrability of the beam, and can be monitored over time to ensure that an X-ray tube is not deteriorating.

3.6 Factors Affecting the Output Intensity and Quality of the Beam

A photon beam produced using high kVp has a high-quality beam, which would be highly penetrating in its clinical application. However, the measure of quality only addresses half of the X-ray beam equation. The number of photons in the beam must be considered, therefore the relationship between quality and quantity must be examined when considering radiographic image production.

3.6.1 Tube Current

Changing the current of the X-ray tube (the milliamps or mA) changes the number of electrons hitting the target. If you increase the mA by a factor of 2 then the number of X-rays emitted at each energy will also increase by a factor of 2. The shape of the output spectrum does not change, only the amplitude. This is illustrated in Figure 3.6, which shows what happens when the mA is doubled and all other factors are kept constant. This shows that $I \propto mA$, where I is the total intensity, shown by the area under the curve. Changing the current of the X-ray tube does not affect the quality of the beam, as the energy spread and hence effective energy stays the same.

The relationship between the number of cathode electrons released during thermionic emission and the production of X-ray photons is very simple: they are directly proportional. Therefore as the operator of a CT simulator increases the tube current, there will a predictable increase in the number of electrons released. This relationship will have no bearing on beam energy or penetrating power, however mA can be used to influence image density.

3.6.2 Peak Tube Voltage

Changing the voltage across the tube increases the kinetic energy of the electrons that reach the target. This means that the amount of bremsstrahlung produced increases, as well as the average energy and the maximum energy of the X-rays produced. This is shown in Figure 3.7, which shows two spectra, one with a peak tube voltage (kVp) of 70 kV and one with 80 kV. All other factors have been kept the same. The output intensity increases by a factor proportional to the kVp², as shown by Eq. (3.5). The quality of the beam has also increased, because the effective energy of the beam has increased.

3.6.3 Filtration

Applying a filter over the exit window will alter the number of X-rays in the useful beam and also their energy. A filter such as aluminium will filter out more of the lower-energy X-rays because these are attenuated more easily by the metal, whereas the higher-energy X-rays will pass through. The beam coming out of the tube will always have some effect from filtering, because the exit window and any inherent filtration will attenuate some low-energy photons. Figure 3.8 shows the effect of adding filtration into the exit beam. The highest energy of the spectrum (the kVp) stays the same, as the maximum energy of the X-rays coming out of the tube

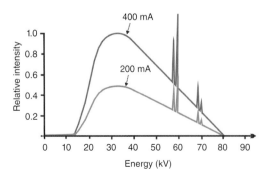

FIGURE 3.6 The effect on the tube spectrum when the mA has been halved.

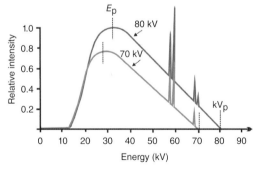

FIGURE 3.7 The effect on the tube spectrum when the kV has been reduced from 80 kV to 70 kV.

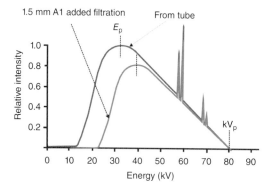

1.5 mm A1 added filtration

FIGURE 3.8   The effect on the tube spectrum when filtration has been added to the exit beam.

has not changed and some of these will always pass through all filtering unattenuated. The effective energy shifts to a higher kilovoltage as the number of lower energy X-rays has decreased. Filtration of the kV photon beam reduces the patient dose, as lower-energy X-rays will always be absorbed by the patient without giving any useful information to the medical image produced.

3.7 X-ray Production and Clinical Practice

The development of new technology has allowed for advances in the acquisition, storage, and mobility of digital imaging.

X-rays have a variety of uses in both diagnostic and therapeutic clinical departments. X-ray energies are used in CT simulation in the 50–120 kVp range, to obtain patient anatomical information when planning the patient's radiotherapy and in the range 60–250 kV, X-ray photons can be used to treat superficial tumours.

The basic concepts of X-ray production are the building blocks to understanding the developments within radiotherapy clinical practice; for example, the advancement of LinAcs featuring OBIs to gain better geometric detail and enhanced image resolution of treatment delivery.

Further Reading

Holmes, K., Elkington, M., and Harris, P. (2013). *Clark's Essential Physics in Imaging for Radiographer.* London: CRC Press Taylor & Francis Group.

Symonds, R.P., Mills, J.A., and Duxbury, A.M. (2019). *Walter and Miller's Textbook of Radiotherapy, Radiation Physics, Therapy and Oncology,* 8e. Edinburgh: Churchill Livingstone, Elsevier.

Washington, C. and Leaver, D. (2016). *Principles and Practice of Radiation Therapy,* 4e. Missouri: Elsevier Mosby.

CHAPTER 4

Radiation Detection and Measurement

Jan Chianese and Fiona Chamberlain

Aim

The aim of this chapter is to provide an introduction to the theory of dose measurement and give an overview of the design and operation of practical dosimeters encountered in the modern radiotherapy department.

4.1 The Unit of Absorbed Dose

There is no definition of a fundamental unit of radiation that causes known responses in different biological models because of the disparate interaction properties of different particles and qualities of radiation. It is possible, however, to relate the damage mechanisms of radiation to the amount of ionising energy deposited in tissues. Although the precise microscopic distribution of this energy deposition has a profound effect on the overall biological response, for particles and qualities producing similar interactions (such as electrons and photons in the range 0.05–10 MeV) the constant of proportionality remains the same. It is impractical to measure microscopic distribution and so a macroscopic assessment of absorbed energy is made quantified by the SI unit of absorbed dose – the gray.

The gray is defined as: 'The absorbed dose (D) is the quotient of $\mathrm{d}e$ by $\mathrm{d}m$, where $\mathrm{d}e$ is the mean energy imparted by ionising radiation to matter of mass $\mathrm{d}m$'.

$$D = \frac{\mathrm{d}e}{\mathrm{d}m}$$

1 gray = 1 joule per kilogramme (1 Gy = 1 J kg^{-1}).

4.1.1 Measuring the Gray

Nationally accredited measuring laboratories will keep specialist equipment that measures absorbed dose under controlled conditions, enabling an absolute standard to be produced (the primary standard). Dosimeters across the country are sent to this centre for comparison and subsequent calibration against this standard and are therefore known as secondary standards. Dosimeters calibrated against secondary dosimeters are termed tertiary standards. Calibration of the local standard against the primary standard is recommended every two years [1].

Practical Radiotherapy: Physics and Equipment, Third Edition. Edited by Pam Cherry and Angela M. Duxbury.
© 2020 John Wiley & Sons Ltd. Published 2020 by John Wiley & Sons Ltd.

4.1.2 Calorimetry

Calorimetry is one method of measuring absorbed dose whereby the precise quantification of minute temperature changes in irradiated samples are used to produce direct evidence of the energy absorbed during the process, because the heat energy absorbed by a sample is proportional to the absorbed dose. Calibration of local ionisation detectors against a national calorimetric standard also exists for a range of megavoltage photon qualities; however, calorimetry is not always practicable because it suits the measurement of large absorbed quantities of radiation under very controlled conditions. Therefore there are other preferred methods for less energetic X-rays and electrons.

The first step is to specify a unit of ionisation that is compatible with absorbed dose.

4.1.3 Exposure

Exposure is defined as: 'The exposure (X), is the quotient of dQ by dm where the value of dQ is the absolute value of the total charge of the ions of one sign produced in air when all the electrons (negatrons and positrons) liberated by photons in air of mass dm are completely stopped in air' [2]. The SI unit of exposure is coulombs per kilogramme (C kg^{-1}).

This definition explicitly defines exposure for photons interacting with a defined mass of air and no other radiation particles or irradiated medium. To determine the exposure at some point within any other medium, it is necessary to replace a small part of that material with a volume of air small enough to prevent disruption of the photon field. The process covered by this definition thus comprises two stages. First, photons interact with the air to produce electrons (by photoelectric absorption or Compton scatter) or electrons and positrons (by pair production). Second, these electrons and positrons diffuse though the air causing more ionisation (see Chapter 5 for further details of interaction processes). Exposure is thus the collection of all the ions of one sign when the energy of all subsequent particles has been completely dissipated.

It should be noted that some of the secondary particles will lose a small amount of energy by the bremsstrahlung process, which in turn may cause further ionisation, and this must be excluded from the total charge contributing to the definition of exposure.

As absorbed dose in $(D_{air}) = X\dfrac{W}{E}$, where

E = the charge on an electron and W = the mean energy expended in the formation of one ion pair, and exposure (X)

$$= \frac{dQ}{dm}$$

and $D_{air} = \dfrac{W_{air}}{e} \times \dfrac{dQ}{dm} = \dfrac{W_{air}}{e} \times X$

Absorbed dose in material (D_{mat})

$$= \frac{A_{mat}}{A_{air}} \times \frac{W_{mat}}{e} \times X \tag{4.1}$$

where W_{air} = average energy absorbed in the production of a single ion pair in air (33.85 eV); e = charge on each ion; W_{air}/e = 33.85 J/C; A_{mat} = mass energy absorption coefficient for material; and A_{air} = mass energy absorption coefficient for air.

Although the concept of exposure satisfies the mathematical requirements of the derivation of dose, there are obvious practical problems when attempting to irradiate a defined mass of air whilst leaving a surrounding volume sufficient to attenuate the secondary particles, unirradiated. The practical solution is the free-air chamber that utilises charged particle equilibrium to circumvent this dilemma.

4.2 Free-Air Ionisation Chamber

The theory and operation of this exposure device may be explained by considering the schematic diagram in Figure 4.1. A collimated photon beam enters the chamber through the diaphragms on the left-hand side exiting through the opposite wall. Within the body of the chamber, a parallel

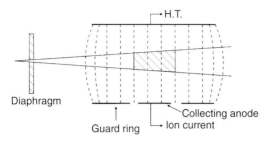

FIGURE 4.1 The 'free-air' ionisation chamber.

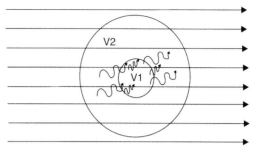

FIGURE 4.2 Principle of the 'air-wall'.

plate electrode assembly is mounted with guard wires and a concentric guard ring arranged to define a volume of air from which secondary charged particles are collected. The separation of the plates is chosen to ensure that any remaining kinetic energy of the secondary particles is dissipated before their arrival at the collecting electrode, whilst being sufficiently close for the applied polarising voltage to collect all the ions produced within the defined volume. In order to satisfy the conditions imposed by the definition of exposure, the ions generated within the collection boundary (shaded area) that are lost to the periphery must be balanced with externally generated ions entering this critical volume. This is the state of electronic equilibrium. Corrections are required for lack of saturation in the ionisation current, the presence of any water vapour, and ionisation resulting from bremsstrahlung and scattered radiation or leakage through the primary collimators.

4.3 Cavity Chamber (Cylindrical or Thimble Chamber)

The free-air chamber is capable of accurately determining exposure for energies up to 300 kV. Above this energy the separation of the electrodes demands prohibitive polarising voltages to collect the charges produced. Although the free-air chamber enables a definitive measurement of exposure, by utilising the concept of electronic equilibrium, it is not a practical piece of equipment for everyday clinical use due to its large size. More portable dosimeters have been designed that are more practical for use in the high-energy ranges used in radiotherapy. These portable devices have small detectors capable of measuring exposure 'in phantom' without agitating the radiation fluence. To achieve this goal the 'air-wall' concept is used (Figure 4.2).

Consider the small volume of air, V_1, completely surrounded by a larger and concentric volume of air, V_2, uniformly irradiated by a photon radiation field. If V_2 is sufficiently large such that the energies of the secondary particles produced within V_1 are dissipated before leaving V_2, then the geometric requirements for achieving electronic equilibrium are satisfied. If V_2 is then compressed to 1/1000 of its original volume, the diameter can be reduced without compromising the electronic equilibrium and, if central and peripheral electrodes are incorporated, an ionisation detector with similar performance characteristics to the free air chamber can be achieved. In practice, V_2 is not actually compressed but is replaced by a material of similar atomic number but greater density, e.g. graphite; this has the added benefit of being a conductor and can therefore act as one of the electrodes. The complete assembly is known as the thimble chamber (Figure 4.3).

Using this device it is possible to extend the estimation of exposure across a greater range of energies (typically the Farmer-type chambers can measure up to 50 MeV) with equipment that is essentially portable and suited to the rigours of practical radiotherapy output measurements.

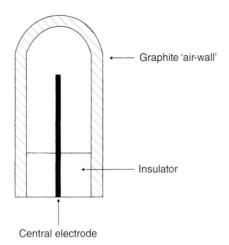

FIGURE 4.3 The thimble chamber.

4.4 Parallel Plate (Pancake) Chambers

Parallel plate chambers, as the name suggests, are constructed of two parallel plates of material (plastic) that form the walls of the chamber. These walls are coated with a conducting layer that forms the positive and negative electrodes. A layer of gas between the walls acts as the collecting volume. The electrodes lie close together so that the air cavity can be constructed very thinly, leading to very little noticeable perturbation. Guard electrodes (rings) create uniform field lines by minimising settling time of the chamber. Parallel plate chambers must be used when the mean electron energy is greater than 5 MeV at any depth [1]. These chambers can measure a range of energies up to 50 MeV electrons. Desirable properties of these chambers are that they should be waterproof and their construction as homogeneous and water equivalent as possible.

4.5 Air Kerma

The term 'kerma' originates from the acronym 'kinetic energy released per unit mass'. This term is not complete without specifying the material concerned.

It is formally defined as: 'the quotient dE_{tr} by dm, where dE_{tr} is the sum of the initial kinetic energies of all the charged ionising particles liberated by uncharged ionising particles in a material of mass dm' [2].

Therefore:

$$K = dE_{tr}/dm.$$

Kerma is therefore an energy equivalent to exposure and is measured in joules/kilogramme and therefore has the same dimensions as absorbed dose, the gray, being related by the expression:

$$\text{Absorbed dose} = \frac{A_{mat}}{T_{air}} \times \text{air kerma (Gy)}$$

where A_{mat} = mass energy absorption coefficient for material; T_{air} = mass energy transfer coefficient for air; and $A_{mat}/T_{air} \approx 1.1$.

The difference between the quantity of energy transferred and the eventual energy absorbed is only 0.4% and is due to bremsstrahlung production.

4.6 Dosimetry of Megavoltage Photons

Unlike the traditional approach to exposure measurement, where the electronic equilibrium conditions are satisfied entirely within the detector body and the unit acts as a 'photon probe', consideration must be given to the charge balance at a single point in a large medium exposed to uniform photon irradiation in which a gas cavity has been introduced. In this case, if the cavity is sufficiently small to prevent the disturbance of the particle fluence within the medium, the same number and energy of electrons traverse this volume, whether gas or medium, and the ratio of the electron energies lost per unit mass of gas to medium is the same as the ratio of the two mass stopping powers (S) to the energy lost (dE) by the charged particles in traversing a small distance (dl) divided by its density (μ), i.e.

$$S = \frac{dE/dl}{\mu}$$

If this absorbed energy in the gas produces a charge J, then the energy required to produce this ionisation is given by JWg/e, where Wg is the mean energy required to produce one ionisation in air and e is the charge on the electron, the equivalent absorbed dose (D_m) within the medium is given by:

$$D_m = S_{mg} \times J \times Wg/e \qquad (4.2)$$

where S_{mg} is the stopping power ratio of medium to gas. This equation summarises the hypotheses proposed initially by Bragg (1912) [3] and then refined by Gray (1929, 1936), [4, 5] and relies for its validity on four basic assumptions:

1. Charged particle equilibrium exists in the absence of the cavity;
2. The particle fluence is not disturbed by the cavity presence;
3. The mass stopping power ratio is constant over the energy spectrum;
4. The secondary particles lose their energy by a large number of small interactions.

Eq. (4.2) is analogous to the low-energy photon version expressed in Eq. (4.1), but with the ratio of the mass energy absorption coefficients replaced by the stopping power ratio S_{mg}.

As discussed previously the ionisation chamber:

- is generally calibrated in terms of air kerma rather than charge itself;
- has a minimal effect on particle fluence;
- disturbs the continuity of the material by its very presence.

Therefore, in terms of the reading, R, of an instrument calibrated in air kerma, the formula [6] for deriving absorbed dose to water (D_w) is:

$$D_w = R \times N \times C\lambda$$

where R is the dosimeter reading corrected for temperature and pressure; N is the calibration factor converting the reading R to grays in air kerma; and $C\lambda$ is the factor converting air kerma to absorbed dose for the photon energy of use.

$C\lambda$ brings together the conversion from exposure to air kerma at 2 MV, the calibration energy, and the variation sensitivity with energy of the secondary standard ionisation chamber for which $C\lambda$ is calculated. So, in summary, $C\lambda$ is the factor that allows a secondary standard to be used instead of the primary one.

Ionisation chambers for megavoltage photons are now calibrated directly in absorbed dose and not air kerma via the NPL (National Physical Laboratory) absorbed dose standard and the Institute of Physical Sciences in Medicine Code of Practice [6, 7]

4.6.1 Electrons

The Bragg–Gray cavity theory is also used in electron dosimetry, but there is a fundamental difference in the way that dose is derived from ionisation measurements compared with that used for photons [1]. The energy spectrum of a photon beam does not change significantly with increasing depth of penetration in water; the factors relating absorbed dose to ionisation remain effectively constant, because electrons are absorbed within a medium. However, the average energy of their spectrum decreases approximately linearly with increasing depth, reducing to zero at their maximum penetration, R_p.

If the mean incident energy of the electrons is denoted E_0 then the approximate mean spectral energy can be calculated at any depth (d) by the equation:

$$E_d = E_0 (1 - d/R_p).$$

Derivation of the dose at any depth therefore involves two stages: first, determination of the mean incident energy from a half-value thickness in water measurement; and second, application of the corresponding correction factors for the particular energy at depth to the ionisation values measured under appropriate clinical conditions.

4.6.2 Calorimetry

Although dose derivation using the Bragg–Gray approach, under conditions of charged particle equilibrium, is accepted, there are several assumptions enshrined within the theory that are difficult to measure directly and will always introduce unacceptable margins of uncertainty. To remove these errors of uncertainty, a more direct measurement of energy deposition is required, which to date has been achieved for megavoltage photons using a graphite calorimeter (Figure 4.4).

Although graphite has a specific thermal capacity some six times greater than that of water, the temperature increase resulting from a typical radiotherapy fraction is still only a few thousandths of a degree Celsius, and certainly negligible compared with the changes in the surrounding ambient temperature. To determine these fluctuations accurately and to improve on the alternative methods of dosimetry, the measuring system must be capable of discriminating temperature changes of one-millionth of a degree. To measure these minuscule temperature changes resulting from absorbed radiation dose the sample, or, in this case, graphite 'core', must be thermally isolated from the local environment. This is partially achieved by mounting the core inside an evacuated 'jacket' of equal mass and material, which is in itself thermally isolated from the surrounding 'mantle' by a vacuum gap.

To compensate for any thermal transfer from core to jacket the system is calibrated by heating the core using a known amount of electrical energy and observing the temperature changes in the jacket. As each component of the calorimeter has both heaters and thermocouples embedded within it, the whole assembly can be heated and maintained at a stable temperature to minimise any thermal transfer to and from the surrounding environment. More recently the NPL has developed a portable calorimeter that can be used on site in clinical departments [8].

4.7 Radiation Detection and Measurement

Table 4.1 lists the effects of radiation that form the basis of various detectors and dosimeters.

Some of the devices are best suited to direct measurement of doses received by patients and clinical staff and others to measurement of doses from treatment machines (at commissioning, acceptance, and routine quality assurance testing).

It is recommended that all patients receiving radiotherapy have their first treatment dose checked with a dosimeter [1] and the most commonly used device for this purpose is a semiconductor device. Other devices used in the radiotherapy department to measure absorbed dose are ionisation chambers, radiochromic film, OSL (optically stimulated luminescence), and thermoluminescent dosimeters (TLDs).

To be useful in a radiotherapy department a detector must satisfy certain basic requirements. It should:

- be accurate;
- be sensitive;
- exhibit a linear response to dose;
- be mechanically robust;
- have a suitable physical size.

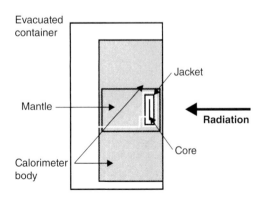

FIGURE 4.4 The absorbed dose calorimeter.

TABLE 4.1   **Properties of radiation which form the basis of measuring devices.**

Effects of radiation	Example of dosimeter/detector
Heat	Calorimeter
Photoluminescence	Optically Stimulated Luminescence dosimeter (OSL)
Ionisation	Thimble chamber, semiconductor detectors, Geiger Muller tube
Chemical effect	Fricke dosimeter
Scintillation	Scintillation counter
Chemical	Radiochromic film
Thermoluminescence	Thermoluminescent dosimeter (TLD)

4.7.1 Semiconductor Detectors

These have three uses in radiotherapy:

1. Relative dosimetry of photon and electron beams;
2. In vivo dosimetry of photon and electron beams;
3. Quality assurance measurements.

4.7.1.1 Principles of Operation

A semiconductor has electrical conducting properties somewhere between those of a conductor and those of an insulator. The most commonly used semiconductor material is silicon, which is a group IV element in the periodic table. Silicon has four electrons in its outer valence band. In pure silicon, these valence electrons are covalently bonded with valence electrons in adjacent silicon atoms to form a crystal lattice. If the crystal absorbs energy, the covalent bonds can be broken, resulting in a free electron and a positive hole where the electron once was. The electron can then move through the crystal. If the positive hole takes up an electron from a neighbouring atom, the hole also moves. If impurities are added to silicon, a process known as doping, semiconductors with excess electrons or excess positive holes can be created (n- and p-type semiconductors, respectively).

A p-type semiconductor consists of silicon to which has been added a substance from group III of the periodic table, such as boron or aluminium. Group III elements have three electrons in their valence band that are able to form covalent bonds with the silicon atoms; however, one bond is not completed and thus a positive hole is created. In an n-type semiconductor an element is added from group V of the periodic table, such as phosphorus or arsenic. Group V elements have five electrons in their valence band. Four of these are able to take part in covalent bonds with silicon atoms, the fifth being free to move though the crystal (Figure 4.5).

If the device is irradiated, electrons and positive holes are created. The electrons are attracted towards the positively charged impurity in the n-type silicon and the positive holes diffuse towards the negatively charged impurity in the p-type silicon. This constitutes an ionisation current that is proportional to the incident dose rate and can be measured using an electrometer.

In practice, semiconductor dosimeters comprise a large portion of one type (p or n) and a smaller part of the other type. The dosimeter is then classified as either a p- or n-type detector according to the larger constituent part; n-type detectors show a sensitivity decrease and become nonlinear with respect to dose rate as a result of radiation damage; p-type semiconductors do not suffer this drawback and also demonstrate a slower sensitivity decrease after irradiation, and for this reason are preferred for most clinical applications.

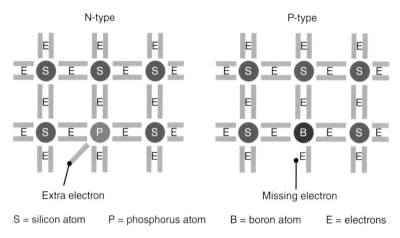

FIGURE 4.5 Semiconductor process.

4.7.1.2 Detector Design

The detector consists of a small silicon detector crystal (external dimensions 2.5 mm × 2.5 mm × 0.4 mm) mounted on a Perspex plate (Figure 4.6). It is connected via aluminium foils to a coaxial cable (wireless detectors are also now available – Figure 4.7), and it is encapsulated in a protective sheath. A build-up cap is also incorporated and the type of material from which it is made and its thickness depend on the radiation quality being measured.

4.7.1.3 Advantages

The semiconductor detector has the following advantages:

- High electrical signal: this means that the device is very sensitive – approximately 18 000 times more sensitive than an ionisation chamber.

- Small physical size: this is possible because of the high sensitivity, which means that the measuring volume can be small. This has the added advantage that the effective measuring point can be located close to the surface of the detector, providing a high degree of spatial resolution.

- Mechanically stable.

- Independent of atmospheric pressure – therefore no pressure correction factor is required.

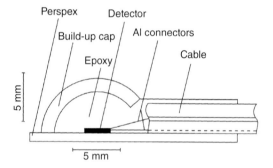

FIGURE 4.6 Scanditronix p-Si patient dosimetry detector. (Source: reproduced by permission Scanditronix Medical AB.)

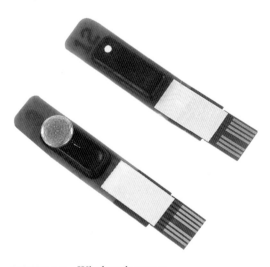

FIGURE 4.7 Wireless detectors.

- The small stopping power variation with energy in electron beams makes the detector suitable for measuring electron beams.

- Immediate readout available.

4.7.1.4 Limitations

The semiconductor detector has the following limitations:

The sensitivity of the detector varies with temperature (in clinical practice, this variation is of the order of 1–3%); this is a consideration when *in vivo* measurements are made. The temperature of the detectors will rise when in contact with the patient's skin. To account for this the detectors may be placed on the patient three to four minutes before treatment starts to allow time for the detector to reach a steady state. A correction factor is then applied to take into account the change in sensitivity due to temperature (usually an increase). Alternatively, the detector may be calibrated at body temperature using a phantom at a raised temperature.

The sensitivity also varies with accumulated radiation dose. Above a certain accumulated dose, the sensitivity stabilises and for this reason detectors are often supplied preirradiated.

Radiation damage is a particular problem in n-type detectors that progressively exhibit a nonlinear response with dose rate; p-type detectors are less susceptible to this effect. The amount of damage inflicted on the detector is related not only to the total radiation dose but also to the quality of radiation.

4.8 Thermoluminescent Dosimeters

These have four uses in radiotherapy:

1. Relative dosimetry of electron and photon beams;

2. In vivo dosimetry of electron and photon beams;

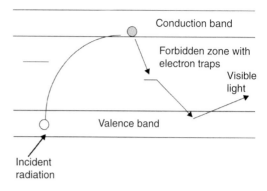

FIGURE 4.8 Principles of thermoluminescence.

3. Personal monitoring;

4. Environmental monitoring.

4.8.1 Principles of Operation

Crystals that have luminescent properties have impurities introduced which create F-traps (electron traps). When the crystal is irradiated, electrons in the valence band may receive sufficient energy for them to be raised to the conduction band. Electrons may then fall back to the valence band or get caught in an electron trap (Figure 4.8). Electrons caught in the traps are unable to escape until the crystal is heated. When sufficient heat is applied the electrons gain thermal energy and fall back from the electron trap to the valence band; in doing so the electrons emit energy in the form of light photons. The total light output is proportional to the number of trapped electrons, which in turn is proportional to the energy absorbed from the radiation beam.

4.9 TLD Detector Types

There are a number of different crystalline materials that exhibit thermoluminescent properties. The most commonly used within radiotherapy are those based on lithium fluoride (LiF) because LiF is approximately tissue equivalent (effective atomic number of 8.2 compared with 7.4 for tissue) and almost energy independent in the range 100 keV– 1.3 MeV gamma radiation. Other TLD materials include those based on lithium borate ($LiBO_4$), calcium fluoride (CaF_3), and calcium sulphate ($CaSO_4$). Each of these materials has specific advantages with regard to sensitivity, measuring range, or tissue equivalence, but LiF has the best overall properties for most purposes within radiotherapy [8].

TLD materials are supplied in powder form and as solid discs, rods, and chips (Figure 4.9). Discs can be encapsulated in Teflon for use in personal dosimeters, which may incorporate built-in filters to enable

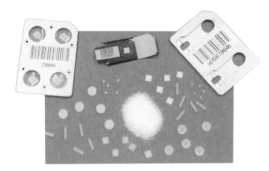

FIGURE 4.9 The variety of physical forms of thermoluminescent dosimeter (TLD) materials available. (Source: reproduced courtesy of Harshaw/Bicon NE Technology Ltd.)

energy discrimination of radiation dose received. The advantages and limitations of TLDs are outlined in Table 4.2.

4.10 Optically Stimulated Luminescence (OSL) Dosimetry

The process is the same as that for TLD, except the stimulus for the luminescence is a light source (usually green light source), rather than heat.

Material: Al_2O_3C
Characteristics for radiotherapy:

- Small size;
- Good reproducibility;
- No correction factors when environmental conditions are met;
- Linear dose response (up to 400 cGy at 6 MV);
- Dose rate independence;
- Not energy dependent;

TABLE 4.2 Advantages and limitations of thermoluminescent dosimeters (TLDs).

Advantages	Limitations and disadvantages
Reusable	Precision can be affected by poor handling and storage
Automated readout	Immediate readout is not possible
Energy independent over a wide range of the energies	'Fading' – unintentional release of trapped electrons, may be caused by exposure to heat or light (particularly ultraviolet)
Similar atomic number to soft tissue (except those containing calcium)	Some types may liquefy if left in humid conditions
Capable of measuring over a wide range of doses	Scratches on the surface of the thermoluminescent dosimeter (TLD) or reduction in mass will affect the light emission characteristics
Small physical size	May become contaminated by grease or adhesives

TABLE 4.3	**Advantages and limitations of Optically Stimulated Luminescence (OSL) dosimetry.**
Advantages	**Limitations and disadvantages**
• High sensitivity	• Sensitivity to light
• High precision	• Non-tissue equivalent
• Size	• Only one material currently available (only one provider)
• Convenience	• Needs to be bleached if re-used
• Fast nondestructive readout	
• Readout flexibility	
• No significant fading	
• No need for annealing (compared to thermoluminescent dosimeter [TLD])	
• Dose is stored permanently but can be reused (see disadvantages)	

- Isotropic response to radiation;
- Can be used in phantom, e.g. IMRT QA;
- In vivo external beam and brachytherapy.
- The advantages and disadvantages of OSLs are outlined in Table 4.3.

4.11 Dosimetry in CT

As treatment planning (and treatment and tumour monitoring) is routinely undertaken using computed tomography (CT), the dosimetry terms and techniques are described. CT dose is usually expressed in terms of CTDI (CT Dose Index) or Dose Length Product (DLP).

CTDI is a standardised measurement of CT scanner output; this is a dose to a phantom from a single gantry rotation. This allows comparison from one CT scanner to another in terms of dose. This does not take into account the areas of the body being scanned, as dose is not equal across a scan plane, so dose is calculated from the centre to the periphery, which gives a weighted dose, $CTDI_w$.

A more useful dose measurement takes into account the pitch of the scan; higher pitch has larger gaps between slices, and lowers the dose. This is volume, $CTDI_{vol}$:

$$CTDI_{vol} = CTDI_W / pitch$$

All of these values are expressed in mGy.

The DLP is the total dose to the patient along the distance scanned:

$$DLP = CTDI_{vol} \times distance\ scanned$$

The unit of DLP is mGy*cm.

Effective dose takes into account the radiosensitivity of different organs; this is measured in mSv (Figure 4.10).

Dose in CT is measured using a phantom with a pencil/thimble ionisation chamber; this gives the CTDI and then subsequent values can be calculated from this value.

4.12 MRI LinAc

The advent of the MRI LinAc has led to research into compatible strategies for absolute beam dosimetry. Preliminary reports have highlighted positive development into the use of portable calorimeters and measurement of Cherenkov light (which is proportional to photon beam emissions), as well as the use of medical oxide semiconductor field or MOSFET as suitable tools for dosimetry measurements for MRI LinAcs [9, 10].

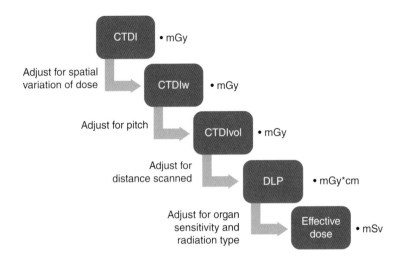

FIGURE 4.10 The Dose Length Product (DLP) is the total dose to the patient along the distance scanned. (Source: reproduced with the kind permission of RadiologyCafe.)

References

1. Institute of Physics and Engineering in Medicine (IPEM) (2003). Code of Practice for Electron Dosimetry for Radiotherapy Beams of Initial Energy from 4 to 25 MeV based on an absorbed dose to water calibration. *Physics in Medicine and Biology* 48: 2929–2970.
2. International Commission on Radiation Units and Measurements. 2014. ICRU Report 90, Key Data For Ionizing-Radiation Dosimetry: Measurement Standards And Applications.
3. Bragg, W.H. (1912). *Studies in Radioactivity.* London: Macmillan.
4. Gray, L.H. (1929). The absorption of penetrating radiation. *Proceedings of the Royal Society* A122: 647.
5. Gray, L.H. (1936). The absorption of penetrating radiation. *Proceedings of the Royal Society* A156: 578.
6. International Commission on Radiation Units and Measurements. Implementation of Recommendations of ICRU Report 90, Key Data For Ionizing-Radiation Dosimetry: Measurement Standards And Applications. Volume 14, Issue 1, 1 November 2014.
7. Institute of Physical Sciences in Medicine (IPSM) (1990). Code of Practice for High Energy Photon Therapy based on the NPL absorbed dose calibration service. *Physics in Medicine and Biology* 35: 1355–1360.
8. McEwen, M.R. and Duane, S.A. (2000). Portable graphite calorimeter for measuring absorbed dose in the radiotherapy clinic. *Physics in Medicine and Biology* 45: 3675–3691.
9. Nusrat H, Renaud J, Entezari N, et al. 2018. AAPM 2018, 60th Annual Meeting Absolute Dosimetry Using a Novel Portable Water Calorimeter Design in MR-Linac
10. Tewatia D, Yadav P, Tanumihardjo I, et al. 2018 AAPM 2018, 60th Annual Meeting Feasibility of MOSFET Real-Time In-Vivo Dosimetry for MRI-Linac Beams Under 0.34 T Magnetic Field.

Further Reading

Khan, F.M. (2014). *The Physics of Radiation Therapy,* 5e. Philidelphia, MA: Lippincott Williams & Wilkins.
Chang, D.S. and Lasley, F.D. (2014). *Basic Radiotherapy Physics and Biology.* Springer.

CHAPTER 5

X-ray Interactions with Matter

Kathryn Cooke

Aim

The aim of this chapter is to outline the principles of the interaction process that occur when ionising radiation interacts with a medium in the energy ranges relevant to radiotherapy.

5.1 Introduction

There are several interaction processes that occur when ionising radiation interacts with matter. These depend on the nature and energy of the primary radiation beam and the structure of the medium through which the radiation beam passes. It is beyond the scope of this chapter to describe all possible interaction processes, so only the three that occur within the X-ray energy ranges utilised in radiotherapy are presented later: photoelectric process, Compton scatter, and pair production.

5.1.1 Attenuation

It is important to understand how the intensity of the X-ray beam is affected when ionising radiation interacts with a medium.

When a beam of X-rays traverses matter, there is a reduction in the intensity of that beam. *Intensity* is defined as the rate of flow of photon energy through a unit area lying at right angles to the path of the beam. This reduction in intensity is referred to as *attenuation* and involves a process of absorption, scattering, or a combination of both.

Absorption is the transference of energy from the primary X-ray beam to the atoms of the medium through which the X-ray beam is passing. It is defined as the energy deposited in the material per unit mass. The transferred energy is converted into kinetic energy of the electrons within the medium, enabling them to move through the medium. The electrons may interact with other atoms in the medium causing *ionisation* and *excitation* (see Chapters 2 and 3). This results in the chemical and biological changes important to radiotherapy.

Scattering occurs following a collision interaction between the primary X-ray beam and the atoms of the medium through which the X-ray beam is passing. The incident photon is deflected out of the path of the primary beam and travels onward in a new direction. This collision may or may not involve transference of energy from the incident photon to the medium.

The size of the nucleus of an atom is extremely small compared with the overall

Practical Radiotherapy: Physics and Equipment, Third Edition. Edited by Pam Cherry and Angela M. Duxbury.
© 2020 John Wiley & Sons Ltd. Published 2020 by John Wiley & Sons Ltd.

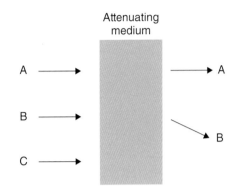

FIGURE 5.1 Process of attenuation. (A) transmission; (B) scattering; (C) absorption.

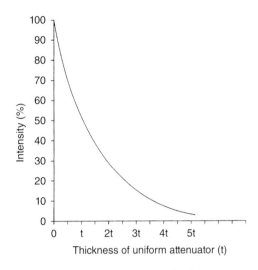

FIGURE 5.2 Exponential relationship between intensity of transmitted radiation and thickness of attenuator for a homogeneous beam of X-rays.

size of the atom and so most of the atom is considered as space.

Therefore, there is a high probability that some X-rays will pass straight through a medium without undergoing absorption or scattering (Figure 5.1). The X-rays are said to be transmitted and it is these X-rays that play a part in the production of a radiographic image and contribute to the exit dose of a beam of X-rays used for radiation treatment.

5.1.2 Exponential Relationship

Although it is impossible to predict which photons will interact with the medium, it is possible to predict the fraction of total photons that will undergo interaction. Experimentally it can be shown that for a narrow, homogeneous beam of X-rays, i.e. a beam of photons of similar energy, the intensity of radiation transmitted is reduced in an 'exponential' manner (Figure 5.2). Equal thicknesses of uniform attenuating material placed in the path of the beam produce equal fractional reductions in the intensity of radiation transmitted, e.g. a thickness of attenuator (t) reduces the intensity of the beam initially by 50% (100% reduced to 50%), then again by 50% (50% reduced to 25%). This is referred to as an exponential relationship and is represented by the equation:

$$I_t = I_0 e^{\mu t}$$

where I_t = intensity with medium of thickness (t) inserted in the path of the beam; I_0 = intensity with no medium in path of beam; e = exponential coefficient; μ = total linear attenuation coefficient; and t = thickness of stated medium.

Due to this exponential relationship it is not possible to attenuate an X-ray beam completely, although the intensity may be reduced to an insignificant level.

5.1.3 Half-Value Layer

An important descriptor known as the half-value layer (HVL) can be related to the exponential relationship between the attenuator and the intensity of the beam. The HVL is the thickness of a stated medium that will reduce the intensity of a narrow beam of X-rays to exactly half of its original value.

The first HVL is indicated in Figure 5.2 by the value of the thickness of attenuator that reduces the intensity of the beam from 100–50%; the second HVL is the thickness that reduces the intensity of the beam from 50–25%. For a homogeneous beam of radiation, these values will always be equal, e.g. referring to Figure 5.2, the HVL is 't'. However, an X-ray beam is heterogeneous and comprises photons of differing energies, so successive values of HVL cannot be the same due to filtration of the lower energy photons in the beam by the initial attenuation. The beam increases in homogeneity as filtration occurs and later values of HVL will become equivalent.

By definition, if the intensity of a beam of X-rays is reduced to 50% of the original intensity by a stated material of thickness HVL, it can be said that:

$$I_0 \div I_{\mathrm{HVL}} = 2.$$

By inserting this value in the exponential equation, it is found that the HVL is related to the linear attenuation coefficient (μ) by:

$$\mu = 0.693 \div \mathrm{HVL}.$$

The HVL and related tenth-value layer (TVL) are terms commonly used when discussing radiation protection materials. TVL is the thickness of a stated medium that will reduce the intensity of a narrow beam of X-rays to exactly one-tenth of its original value.

5.1.4 Attenuation Coefficients

An attenuation coefficient indicates the attenuating ability of a medium. The *linear attenuation coefficient* used previously is defined as the fractional reduction in intensity of a parallel beam of radiation per unit thickness of the attenuating medium traversed and is awarded the SI unit of m^{-1}. It is essential that the beam of radiation is parallel (nondivergent), so that it is not affected by the inverse square law (see Chapter 2).

Attenuation of an X-ray beam involves an interaction between a photon and an atom of the attenuating medium. Therefore, the possibility of an interaction occurring increases as the number of atoms per unit volume of the medium increases; conversely it decreases as the number of atoms per unit volume of the medium decreases. The definition of the linear attenuation coefficient (μ) suggests that it is dependent on the actual thickness of

traversed medium but this does not take into account the actual number of atoms within the traversed thickness. Therefore, any change of state in the same thickness of medium, e.g. solid to gaseous state, involving a decrease in the number of atoms per unit volume, i.e. change in density, is not accounted for by the linear attenuation coefficient.

To relate the dependence of attenuation to the number of atoms present in the medium, the *total mass attenuation coefficient* is used (μ/ρ). This is defined as the fractional reduction in intensity in a parallel beam of radiation of cross-section area per unit mass of attenuating material and is awarded the SI unit $\mathrm{m}^2\,\mathrm{kg}^{-1}$. This coefficient takes account of the possible different densities of an attenuating material and the value is therefore constant unless the elemental composition of the attenuating medium is altered. As presented below, there are several ways in which an X-ray beam may be attenuated, depending on the nature and energy of the primary radiation and the structure of the medium through which the X-ray beam passes. Each attenuation process has a related attenuation coefficient and the total linear or mass attenuation coefficient is the sum of these individual attenuation coefficients.

5.2 X-ray Interaction Processes

There are approximately 12 different interaction processes that may occur when ionising radiation interacts with matter, but within the X-ray energy ranges utilised in radiotherapy only three are thought to be relevant: photoelectric process, Compton scatter, and pair production.

Elastic scattering occurs at X-ray energies below those utilised in radiotherapy but is worthy of note as a comparison to Compton scatter. In addition, an attenuation process known as *photonuclear disintegration* occurs at very high-megavoltage (MV) photon energies, resulting in the ejection of a particle

TABLE 5.1	Relationship of interaction processes to atomic number, electron density, and beam energy.		
	Photoelectric process	**Compton scatter**	**Pair production**
Atomic number	Proportional to Z^3	Not dependent on Z	Proportional to Z
Electron density	Not dependent on electron density	Proportional to electron density	Not dependent on electron density
Beam energy	Proportional to $1\,keV^3$	Proportional to $1\,keV$	Only occurs at energies > 1.022 MeV

(usually a neutron) from the nucleus of the atom. These interactions occur over a small range of high photon energies and are outside the scope of this chapter.

A summary of the main X-ray interaction processes is presented in Table 5.1.

5.2.1 Elastic Scattering

This interaction process occurs at very low photon energies, below those useful for radiation treatment. It involves a collision interaction between the incident photon and an electron orbiting the nucleus of an atom in the attenuating medium. The energy of the incident photon is considered insignificant when compared with the binding energies of the electrons. This inhibits the transfer of energy from the incident photon to the electron. The consequence of the collision is that the incident photon continues to travel through the medium but in a different direction, i.e. it is scattered. The interaction is considered 'elastic' because there is no resultant loss of energy from the X-ray beam.

5.2.2 Photoelectric Absorption

Photoelectric absorption occurs at the X-ray energies utilised for diagnostic imaging, radiotherapy kilovolt imaging, and superficial and orthovoltage radiation therapy. Within these X-ray energy ranges, i.e. 50–500 kV, the energy of the incident photon is equal to or

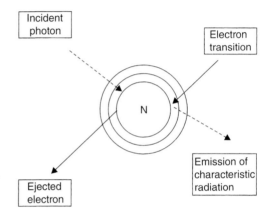

FIGURE 5.3 Photoelectric absorption.

slightly greater than the binding energy of the inner orbital electrons of the atoms through which the X-ray beam passes. This is a requirement for photoelectric absorption, summarised below, to occur:

- Incident photon interacts with an inner shell electron, transferring all of its energy to that electron (Figure 5.3).
- The incident photon no longer exists as a result of this interaction, i.e. it has been absorbed.
- The transferred energy from the incident photon overcomes the binding energy of the orbiting electron, causing it to be ejected from the atom.
- The ejected electrons, referred to as *photoelectrons*, are emitted at all angles. The higher the energy of the incident photon, the smaller the angle of photoelectron emission in order to conserve momentum and energy in the interaction.

- All remaining energy is converted to kinetic energy of the photoelectron, allowing it to travel through the attenuating material.
- The photoelectrons dissipate their kinetic energy in the atoms of the attenuating material until they are brought to rest.
- Ejection of the photoelectron from the atom leaves a vacancy in the inner electron shell, causing the atom to be unstable.
- The vacancy is filled by electron transition from an outer shell (see Chapter 2).
- The atom produces a photon of radiation, referred to as characteristic radiation, the energy of which is related to the binding energies of the two electron shells involved in the transition.
- The characteristic radiation is reabsorbed by the medium.

The characteristic radiation is so called because it is characteristic not only of the transitional shells but also of the particular element in which the interaction has taken place. It usually possesses less energy than the binding energies of the electrons of that medium, so is unlikely to interact further by photoelectric absorption. It is more probable that the characteristic radiation will be reabsorbed very close to the interaction in the same medium. This may not be the case with high atomic number materials because the characteristic radiation emitted will have a greater energy and may be transmitted if produced near to the surface of the medium. This is not of importance in soft tissue, however, and the photoelectric process is usually regarded as one of total absorption as the energy of the incident photon is completely absorbed by the medium.

Conservation of energy in this interaction is shown by the equation:

$$Ep = Eb + (mv^2/2)$$

where Ep = energy of incident photon; Eb = binding energy of electron; m = mass of photoelectron; and v = velocity of photoelectron.

During the photoelectric interaction the atom recoils slightly in order to conserve momentum in the system. It is not possible for the incident photon to interact with 'free' electrons by the photoelectric process as energy and momentum could not be conserved in the interaction.

The probability of the interaction taking place increases with the atomic number (Z) of the attenuating medium and is approximately proportional to Z^3, i.e. if the atomic number of the element is doubled, the probability of photoelectric absorption occurring at a specific energy is increased eightfold.

Given that the binding energy associated with a particular electron orbit is dependent on the atomic number of the atom, the K-shell absorption limit is reached at lower energies in atoms of lower atomic number. Therefore, for materials of low atomic number, e.g. soft tissue (comprising mainly fat, water, and muscle, creating an effective Z of approximately 7.5), the photoelectric process occurs over a lower energy range than for a material of high atomic number, e.g. lead ($Z = 82$).

At very low photon energies, e.g. > 10 keV for tungsten where the binding energy for the L-shell is 12.1 keV, photoelectric absorption can occur only in the outer M and N orbits. As the energy of the incident photon increases and becomes equal to the binding energy of the L-and K-shells, photoelectric absorption preferentially occurs in the inner shells. As the photon energy increases above the limit for the K-shell, attenuation by photoelectric absorption becomes less likely and Compton scatter becomes the dominant process. Indeed, the probability of photoelectric absorption occurring decreases dramatically as the energy of the incident photon increases and in general is considered to be inversely proportional to the cube of the kiloelectron volts (keV^3).

In reality, the above statement is a simplification of the dependence of the photoelectric process on the energy of the primary beam. As previously stated, the probability of M-shell transition decreases, in an inverse relationship to the keV[3], as the incident photon energy increases. This continues until the incident photon energy becomes close to the binding energy associated with the L-shell. Preferential absorption now occurs in the L-shell and the probability of photoelectric absorption and L-shell transition occurring abruptly rises. This is contrary to the general relationship between the probability of photoelectric absorption and the energy of the primary beam. As the incident photon energy continues to increase above the binding energies of the L-shell, the probability of photoelectric absorption occurring decreases, again in an inverse relationship to the keV[3]. This principle occurs within each separate electron shell. The point at which the attenuation suddenly increases is known as the *absorption edge* and is an important phenomenon with implications for the choice of quality filters used in orthovoltage treatment units (see Chapter 8).

5.2.2.1 Practical Relevance of Photoelectric Absorption to Radiotherapy

The differential blackening and great contrast between areas of soft tissue and bone observed on a simulator localisation or verification radiograph occurs as a result of the photoelectric process being the predominant attenuation process at these lower energies, typically 50–120 kV. The partial mass attenuation coefficient of this process is dependent on the atomic number of the medium traversed and, as bone has a higher effective atomic number (approximately 13) than soft tissue (approximately 7.5), the absorption in bone will be many times higher than in soft tissue, resulting in less X-ray transmission reaching the film through bone than soft tissue.

The above principle is again applied at these lower energies when attempting to achieve contrast between specific anatomical structures, e.g. bladder or kidney, and surrounding areas of soft tissue of similar atomic number. An artificial agent possessing a high atomic number, e.g. iodine ($Z = 53$) or barium

($Z = 56$), may be introduced into the body to outline these specific structures. Due to the differential absorption between the 'positive contrast agent' and the surrounding soft tissue, a varied intensity pattern of transmitted X-rays is produced, allowing visualisation of the required anatomy.

Air within the respiratory tract may be considered a negative contrast agent. It possesses a lower density than soft tissue, allowing production of a varied intensity pattern of transmitted X-rays. Air may also be artificially introduced as a negative contrast agent, in addition to positive contrast agents in 'double-contrast' studies such as barium enemas.

When using X-rays in the superficial and orthovoltage energy ranges, it is imperative to remember the dependence of the photoelectric process on the atomic number of the substance. When treating tumours lying directly beneath the bone, the preferential absorption in bone produces a reduced dose at the tumour site itself. When treating tumours arising in cartilaginous areas, e.g. the pinna of the ear, the cartilage may receive a greater dose than planned due to its higher atomic number and consequent preferential absorption, ultimately leading to cartilage necrosis. Electron therapy, which is independent of the atomic number of the material traversed, may be more appropriate in the management of tumours arising in these areas.

A further practical relevance is highlighted in the choice of materials used in the radiation protection of diagnostic imaging and radiation treatment rooms, and this is discussed later with the practical relevance of the other attenuation processes.

5.2.3 Compton Scattering

The interaction process of Compton scattering is also referred to as inelastic or modified scattering and may be compared with the previous description of elastic scattering. The Compton process involves a collision interaction between the incident photon and a 'free electron', resulting in both absorption (transfer of energy from the X-ray beam to the atoms of the attenuating medium) and scattering (path of the incident photon is altered).

As the energy of the incident photon increases, the binding energy of the orbital electrons in the attenuating material becomes almost insignificant in comparison. The electron is no longer bound and is considered to be a 'free electron'. During a Compton scatter interaction the following steps occur:

- The incident photon collides with a free electron and transfers some of its energy to the free electron in the form of kinetic energy.
- The electron recoils from the collision and is ejected at speed from the atom in either a forward or a side direction to travel through the attenuating material (Figure 5.4).
- The electron undergoes many electron–particle interactions, dissipating its kinetic energy before coming to rest.
- Radiation damage occurs as a result of electron–particle interactions.
- The incident photon continues but is deflected from its original path (Figure 5.4) and possesses less energy, as it has transferred an amount to the electron.
- The scattered photon has a reduced frequency and increased wavelength compared with the incident photon.

Given that the total energy in a system must remain constant, it follows that the energy of the electron plus that of the scattered photon must be equal to the total energy of the incident photon. The electron and scattered photon therefore have an inverse relationship, i.e. if the electron recoils with a large kinetic energy then the scattered photon has an associated small amount of energy. This produces a spectrum of electron and scattered photon energies. Momentum is also conserved in this collision interaction by the electron removing some of the momentum of the incoming photon.

It follows therefore that the energy and the angles of travel of the recoil electron and the scattered photon are interconnected by this need for conservation of energy and momentum. In a situation of maximum energy transfer, i.e. a direct hit, the electron is ejected in the direction of travel of the incident photon whereas the scattered photon is deflected through 180°. Conversely, in a situation of minimum energy transfer, the electron recoils at an angle of 90° to the original direction of travel of the incident photon with minimal scattering of the photon. Most collisions lie somewhere between these two extremes.

It is known that incident photons of low energy lose only a small amount of energy on collision and therefore the electron travels through the medium with low kinetic energy whereas the amount of scattered radiation is high. This is in comparison to interactions involving incident photons of high energy where a larger energy transfer ensues, enabling the ejection of an electron possessing a higher kinetic energy. As an adjunct to this, it is important to note that less scattered radiation occurs in interactions involving higher energy X-rays.

In practice, low-energy photons are scattered equally in all directions whereas high-energy photons are primarily scattered in a forward direction. In addition to the effects of differing electron ranges for orthovoltage and MV X-ray beams, this occurrence contributes to a difference in the position of the maximum dose for the respective X-ray beams. Comparison of the isodose curves shows that the orthovoltage beam dose is maximum at the surface of the attenuator, and at a point

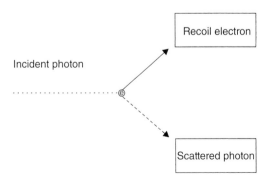

FIGURE 5.4 Compton scattering.

at a depth below the surface of the attenuator (dependent on the actual beam energy) for a MV beam. This is known as the 'buildup region'. The 'backscatter' produced by Compton interaction at orthovoltage energies contributes significantly to the dose at the surface of the attenuator, reaching 50% at its maximum contribution. Thereafter the amount of back scatter decreases as the energy of the primary beam increases, because there is a reduction in the amount of scatter produced and more photons are scattered in the forward direction. At MV energies there is less scattered radiation outside the beam edge and less variation of central axis dose with field size, because the scatter is mainly in the forward direction and its contribution reduced.

This may again be observed through comparison of isodose curves for orthovoltage and MV beams. The isodose curves for orthovoltage are more rounded due to the higher probability of scatter being produced at large angles at these lower energies. Indeed, the scatter contribution at these energies causes the 10 and 20% isodose curves to lie outside the geometrical edge of the beam (see Chapter 9).

The partial mass attenuation coefficient for Compton scatter decreases with energy approximately inversely proportional to the keV^3. However, the relative importance of Compton scatter in the interactional processes increases with increasing energy due to the partial mass attenuation coefficient for the photoelectric process being more dramatically dependent on the beam energy, e.g. inversely proportional to keV^3. It is dependent on both the physical density and the electron density of the medium traversed but is independent of the atomic number because the interaction process only involves 'free electrons'.

5.2.3.1 Practical Relevance of Compton Scatter to Radiotherapy

When employing custom-made blocks to irradiate tissue in an irregularly shaped field or to shield specific structures, it is important to acknowledge that the area directly beneath the shielding block will still receive some dose due to partial transmission through the block and, more importantly, due to the contribution of scatter from tissues outside the shielded area. This increases when the shielded area is central to the path of the beam. In addition, large amounts of shielding may actually reduce the expected scatter component to those tissues that require irradiation. In these instances a revised equivalent square is vital for accurate dose calculations.

Without digital enhancement, verification portal radiographs taken at MV energies exhibit a poor contrast ratio between bone and soft tissue compared with those taken using kilovoltage X-rays. At MV energies, the image is produced as a result of differential absorption due to Compton scatter. Unlike the photoelectric interaction, the partial mass attenuation coefficient for Compton scatter is independent of atomic number and, therefore, there is very little difference in absorption between bone and soft tissue. However, the difference in actual densities of structures in the path of the X-ray beam contributes to the image produced. For example, areas containing air (density $0.3 g/cm^3$) attenuate the beam less than soft tissue (density $1.0 g/cm^3$) or bone (density $1.8 g/cm^3$), therefore allowing more X-rays to be transmitted to the film. In addition, any differences in electron density enhance this effect, e.g. hydrogen contains twofold the average value for electron density and, as soft tissue contains a high proportion of hydrogen, the Compton effect is often greater.

A consideration when using MV X-rays to treat target volumes in the thoracic region is the increased transmission through the lung as a result of the decreased attenuation in air caused by the lower density. The soft tissues beyond the lung subsequently receive a greater dose than is initially expected and an inhomogeneity factor is usually used in the planning process to account for this. The presence of malignant lung tissue further complicates the planning process because the density can be considered to be similar to that of soft tissue and not of air.

A further practical relevance is again highlighted in the choice of materials used in the radiation protection of imaging and treatment rooms (see Section 5.3.1).

5.2.4 Pair Production

Pair production can be considered a two-stage process, although it will become evident that the title is gained from the first stage of the process, which results in the production of two particles. This interaction process provides an excellent example of Einstein's theory of the equivalence and transposition of mass (m) and energy (E) as quantitatively represented by the equation:

$$E = mc^2$$

where c = velocity of light (m s^{-1}).

5.2.4.1 Stage 1: Creation of Mass from Energy

- The protons in the nucleus of the atoms of the attenuating medium carry a positive charge, resulting in an electric field around the nucleus.
- A high-energy incident photon passes close to the nucleus of an atom in the attenuating medium and interacts with the electric field.
- The incident photon spontaneously 'disappears', transposing all its associated energy in the formation of two particles, each having a mass equal to that of an electron but carrying opposite negative and positive charges. These particles are usually referred to as a *negatron* (−) and a *positron* (+) (Figure 5.5).
- The total charge in the interaction therefore remains at zero.
- The positron and negatron move through the attenuating medium.

This is an illustration of the creation of matter from energy. By substituting the mass of an electron (9.1×10^{-31} kg) and the value

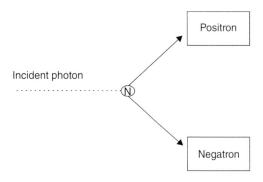

FIGURE 5.5 Pair production stage 1: creation of mass from energy.

for the velocity of light (3×10^8 m s^{-1}) into Einstein's equation, and using the conversion of 1.6×10^{-19} J, being equivalent to 1 eV, it is calculated that the energy equivalent to the rest mass of one electron is 0.511 MeV. As previously stated, during this first stage of the attenuation process, two 'electron' particles are produced, the negatron and positron, and therefore a threshold value for this stage to occur exists and must exceed the rest masses of both particles, i.e. 1.022 MeV. Thus, the pair production process is relevant only at MV energies above 1.022 MeV.

Excess energy of the incident photon above the threshold value of 1.022 MeV is divided between the negatron and positron as kinetic energy. This may or may not be divided in equal amounts between the two particles, resulting in the production of a possible range of particle energies. The particles are gradually brought to rest as they pass through the attenuating material, causing particle interactions as their kinetic energy is dissipated in the medium.

5.2.4.2 Stage 2: Creation of Energy from Mass

- The positron and negatron are brought to rest.
- The positron is very unstable and recombines with a negatron.
- The positron and negatron are annihilated and energy is created from mass according to Einstein's equation.

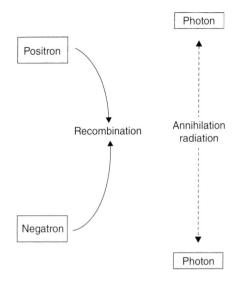

FIGURE 5.6 Pair production stage 2: creation of energy from mass.

- Two photons, referred to as *annihilation radiation* are produced, travelling in opposite directions (Figure 5.6).
- Each photon has energy of 0.511 MeV.

The pair production process is of particular note in the interaction processes discussed in this chapter, because the probability of the process occurring actually increases with increasing incident photon energy once the threshold value of 1.022 MeV has been reached. As described earlier, the probability of the photoelectric process and Compton scatter occurring decreases with increasing incident photon energy.

The electric field of the nucleus of an atom is dependent on the number of protons contained within that nucleus. A higher number of protons, i.e. a higher atomic number, produce a greater magnitude of electric field with which the incident photon can interact. Therefore, it follows that the probability of pair production occurring is proportional to the atomic number of the attenuating material. A practical relevance of this is highlighted in the slight contrast between soft tissue and bone exhibited on a portal radiograph taken using X-rays interacting by the process of pair production.

In summary, attenuation of the X-ray beam by the process of pair production is possible only at MV energies above the threshold value of 1.022 MeV. Even at the most common MV energies used in radiotherapy (4–20 MeV), the predominant process is that of Compton scatter. Indeed, due to the dependence of pair production on the atomic number of the medium transversed by the X-ray beam, this process is of little relevance in soft tissue at the energies stated.

5.3 Electron Interactions and Ranges

Common to each interaction process is the production of a high-speed electron that is able to travel through the medium and produce chemical and biological changes within the atoms. It is unable to pass directly through the medium and follows a tortuous path as a consequence of the induced repulsion caused by the electron cloud surrounding each nucleus and by the induced attraction caused by the positive nucleus. This therefore reduces the actual depth to which the electron is able to travel through the medium.

As it travels, the electron may interact with the atoms themselves causing excitation or ionisation, with an associated rise in temperature depending on the amount of energy transferred to the atom. An 'excited' atom may be chemically reactive or may reradiate the energy given to it by the photoelectron in the emission of ultraviolet or visible light. Ionisation, due to the ejection of an electron, may cause disruptive chemical changes within the atoms because it is the outer electrons that play a major role in the formation of chemical compounds. There will also be an associated emission of characteristic radiation.

If no chemical changes occur due to ionisation and excitation, recombination of the electron with a positive ion rapidly follows and characteristic radiation is emitted. In theory it would be possible for photons to be produced as a result of the electrons being decelerated by the proximity of the electric field of the nucleus, i.e. bremsstrahlung production, as described in Chapter 3, but this is unusual because soft tissue has a low atomic number. Bremsstrahlung production is dependent on the atomic number of the medium and therefore there is a greater possibility of this occurring in materials of higher atomic number.

Although it has been noted that a range of secondary electron energies is produced as a result of the various interaction processes, it is important to be able to indicate the average range of electrons produced by specific photon energies. In practice, this range increases dramatically from lower photon energies to MV photon energies. Photons used in the orthovoltage range produce electrons with a range of < 0.1 cm, insignificant when compared with the average range (in centimetres) for MV energies (approximately one-quarter that of the photon energy [MV]). This partially explains the use of MV X-rays for treatment of tumours at depth within the body. Lower-energy photons that produce electrons with an extremely small range are unable to penetrate deeply, making them suitable for treating superficial lesions only.

A further significant factor is that the electron interactions do not occur evenly throughout the range of the electron. A higher-energy electron produces fewer ionisations per unit length than an electron possessing lower energy. Therefore, the effects of electrons with a low energy and subsequent short range are seen close to their point of origin in comparison to the effects of high-energy electrons which are observed towards the end of the range when they are travelling more slowly. This is represented by the *Bragg ionisation effect* graph (Figure 5.7).

This phenomenon partially explains the dose buildup region and subsequent 'skin-sparing effect' seen with MV energies, approximately equal to the range of the electrons. This is not seen for orthovoltage beams because the energy deposited by the short-range electrons occurs very close to the point of origin, e.g. close to the surface of the

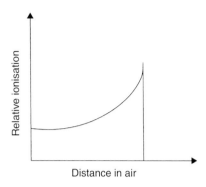

FIGURE 5.7 Bragg ionisation effect.

patient. In addition to this, there is the significant effect of the back scatter mentioned in Section 5.2.3.

5.3.1 Further Practical Relevance of the Interaction Processes

Materials used in radiation protection measures must take into account the energies of the X-rays that they are designed to shield. In general, all radiation protection materials have a high atomic number, density, and electron density, making them suitable to attenuate the beam efficiently by all the interaction processes discussed and, therefore, at all energies used in the radiotherapy department. Although lead is an ideal choice ($Z = 82$, density = $11\,350\,kg\,m^{-3}$) at lower X-ray energies, it is considered impractical at MV energies due to the large thickness required for adequate shielding. Solid concrete (density = $2350\,kg\,m^{-3}$), usefully used in the actual construction of rooms housing MV equipment, offers a practical and less expensive alternative. The effectiveness of any barrier may be related to the alternative thickness of lead required to provide a similar degree of protection and is stated in millimetres of lead (Pb) equivalent, accompanied by the photon energy of the X-ray beam. A review of radiation protection materials can be found in Chapter 12.

Tissue-equivalent materials known as phantoms are used in radiotherapy when simulating the X-ray interaction in the human body for the purposes of radiation measurements. Phantom materials include water, Perspex, and mix D (paraffin wax, polyethylene). Other materials include the use of solid phantom materials such as solid water, virtual water, plastic water, polystyrene, and polymethylmethacrylate for their equivalence to liquid water. They are designed for photon and electron beam calibrations, and eliminate the inconvenience of transporting, setting up, and filling water tanks.

All these materials possess an atomic number, electron density, and physical density similar to those of soft tissue and may represent the interaction of X-rays in the body by the photoelectric, Compton scatter, and pair production processes. Other tissue equivalent materials known as bolus may be used to fill tissue deficiencies such that the X-ray beam does not enter an oblique body surface. Materials such as paraffin wax or 'Lincolnshire bolus' fill any 'gaps' and similarly attenuate the X-ray beam and generate the same scatter radiation and dose distribution as that produced by soft tissue. Bolus material placed over the skin surface eliminates the skin-sparing effect of MV radiation treatment, ensuring that the maximum dose is at the skin surface. This may be useful when treating scar regions but does increase the skin reaction.

Further Reading

Symonds, R.P., Mills, J.A., and Duxbury, A.M. (2019). *Walter and Miller's Textbook of Radiotherapy, Radiation Physics, Therapy and Oncology*, 8e. Edinburgh: Churchill Livingstone, Elsevier.

CHAPTER 6

Principles of Imaging Modalities

Caroline Wright, Katheryn Churcher, and Jonathan McConnell

Aim

The aim of this chapter is to introduce the principles and practice of all of the imaging modalities that are utilised to capture images required for the pre-treatment imaging process.

6.1 Introduction

This chapter presents an overview of pre-treatment imaging. It describes the physical principles of image formation for the range of imaging modalities used in radiotherapy (RT) pre-treatment imaging (conventional plain film and digital radiography [DR], computed tomography [CT], magnetic resonance imaging [MRI], ultrasonography [US], and positron emission tomography [PET]). An overview of the key features of the equipment and techniques used to acquire optimal images for these modalities is outlined, in context with diagnoses for which each modality may be used to image. The associated advantages, disadvantages, and safety considerations are also addressed for each modality. A review of how the modalities can be used independently and in combination with one another (hybrid imaging, and image co-registration)

is presented together with considerations for future applications of the modalities.

6.1.1 Production of a Radiographic Image

Technological advances in radiographic practice have meant that traditional X-ray film is now unseen in the clinical environment. Whilst the technology may have changed, the properties and interaction of X-rays with matter remain the same. Similarly, the principles of film-based image formation remain applicable in the digital context. Before each of the contemporary pretreatment imaging modalities are reviewed, it is necessary to first review the properties of X-rays and how they enable visualisation of anatomy and pathology.

6.1.2 Properties of X-rays

X-rays, discovered in 1895 by Roentgen, possess the properties that are noted in other forms of electromagnetic radiation. It is these properties that make X-rays unique in that they allow internal body structures to be rendered visible in a 'non-invasive' way.

Practical Radiotherapy: Physics and Equipment, Third Edition. Edited by Pam Cherry and Angela M. Duxbury.
© 2020 John Wiley & Sons Ltd. Published 2020 by John Wiley & Sons Ltd.

6.1.2.1 Fluorescence

This property is seen when X-rays excite chemical salts such as calcium tungstate or gadolinium oxybromide, causing them to emit light. In the past, these substances were used to create intensifying screens that amplified the X-ray strength or signal to reduce dose whilst generating an image on film mainly using light rather than ionising radiation.

6.1.2.2 The Photographic Effect

Light-based cameras now rarely use film to capture an image, making the photographic effect difficult to imagine. However, this process is similar to that which occurs with light in the photographic negative, with X-rays producing a *latent image* on photographic film that is revealed when processed. The direct effect of X-rays on film may also be employed in personnel dosimetry as a method of radiation monitoring, though this is now generally acquired using thermoluminescent dosimetry rather than film. Most plain two-dimensional (2D) imaging is

generated electronically via a *photostimulable phosphor* (PSP) *imaging plate*, which is held in a cassette or via an amorphous silicon phosphor or amorphous selenium photoconductor. Section 6.1.2.3 will explain further the physical properties of X-rays and how we use these to acquire and optimise a radiographic image.

6.1.2.3 Penetration

Penetration is the term used to describe the travel of X-rays through substances impenetrable to light. During this process, the X-rays are absorbed to a greater or lesser extent depending on the thickness of tissue they travel through (Figure 6.1). The amount of absorption is dependent on the atomic number of the tissues (Figure 6.2) and the energy of the X-ray photons. Image formation therefore relies upon processes that control the amount of radiation that is absorbed by the different tissues and organs in the body. This is dependent on the kilovoltage (kV) used to generate the X-ray beam.

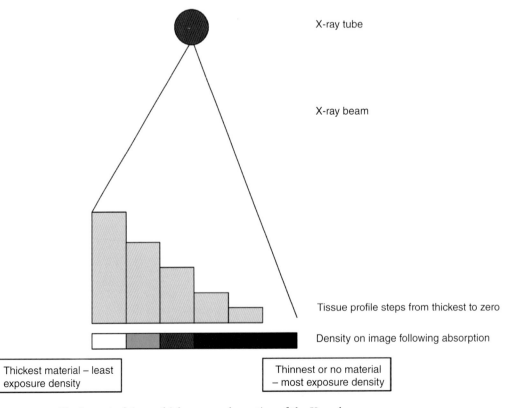

FIGURE 6.1   The impact of tissue thickness on absorption of the X-ray beam.

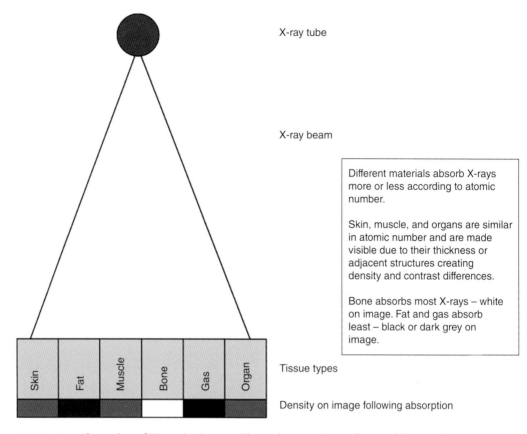

X-ray tube

X-ray beam

Different materials absorb X-rays more or less according to atomic number.

Skin, muscle, and organs are similar in atomic number and are made visible due to their thickness or adjacent structures creating density and contrast differences.

Bone absorbs most X-rays – white on image. Fat and gas absorb least – black or dark grey on image.

Skin Fat Muscle Bone Gas Organ

Tissue types

Density on image following absorption

FIGURE 6.2   Absorption of X-rays in tissues with varying atomic numbers and the resultant greyscale image. Tissues with low atomic numbers (gas and fat) permit transmission of most of the beam, with bone (high atomic number) stopping the majority of the beam with consequent black to white scale of absorption displayed in the image.

6.1.2.4 Ionisation and Excitation

Ionisation and excitation occurs in the atoms and molecules through which the X-rays traverse. The amount of ionisation produced by the X-rays provides a basis for measuring exposure.

6.1.2.5 Chemical Changes

Chemical changes take place when X-rays impart energy to substances. This is particularly important when considering the effect of ionising radiation on body tissues.

6.1.2.6 Biological Changes

Biological changes arise after X-rays have imparted energy to cellular substances. As a result, a proportion of cells undergo changes in their structure.

The combination of these effects allows X-rays to be used in imaging and RT.

Section 6.2 will provide insight into how X-ray images are produced for radiographic purposes. This process provides the basis for an understanding of contemporary image generation and visualisation.

6.2 2D Imaging

6.2.1 Introduction

X-rays are produced from an X-ray tube, following the acceleration of electrons from a hot (usually tungsten) cathode by a voltage difference ranging between 25 and 125 kV. The X-rays are created through photoelectric absorption or bremsstrahlung effects. These occur as electrons from the cathode and are directed at the anode target. Here they either interact with orbital electrons at the atomic level or have their velocity (speed and direction) changed to cause photons in the energy ranges indicated above to be released. The method of plain X-ray image production for *computed radiography* (CR), *DR*, and occasionally *direct digital radiography* (DDR) techniques are consistent with projection radiographic imaging. The way the generated radiation map is then converted into a visible image, recorded, and displayed, however, has progressed in recent years.

Radiographic 2D plain film imaging has been employed for many years in the diagnosis, staging, treatment planning, and verification of RT. It continues to be used in initial investigations at diagnosis, however it has been superseded to a large extent by CT, MRI, PET, and hybrid imaging techniques (discussed later in this chapter). In particular, these modalities are now routinely used for treatment planning, to the point where the 'conventional simulator' (which produced 2D plain film/digital images) is no longer used. However, it remains important to understand the basics of how plain film images are created since this forms the foundation of the modalities in use today.

6.2.2 Production of the Diagnostic X-ray Beam

As discussed above, photons/X-rays are produced by the X-ray tube and have energies in the 25–150 kV range (see Chapter 3). As technology has developed, film-based imaging has been superseded by computed and digital modalities. Irrespective of which system is used however, the steps taken to acquire an image remain similar, beginning with X-ray production and resulting in the formation of a radiation map, which is then converted into a visible image (Figure 6.3).

6.2.3 Interaction with Tissues

X-rays travel through the body tissues and are either absorbed, scattered, or transmitted. Absorption (*attenuation*) creates a variation in the X-ray pattern that exits the patient. This means that there is a reduction in the quantity of the beam, with a change in beam energy or quality. The type and thickness of tissue the beam passes through determines the quantity and quality of the emerging/exiting beam, with high-density materials such as bone reducing the beam quantity far more than with soft tissues such as fat. The emerging *photons* form what is known as a 'map' or 'shadow image'. Film-based systems previously captured the shadow image, however today images are rendered visible on an image receptor (IR) via capture using a CR image plate in a cassette or on a DDR plate.

Scattering of the X-rays via Compton interactions alters the photon direction and velocity, which subsequently affects the energy transmitted to tissues. As a result, the number of X-rays exiting from the patient, and therefore reaching the IR, is reduced. This means that the beam is directed to other areas in the body that do not require imaging. This is best avoided from the point of view of protecting the patient from overexposure to radiation. The scattered photons travel in a direction that will not add to the image. Instead, the scattered photons will hit the IR, resulting in a loss of contrast and a reduction in image sharpness. Photon scattering can occur more than once until all the energy that the X-ray beam possesses is dissipated and the photon is absorbed. The X-ray beam directed towards the patient is called the primary beam, whereas the scattered beam is termed secondary radiation.

6.2.4 Image Contrast and Density

When producing images using conventional radiography, it is important that both the quality and quantity of radiation exposed to the patient is appropriate, so as to ensure the emerging radiation generates a high-quality image with respect to contrast and density.

X-ray beam quantity relates to the number of X-rays that are produced in a given time. It is controlled by altering the milliampere seconds (mAs). Conversely, the quality of the beam or 'penetrative power' is controlled by altering the

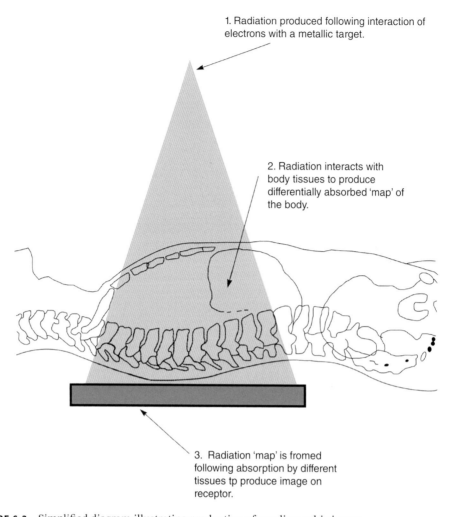

1. Radiation produced following interaction of electrons with a metallic target.

2. Radiation interacts with body tissues to produce differentially absorbed 'map' of the body.

3. Radiation 'map' is fromed following absorption by different tissues tp produce image on receptor.

FIGURE 6.3 Simplified diagram illustrating production of a radiographic image.

voltage/potential difference (kV) that is applied across the X-ray tube. The X-ray beam energy is an important factor in terms of the contrast and density produced in an image. Figure 6.4 summarises the process of interaction and contemporary image processing. The following descriptions and Figure 6.5a–e illustrate the effect of kV and mAs on an image.

The relative impact on the image is shown in Figure 6.5a–e. (Specific exposure factors used are not indicated, since these are dependent upon the type of equipment being used. These are therefore listed as 'standard exposure values').

In Figure 6.5e, high visible contrast enables the liver pathology to be more apparent, however high radiographic contrast does not necessarily equate with good contrast, e.g. high contrast would not allow the detection of a bony metastasis because the bony detail would not be seen. Higher contrast usually equates to less information overall, since there may be many smaller step differences between adjacent parts of the image. This difference in variation is reduced so that the eye is unable to readily identify variation between tissues or identify details. Conversely, high visible contrast with density changes across fewer steps of difference and a narrower range of information is typically seen more readily by the eye due to enhanced contrast between areas of similar tissue composition.

The following descriptions and accompanying diagrams in Table 6.1 compare the

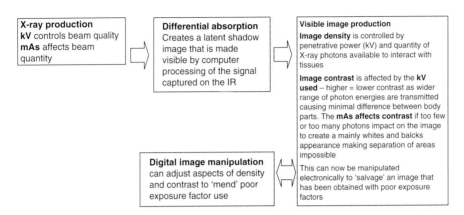

FIGURE 6.4   Summary of X-ray interaction and contemporary image processing.

(a) Standard kVp. standard mAs	In Figure 6.5a, exposure factors were selected such that bone, fat, and soft tissue organs are made visible in the image. This means that the beam has some photons of sufficient energy to penetrate the thinner, less dense portions of bone, and thus reach the IR and make the detail of 'spongy' bone visible. At the same time, the beam has sufficient low-energy photons, which are differentially absorbed by soft tissues (fat, muscle, and other tissues), to vary the amount of radiation passing through them and air. This enables distinctions to be made between the air (minimal radiation absorption) and other tissue types (absorbed according to thickness and or material constructed of). The compact bone is the whitest shade, air is the darkest, and there is a slight but distinctly visible difference between liver and kidney, although the tumour in the liver (represented by a circle) is the same shade as the liver and cannot be seen. The grey scale ranges from white through to black, but the difference between adjacent grey levels is small, so the image contrast is not high.
(b) Increased kVp. standard mAs	In Figure 6.5b, the mAs remains the same but the kV has been raised above the 'standard' value. Therefore; • the beam has more energy • more of it penetrates all tissues, increasing the amount of blackening overall. In this scenario, the fat is black and similar to the air and therefore cannot be seen. The black cannot get any blacker in appearance (to the naked eye), but all the other shades become darker. The grey scale now ranges from pale grey to black, so the contrast is reduced. The differences in grey shades between the liver and kidney are much reduced and it is difficult to differentiate between them.

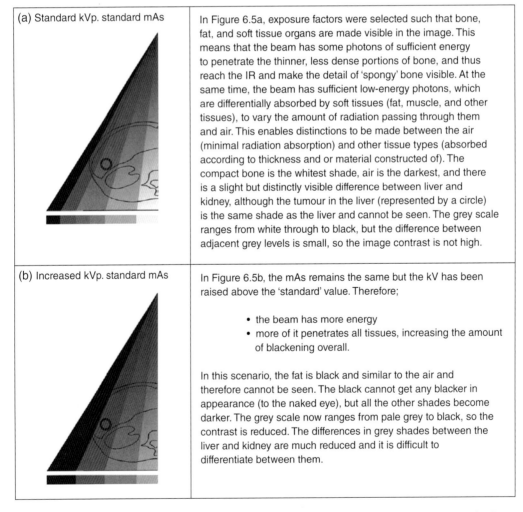

FIGURE 6.5   Effects of exposure type on the plain radiographic image. (a) Standard kilovoltage (kV) and standard milliampere seconds (mAs); (b) increased kV and standard mAs; (c) increased kV and decreased mAs; (d) reduced kV and standard mAs; (e) reduced kV and increased mAs.

(c) Increased kVp. decreased mAs	In Figure 6.5c, the mAs has been reduced below the 'standard' value in an attempt to compensate for the increase in kV. Although the bony tissue is now paler, the increased energy in the beam means that even the densest bone has been penetrated by some radiation, so there are no completely white areas i.e. totally absorbed by the bone. The black is still as black as can be resolved by the naked eye and the shades of grey in the image still range from pale grey to black. However, the palest grey is lighter than that seen in Figure 6.5b. Therefore, *visible contrast* is *increased* compared with Figure 6.5b but reduced compared with Figure 6.5a.
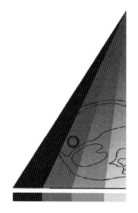	
(d) Reduced kVp standard mAs	In Figure 6.5d, the 'standard' value of mAs has been selected, but the kV is below the 'standard' value. There is: • insufficient penetration through bone to affect the IR so it is completely white. • There is less penetration through fat and air, so those areas are also paler than on the original image. The small differences between the tumour and liver tissue may *just* be visible. The grey scale ranges from white to dark grey so *contrast* is *reduced* compared with Figure 6.5a.
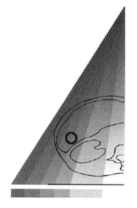	
(e) Reduced kVp increased mAs	In Figure 6.5e, the mAs has been increased to compensate for the reduction in kV. As the energy of the beam is too low to penetrate the bone, there is still no effect on the image in that area, regardless of how much the mAs increases, so the bony areas remain white on the film. However, the beam still has enough energy to penetrate the fat/air and the quantity of the radiation has been increased to whatever is required to make the image black in those areas. Thus, detail has been lost within the bone – it is all white – and the fat can no longer be seen because it is completely black similar to the air. The grey scale ranges from white to black as in Figure 6.5a, but the *visible contrast difference between adjacent tissues* has been increased and the boundary of liver, tumour, and kidney can be seen clearly. Increasing contrast between adjacent parts is helpful BUT in using the term high contrast confusion may be caused.
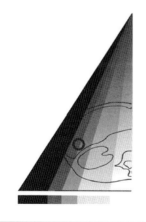	

FIGURE 6.5 *(Continued)*

TABLE 6.1	The impact of exposure factors and image rendition between film and digital receptors.

Film-based responses

Milliampere seconds **(mAs) too low but** kilovoltage **(kV) correct**	**mAs and kV correct**	**mAs too high but kV correct**
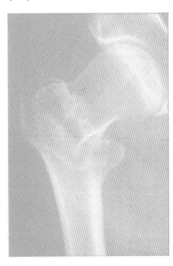	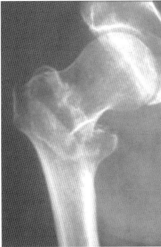	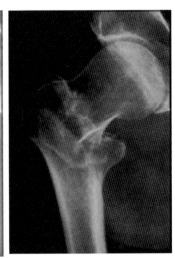

Digital imaging-based responses

mAs too low but kV correct	**mAs and kV correct**	**mAs too high but kV correct**
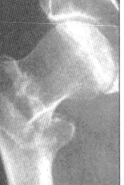	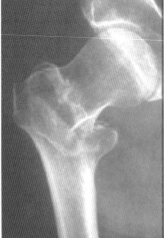	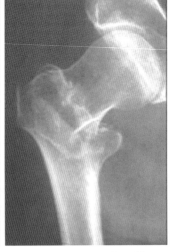
Note the speckled appearance from insufficient signal to generate image. Here not enough mA s and possibly kV was employed.	Good quality image as part penetrated with appropriate density.	Although overexposed on film the image algorithms in digital enable the image to be presented as acceptable image quality.

effect of kV and mAs on contrast and density with respect to plain film and DR.

6.2.4.1 Factors Affecting Contrast

- If the energy of an X-ray beam is too low, then all the energy will be absorbed by the patient, with no exiting photons reaching the imaging device. Thus, there are no density differences to create contrast between adjacent body tissues.
- If the energy of an X-ray beam is too high and the mAs remains the same as above, the image will be too dark with poor contrast.

Where the beam energy is too great, but the mAs is correct, photon scattering occurs and reaches the imaging device, reducing the contrast differences in the image produced and reducing visibility between adjacent tissues in the image. Secondary scatter grids that absorb photons not travelling in a direction perpendicular to the imaging device can improve this problem, preventing image degradation and therefore enhancing the contrast observed between adjacent tissues. This is also now possible with electronic filtration to remove unwanted noise.

6.2.4.2 Factors Affecting Density

- If the mAs is too low but the kV is appropriate, the image produced is considered 'noisy' or 'light'. In these cases, it can be difficult to differentiate between tissues of similar density on the image.
- If the mAs and kV are appropriate, the generated image should have good density and contrast with optimal noise characteristics.
- If the mAs is too high but kV is appropriate, the image density will be too great. In digital images this is less problematic since the computer image can be manipulated. However, the dose delivered to the patient remains excessive.

6.3 Plain Radiography Image Generation

The radiation 'map' produced represents the internal patient anatomy. In order for an image to be visible, the map from the patient interacts with the recording system and is converted to light. The more radiation reaching the recording system, the more light is produced and the greater the degree of blackening on the recording system. In this manner, a radiation map of the body is translated into a visible monochrome (greyscale) image.

In past decades, a film receptor would respond as seen in the left-hand side of Figure 6.6. The diagram shows a relatively narrow band of exposure able to generate an image within an acceptable range of density and contrast. Digital systems are more linear in their response to X-rays and so can provide an appropriate image across a wider range of exposure (depending on the radiation reaching the receptor). The digital response is demonstrated in the digital imaging appearance aspects of Table 6.1 (with associated challenges as described).

6.3.1 Digital Image Formation

The detail that we see in the digital image is controlled by the size of the matrix used to generate the image. This can be explained by using the analogy of a 'chess board'. The squares seen within the image are termed 'picture elements' or *pixels*. Digital image detail is controlled by the number of pixels in this 'chess board'. As the number of pixels increases within an area, so does the potential to visualise detail. Thus, as matrices increase in size they can reveal more information (Table 6.2). This is referred to as increased resolution.

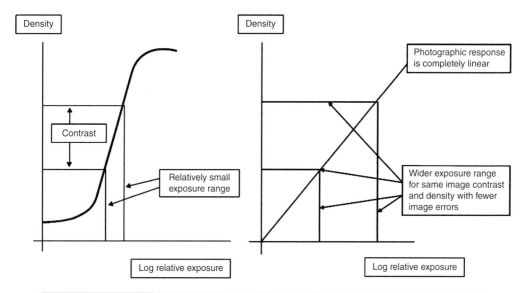

Density

Density

Photographic response is completely linear

Contrast

Relatively small exposure range

Wider exposure range for same image contrast and density with fewer image errors

Log relative exposure

Log relative exposure

Left diagram shows high contrast film and intensifying screen response to exposure

Good contrast difference is achieved in the straight-line portion of the curve but this is at the expense of a narrow exposure tolerance for the body part.

Digital systems (right diagram) operates in the straight-line portion and attempts to extend the linear response to exposure thus effectively widening exposure tolerance range for same contrast and density outcomes.

FIGURE 6.6   A characteristic curve of response as seen in film-based systems compared with the digital exposure response.

6.3.2 Pixel Manipulation

Each pixel in the matrix represents one 'colour'. This is usually a shade of grey between black and white. It is a numerical allocation using 'binary coding' to represent a shade of grey. This matches the amount of radiation hitting that point of the IR. Magnification of the image using a digital system is achieved by 'stretching' the pixels on the screen. The term 'pixellated' is used when this pixel is large enough that its perimeter is visible. The more pixels in a matrix mean that we can stretch the pixel to make smaller items visible but reduce the chance of creating a pixellated image (Figure 6.7). The white to black spectrum is stretched across this greyscale and we can alter the image by raising or lowering the gradient to change contrast. We can also apply 'look-up tables' (LUTs) that enable us to see the useful greys and apply software filters that enhance the edges of objects. It is also possible to manipulate the brightness and contrast levels for greater visibility, which allows a poor

exposure to reveal information without re-exposing the patient.

6.3.3 Computed and DDR Image Capture

CR and DDR are both used to produce digital images, DDR most recently. CR and DDR capture latent/shadow images and project these onto a viewing monitor. The differences in the construction and operation of CR and DDR devices are described in Table 6.3.

6.3.4 Viewing the Image

In the past, images were produced as hard copies and viewed with transmitted light through the film via light boxes. Today, electronic methods of image display are common using computers and monitors to create and display the images and compact discs (CDs) for storage of the image data sets.

TABLE 6.2 Matrix size.

A simple shape is spread on a matrix.	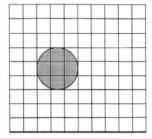
A series of squares represent the shape of the circle.	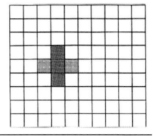
A larger matrix (smaller boxes/ pixels) means more detail within the shape. A greater number of squares would be required to allow an anatomical object to be visualised clearly.	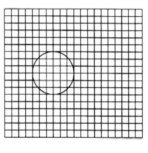

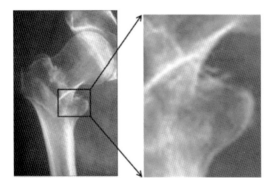

FIGURE 6.7 Pixel enlargement to aid visualisation of a small area.

6.3.5 Liquid Crystal Displays

The monitors which display the image are constructed of liquid crystal. As an electric current is applied across the crystals, they change in shape, each allowing different amounts of light to pass through them; this allows shades of grey and colour to be demonstrated. There are two types of liquid crystal display (LCD) screen, passive and active.

Passive screens use a system that reflects a fluorescent light through the crystals to project the image out of the screen. Disadvantages of using passive screens include;

- reduced brightness;
- a time lag in responding to the changing image;
- low viewing angle (similar to viewing a laptop screen).

Active screens use a light-emitting diode (LED). These are advantageous because;

- the light is much brighter;
- they have superior contrast and resolution;
- they have a similar viewing angle to conventional TV monitors.

6.3.6 Screen Resolution

The resolution of screens is described by the number of dots per inch or the *dot pitch* (DPI). Pitch is measured by the distance between successive colours, thus making monochrome screens inherently sharper. The monitor's resolution of an image may be described by the number of pixels in the image matrix.

6.3.7 Electronic Access to Images

Further advances in technology have enabled images to be viewed remotely and transferred electronically to other remote centres. A system known as *picture archiving and communication system* (PACS) is used to do this.

CR	Direct digital radiography (DDR)
The plate 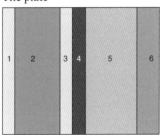 1 = protective overcoat 2 = photostimulable phosphor (PSP) layer 3 = adhesive layer 4 = antihalo (nonreflective) layer 5 + 6 = support layers	Amorphous selenium detector 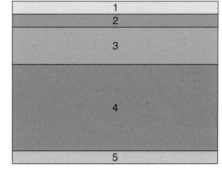 1 = face electrode 2 = dielectric 3 = selenium semiconductor 4 = electronics and signal collecting system 5 = glass plate support
Image plate drawn through 'reader' and sprayed with laser energy.	X-rays that have been differentially absorbed interact with the selenium (or silicon) plate, the energy created as a result of this is converted to an electrical signal used by the thin film transistor (TFT).
Energy is released by 'spraying' with laser light to enable light photons to be generated.	A matrix of TFTs aligns with the selenium layer. Each TFT covers a width of $0:15$ mm and controls the pixel number and size.
Light is directed to photomultiplier tube (PMT) by fibreoptics. Light is amplified as analogue signal through PMT.	Although a thick layer of selenium enhances the electron capture and hence signal noise the selenium thickness is limited to about 1 mm as a larger voltage (over 10 kV) is needed to extract the electrons from the system.
Signal matches TV raster and pixels to generate digital image.	When electrons from the capture layer are released, these activate the TFTs.
Image stored and manipulated via computer.	TFT matrix positions are calculated via the computer to enable the image to be constructed from the signal.
Image plate sprayed with light to clean old information. Plate is reinserted for use into cassette.	Direct digital plates more readily detect the signal and this process does not require the same number of interim stages as required with the CR plate.
Representative diagram of PSP reader	**Representative diagram of TFT digital plate**

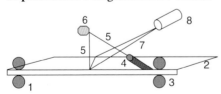

1 = transport roller   5 = path of laser light
2 = PSP plate   6 = rotating mirror – for laser path across PSP
3 = transport roller   7 = emitted light guided to PMT
4 = laser   8 = PMT (creates electrical signal from light)

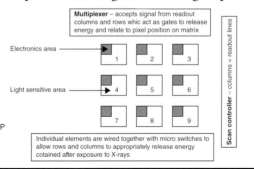

The PACS stores all the patient data, which can be electronically transferred within a hospital upon request. For the transfer of images between hospitals, there needs to be standardisation of the image format. This is achieved using *digital imaging and communication in medicine* (DICOM). If hard copy images are still required, they can be printed using a laser printer. The laser receives the electronic signal from PACS.

6.3.8 DICOM

Imaging data in digital format is produced, manipulated, exchanged, and stored using DICOM protocol, which has been adopted as the universal standard for handling images and associated data. The DICOM standard was jointly developed in the 1980s by the National Electronic Manufacturers' Association (NEMA) and the American College of Radiology (ACR). The standard is now in its third version (DICOM-3) with annual review and revision [1]. Manufacturers of digital imaging systems have adopted the '20 part rule system' whereby they only use the parts of the standard that are responsible for enabling performance of the equipments' assigned task (refer to Carter and Veale for detail on this) [2].

6.3.8.1 DICOM Functions

DICOM uses *object-oriented programming* to define information as 'objects' and considers them in terms of the functions that can be performed on them (such as storing, moving, finding, or printing them). These operations are described as *service classes* and, when defined for a device, inform the user what the device can and cannot do in relation to other systems. This information is contained within the *conformance statement* and includes service classes such as image storage, query/retrieve, print management, and modality worklist, which enables retrieval of patient demographic information.

Each device can exist as either a *service class user* (SCU) or *a service class provider*

(SCP) or both for a given service and object. DICOM always operates between an SCP and SCU that together are known as a *service object pair* (SOP). *SOP classes* link a particular service class with a particular object and are assigned a unique identifier (UID) by DICOM. For DICOM communication to occur, the UIDs of both devices must exactly match.

6.3.8.2 The DICOM Conformance Statement

When considering introducing an imaging or RT device the DICOM conformance statement supplied by the manufacturer is crucially important, because this document provides information on which parts of the standard are supported and for which modality or services. The statement is therefore used to assess whether two devices could transfer information (the device sending the data implementing as a SCU whilst that receiving implements as a SCP).

6.3.8.3 DICOM RT

This is an extension of the protocol handling the RT modality that has a working group overseeing its development. DICOM RT specifies five RT objects:

- RT image: concerned with digitally reconstructed radiographs (DRRs), portal, and simulator images.

- RT plan (RTP): contains geometric and dosimetric data for external beam RT and brachytherapy. An RTP is usually linked to an associated RT structure set (RTSS).

- RTSS: contains information relating to patient anatomy, e.g. structures, markers, and isocentres that are usually defined on treatment planning system (TPS) or VSim workstations.

- RT dose: concerned with dose data such as dose distributions, dose volume, histograms, isodose curves, and dose matrices.

- RT treatment record: contains data obtained from treatment sessions, historical records of the treatment.

A practical example demonstrates how DICOM might function within the RT process:

- When a patient is scanned a DICOM **CT image** study is produced.
- The VSim application query/retrieves the image study.
- Virtual simulation is performed, producing **RTSS**, **RTP**, and DRRs as **RT image** objects.
- The TPS query/retrieves the **CT image**, **RTSS**, and **RTP** and calculates a dose plan. New **RTSS**, **RTP**, and **RT images** may be produced at this stage. The R&V query/retrieves the **RTP data**, initialising a treatment.
- The EPID system creates its own **RT images** for verification.
- During treatment **RT treatment records** are produced for each session.

6.3.9 Challenges of DICOM

6.3.9.1 The DICOM Conformance Statement

The DICOM conformance statement provides information concerning the ability of devices to establish connections and exchange data. It does not guarantee that a device will be able to process and manipulate that data as required. A distinction must therefore be made between *DICOM connectivity* and *application operability*, which can be proved only through rigorous testing in a clinical setting.

6.3.9.2 Integration with PACS

Introduction of PACS, entailing central archiving and record sharing, presents specific difficulties for the RT process. As these systems were developed for radiology they offer limited support for handling the complex mix of DICOM RT images and associated objects. PACS versions of equipment are designed to integrate primarily with *radiology information systems* (RIS), which create and schedule patient orders for an image study. This order allocates a unique accession number, sending messages to the PACS and imaging modalities that update and maintain the accuracy of patient demographic details. Consequently a problem arises because:

1. accession numbers are not a key field in the DICOM standard; and
2. accession numbers have no meaning in an RT context.

One solution is to introduce an independent DICOM RT archive, able to store and distribute data and that can assemble RT objects ready to send to the PACS (using Health Level 7 [HL7] messaging), allocating accession numbers in the process.

6.3.10 HL7

HL7 provides a standard interface for exchange of clinical and administrative data such as patient demographics and reports. It is used for communication between *hospital information systems* (HIS) and the RIS. HL7 ensures that textual information is encoded in a way that allows other computers to correctly read and decipher strings of text. Some parts of HL7 have been used as the basis for textual information storage in the DICOM 'header' that accompanies all images or clinical data saved by this method.

6.3.11 Image Storage

Apart from the easy access to images discussed in PACS, digital imaging systems can readily store a vast amount of images. The images can be stored on CD or DVD (digital versatile disk) or alternatively in a portable memory stick or external hard drive that can hold from 2 GB to over 1 TB of data. Information is usually added to external recording media as a download from the hard drive of the computer.

By comparison, the computer hard drive uses magnetic material impregnated with polished aluminium to enable more information to be stored. Information stored to the hard drive is safe even when there is no power to the system, unlike random access memory (RAM), and loses the stored information only when you deliberately remove or change it. When material is stored to a disk this is logged and a code is provided to enable the machine to select information from the appropriate disk when information is requested from the system. Usually a 'jukebox' system is employed in departments whereby multiple large optical disks are stored together as a library. As data banks grow, more 'jukeboxes' are connected to the system to enable storage capacity to increase.

6.3.12 Processing and Manipulating the Digital Image

The use of digital images provides an opportunity to extract more information or correct for problems in the original data generated by the exposure. When an image is generated, a vast array of grey values is represented in the DDR panel. This is known as the system 'fidelity'. It is a requirement of the system that this is as faithful as possible. This material is stored as *raw* data and forms the basis from which the image can be manipulated. Several approaches such as histogram analysis and exposure control may be adopted to achieve this, with the view to improving image rendition for the human viewer and to ensure maximum information is retrieved from the examination.

6.4 CT

6.4.1 Introduction

CT is an imaging modality that uses X-rays to produce image slices through selected planes of the body. This means that the images are cross-sectional in nature and may be oriented along any of the standard anatomical planes throughout the body (axial, coronal, and sagittal). Through advanced computer technology, CT scanners can now reconstruct images in any direction. CT has long been used in RT and oncology imaging and remains the modality most often used in RT planning. Before we look at the equipment and physical principles of CT we will briefly discuss its use in RT and oncology.

Cancer diagnosis and staging: The diagnosis and initial imaging investigations for patients with a variety of cancers are undertaken using CT. The images allow for identification of pathology and positive lymph nodes, loco-regional and distant spread of disease. Depending on the type of tissues and organs being imaged CT may be used in combination with other modalities to enhance identification of tumours and metastatic disease, for example PET and MRI.

Pre-treatment imaging: The use of CT in the pre-treatment process is currently standard practice, with many RT departments having their own dedicated CT scanner as well as, or in place of, a conventional simulator. The data from CT scans can be transferred directly to RT planning systems, where the electron density information from the scan can be computed (using algorithms) and translated into dose distribution data. Anatomical data from the CT scan is used to produce DRRs which are used in treatment verification and image matching. This section will provide an overview of the physical principles of CT.

6.4.2 The Evolution of CT

Godfrey Hounsfield is credited with the invention of CT in 1972. The first scanner took several hours to collect the raw data required to generate a single image slice. It took several days to reconstruct the image into the form that is so familiar to us today. Since this time, several generations of scanner have been developed, with changes to the detector configurations and X-ray beam in each subsequent generation.

6.4.2.1 Scanner Components

A CT scanner consists of a table, a gantry that houses an X-ray tube, a series of detectors with X-ray filters, and collimators between the source and detectors. A large computer is employed to reconstruct the image. These systems have also allowed for the emergence of image fusion and coregistration, where the properties of all imaging modalities can be exploited for RT planning purposes. The CT image can be combined (fused) with other imaging modalities to enhance anatomical detail and assist in delineation of the target for treatment planning.

6.4.2.2 First and Second-generation CT Scanners

First-generation scanners had a single (pencil) X-ray beam that was projected onto a single detector. It took the early scanners 20 minutes for each slice to be produced, but this eventually reduced to about 5 minutes. In second-generation CT scanners, rather than using the pencil beam, these scanners used a fan beam and several detectors (Figure 6.8), allowing for a larger area to be imaged in a shorter amount of time (approximately 20 seconds per slice). The advent of computer technology significantly improved the time that it took for images to be reconstructed.

6.4.2.3 Third-generation CT Scanners and Beyond

The principles of first- and second-generation scanners underpin the current systems in operation today. In third-generation scanners,

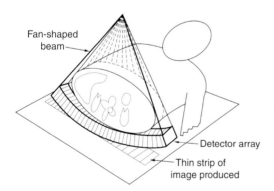

FIGURE 6.8 Fan beam of radiation in a computed tomography (CT) scanner.

both the X-ray tube and the detector array rotate around a gantry. Third-generation scanners have an arched bank of detectors opposite the X-ray tube. These rotate at the same time through a connection in the CT scanner gantry. This means that both the X-ray tube and detectors rotate around the patient during an exposure, which allows the scan data to be collected according to the speed at which the gantry system rotates (Figure 6.9). There is a drawback involving the cables in the gantry. As the system rotates, it would result in crossing of the cables, which means that the unit needs to 'unwind' itself by performing each scan slice in an opposite direction. However, the system enables scans to be generated in just a few seconds per slice for data acquisition.

Fourth-generation scanners have stationary (fixed) detectors in a complete ring around the patient. The X-ray tube rotates around the patient within the ring of detectors, so the distance from tube to skin surface is shorter and geometric un-sharpness potentially greater. As there are a greater number of detectors, the failure of one may have a less noticeable result on the image.

Fifth-generation scanners enable helical slices to be produced. Spiral or helical scanners use slip rings, rather than cables, to provide the coupling between power supply and control/data transfer. These allow for continual rotation of the X-ray tube and detectors whilst the patient is moved through the beam. This technology allows the tube and detectors to rotate as the table moves continuously, to corkscrew through the area of interest (increasing the speed of the image acquisition process). Not only does helical scanning allow faster scanning, but also the dataset acquired relates to a large volume of tissue, giving greater reconstruction possibilities.

Multi-slice CT incorporates multiple rows of detectors that enable several slices to be imaged at the same time. It is possible for these detectors to be either the same size or a variety of sizes. The size of the detector determines the slice thickness, therefore for

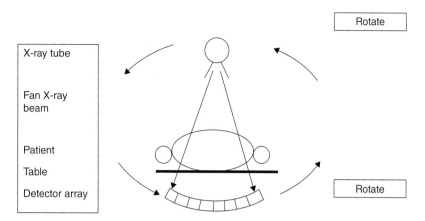

FIGURE 6.9   The third-generation rotate–rotate system with a fan beam and curved array of detectors that both rotate around the patient.

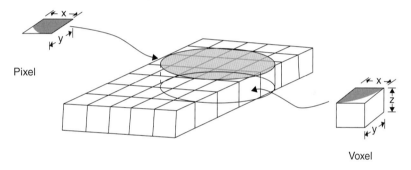

FIGURE 6.10   Differences between a pixel and voxel in a computed tomography (CT) image.

scanners with detectors that are thin in width, the slice thickness can be increased by merging information from adjacent rows. Ultimately, the beam width and number of detectors will control the time taken for a scan and the spatial resolution achievable.

In the older scanners, the slices of the body that were imaged were thicker than those that can be achieved today. Slice thickness related to the detector type and, as a result, anatomical detail was limited. Technological developments in the positioning and array of detectors has enabled acquisition of thinner slices which offers enhanced image resolution, as well as accelerating the process of image acquisition.

The speed of image acquisition is important in the localisation process because

patients need to be placed in the treatment position for the duration of the scan, which may be difficult to maintain for long periods of time.

6.4.3 Image Formation

The images that are generated from third- and fourth-generation scanners take a standard digital format of picture elements or pixels. As each slice has a finite thickness, each pixel also represents a depth or thickness of image slice and this is termed a 'volume element' or *voxel* (Figure 6.10). Each voxel is projected as a shade of grey on the monitor. The spatial resolution of the voxels varies according to the slice thickness and the number of voxels in an image matrix. Essentially this means that the best representation of anatomical information is gained when imaging with a thin slice thickness and there are a greater number of voxels per image.

6.4.4 Image Reconstruction

To construct an image, it is necessary to have several views or projections (at 180° of rotation). Within each view, a series of values equivalent to total absorption of an X-ray beam along a path at a given angle are obtained, relative to the rotation of the X-ray tube and detectors around an object. This value is the *ray sum*, which needs to be maximised to create an image that represents all the structures inside the object. Data processing algorithms are used to reconstruct this information into an image.

6.4.5 Windowing

When a CT image is produced it has a range of grey shades that represent different tissue types and their respective densities. The actual breadth of the steps of grey shades acquired is far beyond the range of the human eye. To counteract this, a technique termed *windowing* is used to manipulate the image. Windowing allows tissues to be represented across a range of grey values that are discernible to the human eye.

The greyscale matches what is known as the *Hounsfield unit* (HU) or *CT number* for specific tissues. These are a set of nominal values that represent different materials. Water is given an HU or CT number of zero (0) and the value for gas is −1000. The grey value for bone is +1000 (or greater). Each of these grey values represent the transition from black through the various shades of grey to white (i.e. from air to water and then to bone). Thus, where there are subtle differences between tissues, selecting a particular window level (WL) when viewing an image can enhance the visibility of soft tissues or delineation of detail in a high-density object,

such as bone, so that greater information can be represented through high-contrast resolution. It is this property of CT data that means that there is excellent contrast resolution. However, due to the limitations in slice thickness discussed earlier, CT images are also considered to have relatively poor spatial resolution.

6.4.6 Image Display

6.4.6.1 Window Width and Level

Windowing techniques allow tissues within a certain grey scale range to be reviewed. In the case of CT, the *window width* (WW) and *WL* may be adjusted to improve tissue visualisation. The WW is the range of HUs displayed on a projected image. The width selects how many HUs are displayed and the level selects which ones are presented. Wide windows (ranging between 400 and 2000) are used when tissues in the image vary greatly in density, for example in the thorax. Narrow WWs (ranging between 50 and 400) are used when tissues of similar densities are to be displayed, for example in the brain.

Increasing the WW results in suppression of 'noise' within the image, so can be useful in improving the image appearance for obese patients or where metal artefacts, such as dental fillings or prosthetic limbs, may be present. The disadvantage however, is that increasing the WW also provides less discrimination between tissues of a similar density. However, a narrow WW can result in overinterpretation of tissues in certain areas, where the contrast of 'noise' in the image can be enhanced and generate unrealistic and confusing tissue edges and shading.

The WL is set at the midpoint for the range selected by WW, for example a WW400 at a level of 100. This would mean 200 HU/CT numbers are displayed above and below that point, so that actual HU/CT values of −100 to +300 would be visible in the image. The optimal WW and WL for reviewing images can vary enormously from one individual to another depending on patient size and body composition. There is a large degree of variance in areas such as the abdomen, with less

TABLE 6.4   **Window width (WW) and window level (WL) in action.**

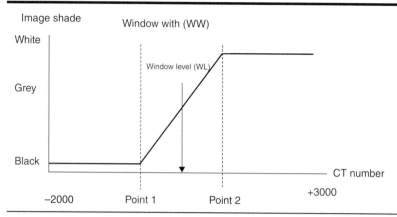

The level is the computed tomography (CT) number that marks the centre of the window of a given width. Narrow windows give high contrast as CT numbers inside the window width are spread across the black-to-white continuum seen on the y axis of the graph. Conversely a wide window at a given level creates a shallow gradient. The interplay between level and widow enable a range of contrasts to be seen so more information is extracted from the image as seen below:

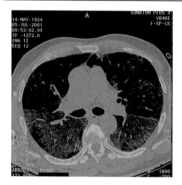

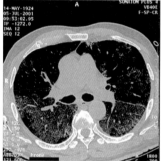

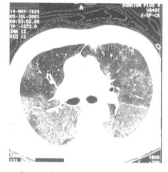

Wide window width and high level allows bone to be seen but does not give a good soft tissue image:

WW = 2950

WL = 1100

Mid-range WW and level gives good contrast (especially when contrast media is used in CT), so the mediastinum and vessels are clearly visible:

WW = 650

WL = −100

A lower level and narrow width will enable high contrasts to be seen. Where large tissue differences evident, e.g. lung alveoli and branching bronchi, this is good:

WW = 750

WL = −700

variance observed when imaging areas such as the brain. Consequently, there is no definitive WW and WL that encompasses all situations and both require some level of modification between individual patients. It is important also to note that different CT scanners can also generate different WW and WL settings requirements in order to provide comparable images (Table 6.4 illustrates the effect of WW and WL on an image).

6.4.6.2 Enlarging the Image

In some cases, it may be necessary to review large areas of the body that cannot be seen all at one time. In this case, one of two approaches can be taken to facilitate viewing:

1. Magnification: this effectively stretches the information from one point across the whole screen. Unfortunately, image clarity is lost during magnification

because the number of pixels covering the initial scan area is stretched across a larger image.

2. All the scan information of a small area can be transferred into a whole matrix. This is possible because each voxel and subsequent pixel are made up of many thousands of data points, which contribute to the pixel at those coordinates in the image. Therefore, a larger amount of information is available to spread across the 'new' pixels, avoiding loss in image clarity.

6.4.7 Identifying the Tissue Composition of a Given Point

When we are uncertain about the tissue composition of a point within the image, we can apply a cursor that is a directed segment over the area of interest. This is called the *region of interest* (ROI). It allows us to obtain a finite measurement for that specific area so that definitive CT numbers can be established. In doing so, a clearer representation of the image (and the tissue types within the image) is achieved, so that we can be certain of the tissue type at a certain point linked to the Hounsfield scale.

6.4.8 CT Simulators

A CT simulator is a dedicated RT CT scanner equipped with a wide bore/aperture, a flat couch top, and moving laser positioning system. The term may also be used when referring to dedicated CT scanners that have integrated virtual simulation software; once a popular method of simulating RT treatment fields, establishing treatment reference points, and/or an isocentre. In clinical practice, such systems tend to be less common now, with most radiation therapy departments employing a dedicated CT scanner with direct transfer of image data to an independent TPS. This

section will discuss the main features of a CT scanner dedicated for RT localisation.

6.4.8.1 CT Aperture

A key feature of a CT simulator is the wider bore/aperture, compared to a diagnostic CT scanner. A standard CT aperture is 70 cm, with a maximum field of view (FOV) of 50 cm. In contrast, the size of the aperture with a wide bore is typically 80–85 cm, with a maximum FOV of 65 cm. The larger FOV offers increased flexibility to scan patients in the optimal position for treatment, as well as accommodate any desired immobilisation equipment. Inclusion of immobilisation equipment within the scan is important so that the impact of equipment that may be present in the treatment beam path is correctly accounted for in the dose calculations performed later.

Reconstruction algorithms available within the CT software can also be used to extend the FOV further to be as large as the physical size of the aperture itself. It is important to note however, that the quality of image data in the extended FOV region is typically reduced, since this data has been generated through the reconstruction of partial projection data, rather than full projection data. Additionally, the electron density of tissues presented in the extended FOV may also be inaccurate. It is therefore important that dose calculations performed in these regions are reviewed, with the understanding of potential dose uncertainty and error.

Whilst a larger CT aperture is clearly advantageous in the RT setting, it is not without disadvantage. There is a reduction in high contrast resolution, increased noise within the images and a higher radiation dose compared to a standard bore scanner. In the RT context however, these factors are considered to be outweighed by the overall benefits gained.

6.4.8.2 CT Couch

Provision of a flat, stable couch is essential for RT planning and, like the wider CT aperture, is a key component. The CT couch should be consistent with the linear accelerator couch that will be used for treatment in several ways. Firstly, it should be of the same material and dimension to allow for accurate treatment dose calculations. Secondly, its design is important; there should minimal adjoining sections, metal supports, or screws that will create image artefact and/or restrict the potential treatment planning options available.

The couch should employ the same indexing system, so that the attachment of any immobilisation equipment/localisation devices can be maintained from planning and throughout the treatment course for improved setup reproducibility. Finally, the couch sag and weight-bearing capacity should also be comparable to that of the linear accelerator couch.

In situations where the CT couch is not consistent with that of the linear accelerator, a CT couch overlay (insert) that replicates the treatment couch may be used. Alternatively, a virtual couch structure may be incorporated into the CT image dataset later during the treatment planning stage.

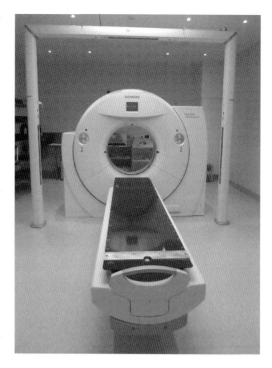

FIGURE 6.11 Computed tomography (CT) Simulator and external laser system. (Source: courtesy of Siemens Healthcare and Sunshine Coast University Hospital.)

6.4.8.3 External Laser Positioning System

Dedicated RT CT simulators have an external laser positioning system in place, which comprise one or more moveable lasers on an external rail system (Figure 6.11). The lasers form crosshairs on the patient's skin that enable the marking of references, landmarks, and baselines. The location of reference marks to be placed on the patient may be changed as desired by adjustment of the laser(s) coordinates using a remote control pad, adjustment of the CT couch vertical and longitudinal position, or alternatively through a combination of both laser and couch adjustment depending upon the individual clinic setup in place. Irrespective of clinic setup, the overall purpose is to define the scan reference point, often referred to as position zero (0) or CT zero (CT0). It is from this scan reference point that the treatment beam(s) isocentre coordinates will later be defined.

6.4.8.4 Lasers Incorporated within the Scanner

It should be noted that all scanners have the addition of an internal laser, housed within the CT gantry itself. This laser identifies the scan plane. However, due to the relative 'inaccuracy' of this laser, it is not generally used for marking patient reference points.

6.4.8.5 Equipment for the Administration of Intravenous Contrast

The injection of intravenous (IV) contrast media during image acquisition assists in differentiating blood vessels from surrounding anatomical or pathological structures. As such, the addition of IV contrast in RT CT simulation has assumed increasing importance in the past few decades, aiding accurate delineation of the treatment target volume for some specific tumour sites.

Delivery of contrast media is typically via a remote contrast injector that operates either as a stand-alone unit, or is coupled to the CT scanner, enabling automatic bolus delivery. The remote injector consists of either a pedestal or ceiling-mounted injector head, containing one to two syringe barrel(s) and a syringe drive or plunger which injects the contrast media at a preprogrammed rate. A local control console, plus a remote-control console, allow for the infusion volume, flow rate, and any required time delays to be programmed.

Alternatively, an automatic bolus tracking method is possible for CT coupled contrast injectors, whereby a desired anatomical ROI is defined (e.g. arch of the aorta) and the CT scanner then takes a single axial image through this region and reads the HU number measured. Single axial slices are automatically acquired until the HU within the ROI reaches a defined threshold limit (e.g. 100 HU). Once the threshold HU is met, the CT couch will then automatically move to the required scan start location and the spiral scan will commence.

6.4.9 4DCT

Respiratory correlated CT, or 4DCT as it is more commonly referred to, plays a significant role in the pretreatment imaging process, reducing the uncertainties associated with respiratory motion, particularly in the thorax and abdomen. If this motion is unaccounted for, motion artefacts are commonly seen, which can lead to errors in both target volume and normal tissue delineation, potentially impacting on the overall volume of tissue to be irradiated, as well as accuracy of RT dose calculations [3, 4].

The aim of any 4D imaging process is to obtain breathing synchronised image information (i.e. image information that tells us where anatomy is in space at different time points in the patient's breathing cycle). Information regarding tumour and organ motion can then be used for the purposes of treatment planning and treatment delivery, as well as treatment verification.

There are three key components to 4DCT acquisition;

1. monitoring of respiratory trace;
2. CT data acquisition;
3. data processing.

6.4.10 Monitoring of Respiratory Trace

Information regarding the patient's respiratory cycle is fundamental to 4DCT; it is the temporal (time) information gained simultaneously with image acquisition that distinguishes a 4DCT process from a standard 3DCT process. Respiratory information is most commonly gained by using an external surrogate that records changes in chest wall or abdominal movement during the breathing cycle. The use of internal surrogate methods that consider changes in lung area, air content, and lung density have been explored, but with varying accuracy compared to external surrogate methods [5].

External monitoring systems use either reflective surface markers, pressure sensitive abdominal belts, spirometry, or deformed surface images in order to determine the patient's breathing cycle and subsequently generate a respiratory signal that can be used to sort the CT image data. The following sections will briefly describe the most common types of equipment currently available to monitor the respiratory cycle.

6.4.10.1 Reflective Surface Markers
These systems employ the use of a reflective marker box and video-based tracking camera to record chest wall/abdominal motion. The tracking camera attaches to the foot of the CT couch and is equipped with an illuminator ring that emits infrared light (Figure 6.12). The reflective marker box, which is made of a lightweight plastic, is placed on the patient's skin surface in a region where chest wall/abdominal motion due to respiration is visible. The motion of the marker is detected by the tracking camera as it reflects the infrared light from the illuminator ring back

(a)   (b)

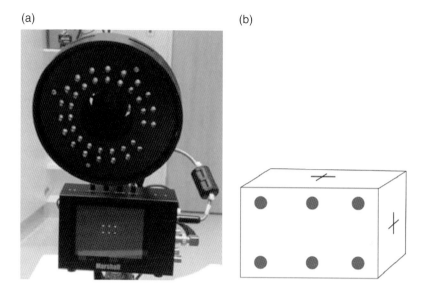

FIGURE 6.12 (a) Tracking camera with illuminator ring and liquid crystal display (LCD) monitor; (b) reflective marker box. (Source: courtesy of Varian Medical Systems, USA and Sunshine Coast University Hospital.)

to the camera. This motion enables transfer of a video signal from the camera to the monitoring computer system.

6.4.10.2 Pressure-sensitive Abdominal Belts

This method uses a latex belt that is placed around the patient's abdomen. As the patient breathes, the belt expands and contracts and the changes in belt pressure are recorded. The pressure changes are subsequently converted by a transducer into a voltage signal that is sent to the CT scanner (Figure 6.13).

6.4.10.3 Surface Tracking

This method does not employ marker boxes or belts in order to record respiratory motion, but instead uses a ceiling-mounted camera and surface patch to track points on the 3D patient surface during breathing (Figure 6.14).

6.4.10.4 Spirometry

Spirometers can be used to measure the tidal volume of air that is displaced during inhalation and exhalation at the time of CT. A turbine-shaped fan is encased in tubing, and the rotation rate of the fan during respiration

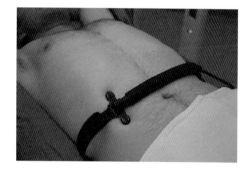

FIGURE 6.13 Example of a pressure-sensitive abdominal belt being used in conjunction with and reflective surface marker for respiratory monitoring. (Source: courtesy of Brayden Geary B.App.Sci.)

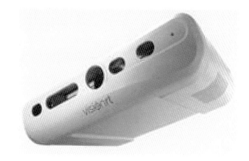

FIGURE 6.14 Example of a surface tracking system for respiratory monitoring. (Source: courtesy of VisionRT, UK.)

determines the flow rate of air. This creates a respiratory waveform that is correlated by software with the CT image data.

Irrespective of the monitoring system in place, quality assurance is paramount to ensure the generated respiratory waveform is representative of both the amplitude and temporal (time) pattern of the patient's breathing cycle in order for accurate correlation with the CT image data.

6.4.11 CT Data Acquisition

4D data can be acquired using one of two methods: axial cine scan or slow helical scan. In an axial cine scan method, images are acquired with a static couch position for at least one breathing cycle. Radiation exposure then temporarily stops whilst the couch moves to the next location and exposure resumes for another full breathing cycle. These steps are repeated for the entirety of the required scan length (Figure 6.15).

In a slow helical scan, the couch moves continuously, but at a low pitch, as image projection data is acquired. The optimal pitch is determined by having first monitored the patient's breathing pattern, prior to image acquisition. Once the average time taken for one full breathing cycle is established, the most suitable scan pitch can be selected. Multiple images of overlapping anatomical information are obtained due to the low scan

pitch and thin slice thickness used. This is often referred to as *oversampling*. Whilst both scan methods provide image data across all phases of the breathing cycle, this is not without disadvantage; in both cases the longer exposure times result in a higher radiation dose to the patient in comparison compared to 3DCT. Furthermore, 4D datasets have a greater impact on CT data storage availability.

6.4.11.1 Data Processing

Following scan completion, each image acquired is tagged with the corresponding respiratory signal that was received from the respiratory monitoring system. It is then possible to reassemble (or process) the entire CT dataset into groups or *bins*, with each bin representing a different moment in time, or more specifically a different moment in the patient's breathing cycle. Since the CT data is processed after scan completion, it is referred to as *retrospective data processing*.

It is important to note however, that prior to any data processing, a crucial quality assurance step in any 4DCT process is to first evaluate the respiratory trace signal. A visual check of the respiratory waveform is essential in minimising the risk of image data being incorrectly tagged to a wrong part of the patient's breathing cycle.

An example is illustrated in Figure 6.16 where some of the inhalation peaks on the respiratory waveform have been incorrectly assigned. These points require manual

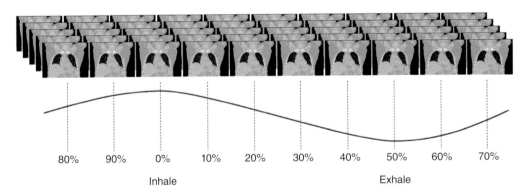

FIGURE 6.15 A 4DCT dataset is a series of 3DCT images, each representing the same volume of anatomy in a different phase of the breathing cycle. (Source: courtesy of Dr Nick Hardcastle PhD.)

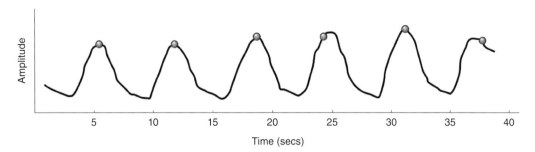

FIGURE 6.16   Incorrect assignment of maximum inhalation on respiratory waveform.

(a)

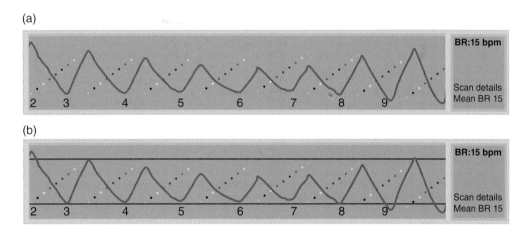

(b)

FIGURE 6.17   Differences in bin determination between phase and amplitude based sorting. (a) In phase based sorting, the data is split into bins of equal 10% time increments. (b) In amplitude based sorting, the data is sorted into 10 bins based on the average maximum inhalation and exhalation amplitudes. (Source: reproduced with permission Elsevier [7].)

adjustment prior to data processing to ensure that each image is tagged appropriately.

4D image data may be sorted according to breathing amplitude or according to phases of the breathing cycle. In amplitude-based sorting, the depth (amplitude) of the patient's breathing is considered, with specific datasets being created according to the corresponding amplitudes of the respiratory cycle. Amplitude-based sorting can be a suitable method of image data sorting where irregular breathing patterns exist, since it typically generates less motion artefacts than observed in phase based sorting [6].

In phase-based sorting, the end-point of inspiration is determined and then the entire respiratory cycle is divided equally into 10% time increments. The end of inhalation equals the 0% phase bin, with the end of exhalation being represented by the 50% phase bin

(Figure 6.17). The advantage with this method of sorting is that the full range of respiratory motion is accounted for, unlike in amplitude-based sorting where the average peak and average troughs/valley amplitudes are used.

Following data processing, a review of the 4DCT dataset to assess overall tumour/organ motion, and for the presence of any image artefacts, is important in validating the dataset prior to treatment planning. The direction and magnitude of tumour motion when the dataset is reviewed as a movie (cine loop) should look be reasonable with respect to inhalation and expiration. Unexpected or erratic tumour motion and/or the presence of image artefact(s) may indicate errors in the processing of data, usually due to a non-uniform breathing pattern, and warrant further investigation (Figure 6.18).

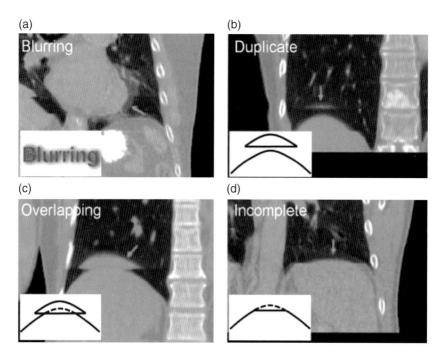

FIGURE 6.18 Examples of the types of image artefacts seen on 4DCT: (a) blurring of anatomical borders; (b) duplication of anatomy; (c) overlapping of anatomy; and (d) incomplete anatomical boundaries. (Source: reproduced with permission Elsevier [8].)

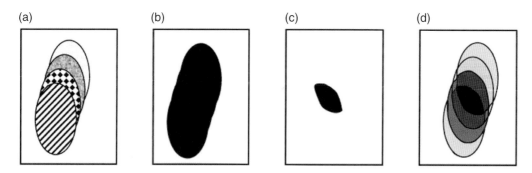

FIGURE 6.19 Pixel-based intensity projections used in 4DCT demonstrating (a) different phases of the 4DCT; (b) maximum intensity projection; (c) minimum intensity projection; and (d) average intensity projection. (Source: reproduced with permission Elsevier [9].)

6.4.12 Clinical Application of 4DCT

The rationale for acquiring 4DCT data is to generate a model of tumour/organ motion that can then be used to inform the treatment planning process. For the purposes of treatment planning, additional datasets can be generated from raw CT data using algorithms. These may include the *maximum intensity projection (*MIP*), average intensity projection (Average)* and the *minimum intensity projection (MinIP)* (Figure 6.19a–d).

6.4.12.1 MIP

The MIP displays the maximum or highest voxel intensities in the stack of axial CT

(a)   (b)   (c)

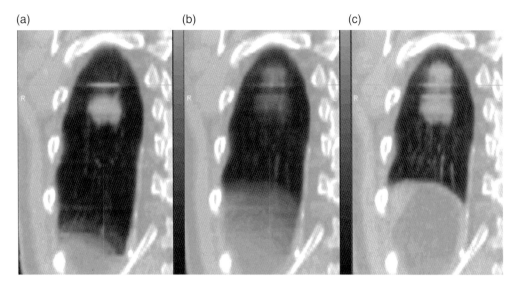

FIGURE 6.20 Coronal computed tomography (CT) images to demonstrate visual difference in lung tumour when viewed (a) single inhale phase; (b) with an average intensity projection; and (c) with a Maximum Intensity Projection (MIP). (Source: courtesy of Dr Nick Hardcastle PhD.)

images. The MIP is useful in regions where the volume of interest is of a higher intensity than the surrounding tissue, for example a lung tumour, where a solid tumour volume is surrounded by air.

Using the example of a lung tumour, the MIP dataset can be considered to provide an overall summary of the tumour position across all phases of the respiratory cycle, illustrating the full extent of tumour motion. The MIP dataset makes delineation of an internal target volume (ITV) more efficient, since contouring can be performed on a single dataset rather than being performed on up to 10 individual datasets, which is a time-consuming and labour-intensive process. However, due to electron density uncertainties associated with MIP datasets, these scans are generally used for contouring purposes only, rather than RT dose calculations.

6.4.12.2 Average Intensity Projection

An average intensity dataset is a single scan displaying the average voxel intensities in the stack of axial CT images across the breathing cycle. The accuracy of voxel electron density in an average dataset is considered to be equivalent to that of a standard 3DCT scan, therefore making it suitable for dose calculation purposes.

6.4.12.3 MinIP

The MinIP displays the minimum or lowest voxel intensities in the stack of axial CT images. This dataset can be useful in identifying structures where there is low contrast between different tissues (Figure 6.20). An example is where tumours are located adjacent to anatomy of similar intensity, such as those in the mediastinum and abdomen.

In summary, 4DCT is beneficial for thoracic, abdominal, and pelvic tumour sites [3], particularly where tumour motion exceeds 5 mm. It plays an important role in the planning of stereotactic and gated treatment techniques, reducing potential dose errors associated with organ motion and movement of multi-leaf collimators (MLC), commonly referred to as the *interplay effect*.

6.5 MRI

6.5.1 Introduction

The MRI scan is similar to a CT scan in that it enables us to see the body in different slices/planes (axial, sagittal, coronal, or oblique). Unlike CT, MRI does not use ionising radiation in the imaging process, however it uses the magnetic properties of hydrogen atoms (the most commonly occurring element in the body, contained in water and fat) to generate images. The phenomenon of nuclear magnetic resonance (NMR) is described as a resonance transition between nuclear spin states of certain atomic nuclei when subjected to a radiofrequency (RF) signal of a specific frequency, in the presence of a magnetic field. MRI images are advantageous because they have higher contrast and allow optimal soft-tissue imaging. This is why they are of use for the diagnosis and pretreatment imaging of specific tumour types.

Cancer diagnosis and staging: In recent years MRI use has seen improved accuracy of diagnostic assessment for prostate cancer [10]. It has also been investigated and used for assessing extra-prostatic extension [11]. MRI is also used in many sites to diagnose and stage tumours, for example in uterine and gynaecological cancer [12] and brain tumours, where it allows clear visualisation of tumour size, boundaries, and location [13].

Pre-treatment imaging: MRI use in the pre-treatment process is becoming increasingly prevalent, where patients can enter the magnetic field and tolerate the scanning equipment. MRI is most useful when the target volume has adjacent soft tissues of low and similar density to each other (such as those of the central nervous system, particularly the posterior fossa and brain stem, head and neck, abdomen or pelvis). MRI is often used in conjunction with other modalities such as CT and PET to optimise tumour visualisation for planning purposes. MRI images are also used to plan brachytherapy (pelvis and thorax) and stereotactic treatments.

6.5.2 Physical Principles of MRI

6.5.2.1 The Spinning Nucleus

It has already been established that hydrogen atoms are responsible for producing MR (magnetic resonance) images. So, how does this occur? Atomic nuclei are:

- either isotopes of elements with an even number of protons and neutrons in the nucleus such as carbon (^{12}C) or oxygen (^{16}O);
- or an uneven number of protons and neutrons such as hydrogen (^{1}H) or sodium (^{23}Na).

Both protons and neutrons have the ability to spin. When there are the same number of protons and neutrons in the nucleus, the spins cancel each other out, so the net effect is zero nuclear spin. A *net spin* therefore occurs only in isotopes that have uneven numbers of protons and neutrons. As hydrogen nuclei consist of one proton only, there is a net spin. As the hydrogen nuclei spins it also wobbles a little (*precesses*) about its axis of spin, rather like a spinning top (Figure 6.21).

The velocity of spin of the hydrogen nucleus is constant as is the precessional frequency (number of rotations [wobbles] in a given period about the precessional axis),

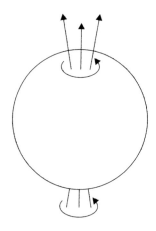

FIGURE 6.21 Precession of hydrogen atoms about an axis.

also termed the '*Larmor frequency*'; however, the direction of axis of the spin can change. Just as with any charged particle that has an uneven number of protons and neutrons, the spin of the moving proton in hydrogen generates a magnetic field. These properties enable us to image the human body.

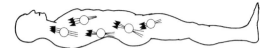

FIGURE 6.22 Protons in longitudinal alignment within patient.

6.5.2.2 Magnetism in the Body
The human body is composed of about 65% water (H_2O) and so is hydrogen atom rich. Hydrogen atoms possess the simplest atomic nucleus and have the strongest magnetic signal of all the elements because they have a single positive charge. Because of the magnetic spin qualities of hydrogen atoms, they are best to use for MR-generated images.

Imagine that each proton in every hydrogen atom is like a small bar magnet that has a magnetic north pole and a magnetic south pole. The term 'spin magnet' is used to describe them because they are in constant motion. Even though each of the individual protons is spinning and creating a magnetic field of its own, there is no net magnetisation in the body, because in their 'normal' state, the axes of the protons are aligned randomly in different directions to cancel out the total magnetic effect. Therefore, rather than using the effect of individual protons spinning and creating their own magnetic fields in a given volume (voxel) of tissue, MRI utilises the total combined magnetic effect of the group of protons in the voxel to create an image.

6.5.2.3 Introduction of the Body into a Magnetic Field
The randomly aligned, spinning protons have the ability to alter their direction in the presence of a magnetic field. When the patient is placed in the magnetic field of the MR scanner, the protons align in one direction. This results in a small net magnetisation (paramagnetism) in the long axis of the patient (Figure 6.22). The precessing spin magnets emit RF waves/signals that are specific to each isotope of an element. This signal in the body is relatively weak because the direction of magnetic field of each proton is slightly different due to its *non-synchronous precession*.

6.5.2.4 Introduction of a Radiofrequency Pulse During Magnetisation
If we want to change the orientation of the spin magnets (which are not truly unidirectional because of their non-synchronous precessions) when the hydrogen atoms are in their magnetised state, an RF pulse can be introduced. This RF pulse is introduced perpendicular to the long axis of the magnet and the patient so that it 'cuts through' the magnetic field. This results in an interruption of the magnetisation effect. If this RF pulse is the same *resonant frequency* (equivalent to the Larmor frequency) as the ¹H protons, 42.6 MHz per tesla (SI unit of strength of magnetic flux density), they change direction. This change in direction occurs because they absorb the energy from the RF pulse. The effect of this is that the spin magnets flip through 90°, which in turn causes two distinct and separate effects:

1. Enough hydrogen protons flip through 90° to reduce the net magnetisation in the longitudinal direction to zero and to cause some magnetism to be established in a transverse direction.

2. The pulse that flips them through 90° has the effect of starting them all off from the same point of spin and for an instant (a few milliseconds) they *resonate*, i.e. they precess in synchrony (in phase) with each other. This causes the transverse magnetic signal to be relatively strong and a 'true' unidirectional field is created.

It is this process which allows the MR signal to be produced. Upon the introduction of a conductor (*the coil*) into the constantly changing magnetic field an electromagnetic effect is produced (refer to Faraday and Lenz laws). This means that a current of a specific voltage is created and runs through the coil. When the RF pulse ceases, the two effects also cease, in the following ways:

1. The energised protons lose the energy that they had gained from the RF pulse and relax back to the 'more-or-less' longitudinal alignment.

   a. This causes the transverse component of the magnetism to decay.

   b. As a result, the longitudinal component of the magnetisation is re-established (Figure 6.23).

   c. The effect is exponential with time (decays rapidly then more slowly) and the time constant for the return of the longitudinal magnetism is known as **T1**.

2. The protons precessing in phase (Figure 6.24) experience interference from other

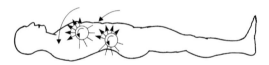

FIGURE 6.23 Longitudinal alignment re-establishing.

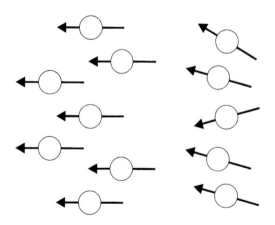

FIGURE 6.24 Illustration of one group of protons in phase and one out of phase, showing perfectly versus imperfectly aligned magnetism.

protons in the vicinity (spin–spin interactions) and rapidly lose the synchronisation.

   a. This results in the *magnitude* of the transverse magnetic component rapidly decaying.

   b. Orientation of the protons once again becomes more generalised within the patient (as they were before the RF pulse was applied).

   c. In a perfectly homogeneous magnetic field this is also exponential with time and the time constant is known as **T2**.

6.5.2.5 Utilisation of T1 and T2 Relaxation in Scanning

The term relaxation relates to the magnetic effect returning from a state of non-equilibrium to a state of equilibrium. The relaxation process has two components, which are exploited when scanning different tissues.

The recovery rate for realignment in the longitudinal direction (T1) occurs more slowly than the decay rate of the magnetic field created in the transverse direction (T2) (i.e. transverse magnetism is lost more rapidly than it takes for reinstatement of longitudinal magnetism).

1. In the case of T1 relaxation this is exponential in that at the start of the process the longitudinal realignment occurs rapidly. However, as time progresses and the closer all the spin magnets get to the point of realignment, the longer it takes to reach the end point.

2. In the case of T2, the decay of the transverse magnetisation is rapid at the start (when the RF pulse is removed) and it then slows down towards the point at which zero transverse magnetisation occurs.

The amplitude of the voltage signal which is created as a result of electromagnetic induction in the coil placed close to the patient's body depends on the T1 and T2 times. These times vary for different tissues for example T1 and T2 for fat is shorter compared with water (this will be further explained).

The variation in T1 times for different tissues is related to molecular motion. As molecules move, tiny magnetic fields are created in local field area (fluctuations of this local field in the range of the Larmor [resonant] frequency have the strongest effect). The larger, slower moving molecules such as fat feel the 'pull' of these tiny magnetic fields more readily than water. Thus, their protons realign more rapidly. The relaxation times for T1 are in the order of seconds.

White matter is the fastest to return to longitudinal alignment, grey matter being next, and cerebral spinal fluid (CSF) taking the longest time. It is this difference in T1 times of tissues that affords the sharp contrast in MRI. For the purpose of RT imaging, it is the water content of tumours and different tissues that gives them different T1 times, which results in the difference in contrast and thus different appearance on MR images.

At the time of T2 relaxation, the spin magnets that were aligned and spinning in synchrony in the transverse direction begin to spin 'out of phase' with each other. They then revert back to their initial (individually spinning) state, which was observed before the RF pulse. The flow of current in the coil is temporarily suspended for this short period of time and thus there is no MR signal. The T2 times are much faster than those of T1 and are in the order of tens of milliseconds. CSF has the longest relaxation time and white matter the shortest. It is the interaction of the 'spin–spin' between the protons and the process of the longitudinal relaxation that allows more rapid decay. The alteration in spin also changes the local field, which affects the precessional frequency. This means that the spin magnets are out of synchrony with each other. As each body tissue has a different T2 relaxation, these can be seen as MR image contrast.

6.5.2.6 Pulsed RF to Create an Image

The image cannot be produced by the application of a single RF pulse, however. A series of pulses, known as a *pulse sequence*, is required. Pulse sequences used in clinical practice vary in sophistication, but two of the simplest are described here.

A *saturation recovery sequence*

- consists of a series of 90° pulses; and
- the time between pulses is known as the *repetition time* (TR).

It has already been said that tissues have different T1 times. For the same TR, tissues with shorter T1 times will give larger signals than tissues with longer T1 times.

If the TR is kept short (about 500 ms) relative to the T1 under investigation (i.e. tissue type), there will be insufficient time for the longitudinal component of the magnetism to be re-established between pulses, and so fewer protons will be tipped through 90° by the next pulse. This is particularly so for tissues with a long T1 time and the TR effectively emphasises differences between the tissues with different T1s. These images are known as *T1-weighted images*. In a T1-weighted image, white matter has the brightest shade (fat) and CSF (fluid) the darkest (Figure 6.25a and c).

A *spin-echo sequence* may consist of

- a 90° RF pulse;
- followed by a 180° RF pulse (Figure 6.26).

As the protons relax back into the longitudinal alignment and have begun to de-phase (lose their synchronisation), they are flipped through 180°. Thus, they continue to precess in the same plane but in the opposite direction. This brings them into line again so that for another brief instant they precess in phase again, giving rise to a second strong signal, called an echo. The interval between the 90 and 180° pulses is called the *echo time* (TE). A series of 90 and 180° pulses constitute the pulse sequence, and the time between each *pair* of pulses is the TR.

Again each tissue has its own unique TR due to this process. If both the TE and TR are kept relatively long, the differences between tissues with different T2 values are enhanced. This results in a T2-weighted image in which CSF (fluid) appears as the brightest grey level

(a)

(c)

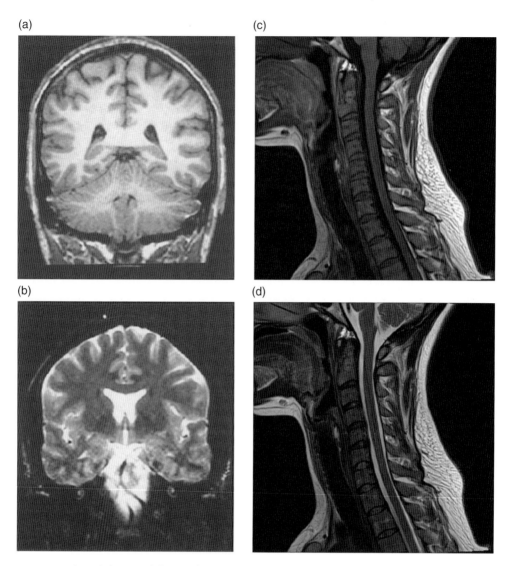

(b)

(d)

FIGURE 6.25   (a and c) T1- and (b and d) T2-weighted scans.

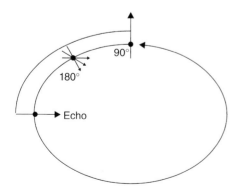

FIGURE 6.26   Relaxation plane with protons after 90° and 180° pulse.

on the image and white matter (fat) as the darkest (Figure 6.25b and d).

As there is a choice of relaxation processes, the patient contrast (differences between body tissues) is not fixed as it is in imaging using radiation. In addition, the pulse sequences can be varied to suit the clinical requirements of an individual investigation. It is this flexibility and lack of ionisation of tissues that gives MRI a major advantage over other imaging modalities.

6.5.2.7 Variation of Body Section Imaged

To be energised, protons must experience an RF pulse that is at their resonant (Larmor) frequency (42.6 MHz T^{-1}), and therefore the strength of the magnetic field affects the frequency of the RF pulse required. If the magnetic field is graduated along its length, there will be only one specific section or 'slice' of the patient's body in which the protons will be energised by the pulse, so only that slice will be imaged. The field *gradient* can be varied to alter the slice imaged. Other field gradients are employed that affect the frequencies of the signals *across* the selected slice and the phases of signals vertically *along* the slice so that the signals from each voxel can be separately identified and represented in the final MR image.

We have already seen that with 'plain radiography' and CT, soft-tissue contrast is relatively poor and this is where MRI excels. With MRI, superior soft-tissue contrast and image resolution are seen and excellent quality images can be produced in any plane throughout the body (transverse, sagittal, coronal, and oblique), whereas in the case of CT (which is dependent on tissue electron density), sagittal and coronal image planes have to be reconstructed from the series of axial slices. In the RT planning process MRI provides an excellent means of enhancing visualisation of the interfaces between adjacent tissues themselves and between tissues and tumours. The images also prove useful in gross tumour volume (GTV) margin delineation and in contouring organs at risk, particularly in the craniocaudal plane. However, the scan sequence can be lengthy and the patient may not be able to tolerate this – see safety notes in Section 6.5.5.

6.5.3 Functional MRI

Functional MRI, or fMRI that is blood oxygen level dependent (BOLD MRI), allows blood flow in regions of the brain to be imaged through changing metabolic activity. When an area of the brain is active, the blood flow increases through the capillaries in order for oxygen and glucose to be deposited there and metabolised by the neurons. This increased metabolic activity and resultant oxygen uptake of the active neurons are markedly different to that of inactive neurons. The small magnetic difference between oxyhaemoglobin (which is diamagnetic) and deoxyhaemoglobin can be detected as changes in MR signals. It is this difference between magnetic effects of oxyhaemoglobin and deoxyhaemoglobin that allows for cortical activity to be captured. This technique is useful in visualising tumours of the CNS and the surrounding active brain tissue. It is anticipated that in the future many more uses of physiological and biochemical MRI imaging (see Chapter 13) will be developed.

A technique known as *diffusion-weighted MRI* (DW-MRI) is one of the newest procedures for tumour imaging. Its mechanism of action is related to the diffusion of water across cell membranes, which is different in normal and tumour cells. The most common use of DW-MRI is for the identification of brain tumours. However, it is also used to detect the response of brain tumours to RT and predict treatment outcome.

6.5.3.1 Limitation to the Use of MRI

There are limitations with the use of MRI in the pretreatment process, such as resource issues associated with the availability of scanners. There is also the suboptimal ability of MRI to image bone and high-density tissues/structures. This is because it does not depend on the electron density of tissues (as is the case with CT). This property of MRI results in challenges associated with achieving accurate dosimetry, because planning algorithms depend on the interface with bone and soft tissue to formulate isodose distributions in a target volume. In addition, MRI does not provide accurate images of the external contour of the patient, which is again vital for planning purposes. The use of MRI for planning purposes is now being explored as manufacturers have developed MRI-only RT packages for use in treatment planning. In current practice, MRI is used with CT. This affords exploitation of the advantageous aspects of both imaging modalities, in accurate volume delineation, as a result of using MRI and superior dosimetric calculation resulting from the properties of CT. The process of using a combination of modalities (also including PET when necessary) is termed 'image fusion/registration' (explained later in this chapter).

6.5.4 Safety

It is important to note the issues related to safety of patients and personnel when using MR scanners. The magnetic field of the MR scanner has to remain constant in order to ensure image accuracy. This means that patients and personnel should ensure that they do not have any magnetic materials/objects within them (e.g. pacemakers, aneurysm coils, tattoos of unknown source material as skin burns are possible). It is also necessary to ensure that any metallic objects such as hairpins and watches are not worn because this can result in serious injury and damage to the equipment. A rigorous routine should therefore be employed by staff to ensure that anyone entering the vicinity of the scanner conforms to the safety regulations. In the case of planning, the immobilisation devices used must be checked to ensure that they do not contain any magnetic substances. Referral to any catalogues listing the magnetic properties of implants in the body of patients is a key component of scanning and without complete certainty of the construct of an object then MRI should not be used.

6.5.5 MR Simulators

The superior soft-tissue definition associated with MR compared to CT has led to an increasing demand in the use of MRI for RT planning purposes. As discussed earlier in this chapter, with limited MR resources, this has driven the development and implementation of MR simulators, dedicated to RT

planning. Whilst the lack of tissue electron density from MR continues to exclude dose calculations on these datasets at present, the ability to acquire MR images in the desired treatment position is clearly advantageous.

Similar to CT simulators, a key feature of an MR simulator is a larger bore/aperture. The standard aperture of a MR scanner is 60 cm; this is typically extended to 70 cm for MR simulators. Increasing the aperture beyond this size has a negative impact upon the quality of images generated due to a reduction in the *signal-to-noise ratio* (SNR) with increasing patient to coil distance. Whilst the MR simulator aperture size is not as large as that of a CT simulator, there still remains increased flexibility to scan patients in the optimal position for treatment, as well accommodate immobilisation equipment. Inclusion of immobilisation equipment within the scan is desirable so that there is consistency in patient position between the CT and MR images. This consistency in patient position is beneficial to reducing potential image registration errors at the time of treatment planning.

MR simulators have an external laser positioning system in place, which comprise moveable lasers on an external rail system (Figure 6.27). As in the case of CT simulators, these lasers form crosshairs on the patient's skin that enable the marking of references, landmarks, and baselines and are used to define the scan reference point.

A flat, indexable couch that is MR compatible (i.e. does not contain ferromagnetic material) is a further key component. MR simulators (as well as newer diagnostic MR scanners) typically have a dockable table that aids both a safe environment as well as supporting efficient patient preparation and workflow.

6.5.6 Maintaining Signal-to-noise Ratio

As with all imaging modalities, maintaining a high SNR is important for optimising image quality. In the case of MR simulators, the

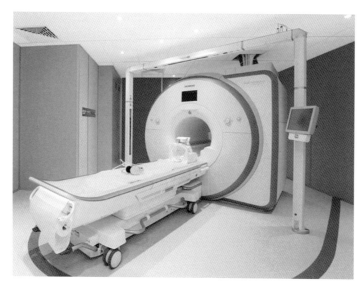

FIGURE 6.27 3T Siemens Skyra with external laser positioning bridge and 30 gauss line demarcation on floor. (Source: reproduced from Rai et al. [9].)

larger FOV required for flexible patient positioning unfortunately has a negative impact on the SNR, reducing image quality. In order to improve the quality of images obtained, MR simulators are equipped with built-in high-density coils which seek to maintain a high SNR. Signal can also be improved by the use of additional RF flexible coils at the time of scanning.

In any simulation process, whether a CT or MR process, establishing a reproducible patient position is paramount. In the case of MR simulators, the SNR is more affected by the larger FOV size than is the case for CT simulators. As such, it is often necessary to consider varying the scan slice thickness, scan parameters, or the magnetic field strength in order to further maintain the SNR. It is however important to be aware of the associated safety considerations when varying these parameters, such as the specific absorption rate and potential heating of tissues that may occur.

6.5.7 Safety

The safety considerations discussed earlier in this chapter for MRI remain applicable for MR simulator suites as well. The zoning of controlled and restricted areas is recommended, as well as demarcation of 30 gauss area adjacent to the magnet, where there is the highest risk of projectile hazards in this region (Figure 6.27). The labelling of all equipment should also be undertaken to clearly identify whether it is MR compatible and can safely enter this area.

The advent of MR simulators is an exciting development, one that promises to change the future of RT localisation and planning from what we are currently familiar with today. However, this imaging modality and the associated safety regulations are largely unfamiliar to therapeutic radiographers, highlighting the need for education, training, and inter-professional collaboration with MR specialist radiographers for safe and successful integration into practice.

6.6 Ultrasound

6.6.1 Introduction

Ultrasound (US) uses high-frequency, short pulsed sound waves to create an image of organs, tissues, and pathologies within the body. The unit of measurement for sound waves is the Hertz (Hz – frequency of one cycle/vibration per second). The frequency of audible sound ranges between 20 Hz and 20 kHz, whereas in medical/diagnostic US (sonography) the frequency range is between 1 and 20 MHz. These higher frequencies are well beyond the range of normal human hearing, however this property allows for detailed imaging of structures within the body.

An US image is formed when the high-frequency sound waves created by a transducer (within the US probe) are emitted in pulses and interact within tissues and at tissue interfaces. As a result, echoes are produced. The echoes are detected by the transducer probe, which is connected to the US machine. These echoes are then processed to form a visible image. This image distinguishes different structures and the function of tissues by virtue of their unique acoustic properties. Thus, the image is created as a result of reflected echoes, rather than transmitted photons (X-ray images).

US has become increasingly utilised in RT and oncology because of its non-ionising properties and non-invasive nature. This means that it is safer to use because it does not involve the emission of X-rays, which are potentially harmful. US is also painless which is advantageous and preferable from a patient's perspective.

US is used in all stages of the cancer imaging process from diagnosis, staging, and treatment planning to treatment verification in external beam RT and brachytherapy. It can also be used to investigate physiological processes such as blood flow using a technique called Doppler US. Before we look at the equipment and physical principles of US we will briefly discuss its use in RT and oncology.

Cancer diagnosis: US has been used for a number of years in the diagnosis of cancer and is the modality of choice when differentiation between cystic/benign and malignant lesions is required. For example, it is used in the diagnosis of breast cancer together with mammography [14] to differentiate between cystic lesions, which are visualised as homogeneous fluid, and malignant lesions, which appear solid. One advantage of US imaging over conventional radiography is that the internal structure of a lesion can be demonstrated. Transrectal US has been identified as a cost-effective method of diagnosing rectal cancer [15]. US is also used in imaging organs such as the uterus, ovary, prostate, liver, and kidney. For example, biannual liver US of high-risk patients allows for early detection of Hepato-cellular Carcinoma [16]. Using US to guide biopsies is an important part of the diagnostic process, for example in prostate cancer US has been fused with MRI (multi-parametric MRI) to target biopsies, however to date there is no conclusive evidence as to its increased capacity to detect cancer. In lung cancer, diagnosis and staging using trans-bronchial needle aspiration guided by endobronchial US has been indicated to reduce time to treatment decisions compared to conventional diagnosis using CT and bronchoscopy [17].

Cancer staging: US is used in the staging of malignancies, for example in head and neck cancer in the identification of cervical node lymphadenopathy. Endoscopic US is now a routine method of evaluating the preclinical staging for gastric cancer [18] and in combination with CT for staging of rectal cancer [19].

Pre-treatment and treatment verification: US has seen heightened popularity in pre-treatment verification (see Chapter 10), for example in verifying bladder volumes at the time of CT simulation and prior to daily radical RT to the prostate gland, rectum, and gynaecological cancers [20, 21]. The position of the prostate gland can also be acquired prior to daily RT using US, where transperineal positioning of the US probe is used to determine the location of the prostate whilst the patient is on the treatment couch. The same technology has also been investigated for evaluating real-time prostate motion during hypofractionated RT [22].

6.6.2 Physical Principles of US

6.6.2.1 US Equipment

The US machine consists of a number of components which are key to image production, display, and operational safety. The equipment

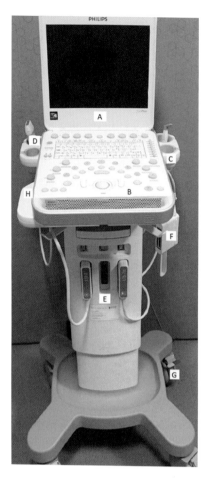

FIGURE 6.28 Portable ultrasound machine. (Source: courtesy of Philips, Monash University.)

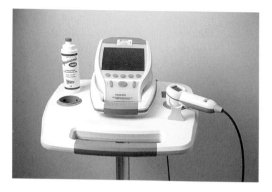

FIGURE 6.29 Radiotherapy (RT) bladder scan ultrasound machine. (Source: courtesy of Peter MacCallum Cancer Centre, Gerard Hynes, Hynesite Photography.)

depicted in Figure 6.28 is an US machine which is docked onto a stand. It is also a portable device, which facilitates access to US scans for patients in other departments of the hospital or even outside of the hospital environment in external clinics.

The monitor (Figure 6.28A) displays the processed image as visible dots, which represent anatomy and pathologies. The control panel (Figure 6.28B) enables image acquisition and manipulation. The transducer holder (Figure 6.28C) allows storage of the probe (Figure 6.28D) and facilitates easy access to a variety of shapes and sizes of probe. The multi-port adaptor transducer receptacles (Figure 6.28E) connect the transducer to the US machine via a cable. The wheel controls (Figure 6.28F) allow the machine to be manoeuvred safely and with ease; each wheel has an independent brake to secure the machine in position prior to use. On the side of the machine (Figure 6.28G) is a DVD drive to allow recording of the US scan images. Printers can be connected to the US machine to produce hard copy images.

As can be seen in Figure 6.29 the US machine used in RT to scan bladder volumes prior to simulation and daily treatment only has one transducer probe because the aim of scanning is to establish the volume of fluid in the bladder rather than differentiate between differing tissue interfaces and identify pathologies.

6.6.2.2 Vibrating Particles

There are a number of different interactions that occur when sound waves come into contact with body tissues. In a similar way to light, US can be absorbed, reflected, and refracted in a medium. The principal difference between US and light is that US waves and the resultant particle motion are propagated in the longitudinal direction. This is different to light particle motion (electromagnetic radiation), which is directed in the transverse direction, at right angles to light wave motion. Thus, sound waves travel through tissues by vibrating in the longitudinal direction. As a sound wave enters a tissue it starts a 'chain reaction' of vibrations as it travels through. As each particle vibrates it comes into contact with the next, which then starts to vibrate; this effect moves (propagates) through the tissue. As the tissues in the body differ, so do the acoustic properties of each tissue; it is this property that is exploited with US.

6.6.2.3 The Production of US Images

When an US examination is undertaken, a uniquely designed handheld probe (*transducer*) which houses a special crystal made of *piezoelectric material* (Figure 6.30) is placed next to the patient's skin. This probe has the ability to convert an electrical signal into ultrasonic energy which then propagates through tissues. As the waves of sound are travelling through the tissues an *echo effect* is generated from some of these interactions. The echo reflects the sound waves back in the direction from which they were initially generated towards the transducer. As well as generating the electrical pulse that converts to sound, the transducer can also convert the echo of sound that travels back through the tissues into electrical energy. It is possible to record the time between the initial pulse of

the US and the resultant echo. This time indicates the distance between the transducer and the tissue (depth of the tissue in the body) that created the echo, which in turn can be used to generate an image.

6.6.2.4 Piezoelectric Crystals

The piezoelectric layer is a thin (about 0.5 mm) disc of *lead zirconate titanate* (PZT) crystals located near the front face of the transducer. The frequency of vibrations of the crystals is determined by the thickness of the piezoelectric layer. These crystals have special properties in that when a voltage is applied to them (via an electrical power source) they change shape. An electrical conducting material is used to coat the front and back surfaces of the crystals through which a potential difference is created for pulsing the crystals. The front conductor is used to earth the transducer and the back one is the live connection. Depending on the polarity of the charge applied, the crystal either contracts or expands. If the current changes direction regularly (an alternating current is generated) the crystals contract and expand according to the changes in the direction of the applied current. The net effect of this contraction and expansion of the crystals is that the surface in contact with the patient effectively delivers a tiny 'punch', in the form of a mild vibration, to the patient's skin. This 'punch' causes the molecules in that area to be compressed, so there is a localised increase in pressure within the medium. The momentum of those molecules is passed on in the same way that a line of carriages run into the back of each other when one is hit by a shunting engine, so the pressure wave is transmitted though the patient (Figure 6.31).

6.6.2.5 Amplitude, Intensity, and Attenuation

The strength of sound can be described in terms of amplitude and intensity. The amplitude indicates the variation between the undisturbed value of an acoustic variable (without sound applied to it) and the value when sound is present. The intensity is the power in a sound wave divided by the area of

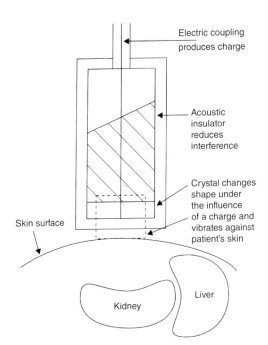

FIGURE 6.30 Ultrasound probe.

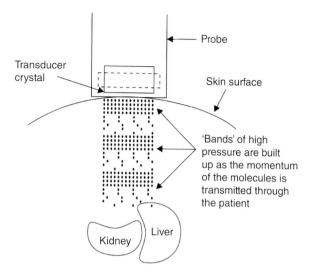

FIGURE 6.31   Transmission of an ultrasound pulse through the patient.

the beam (determined by how the transducer focuses the beam). The intensity of a beam increases as the power of the beam increases. As sound waves propagate, they weaken and as such may limit the depth of imaging; this is as a result of attenuation. Both the amplitude and intensity of an unfocussed US beam will decrease as it travels through a medium. When sound travels it is absorbed and converted to heat (this is the primary type of attenuation when US passes through soft tissues).

6.6.2.6 Transmission and Reflection

When the wave strikes an interface between two types of tissue, some of the wave continues through the new medium (*transmission*) and some is reflected back towards the probe (*echo*) (Figure 6.32). The returning pressure wave impacts on the face of the piezoelectric crystal and the mechanical force causes an electric charge to be produced on the surface. A short pulse of US is generated and the returning waves, or echoes, are detected and measured before the next pulse is applied. This is known as the *pulse-echo technique*.

6.6.2.7 Acoustic Impedance

The amount of sound which is either transmitted through the tissue or reflected back to the transducer depends on the properties of

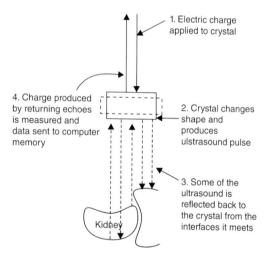

FIGURE 6.32   Generation and detection of an ultrasound pulse.

the two tissues that are adjacent to each other. The acoustic impedance (Z) of tissues is a function of the density of the tissues and the speed of sound within them. If there is a large difference in Z between two adjacent tissues more of the sound will be reflected rather than transmitted; thus, US does not provide good images of bone or air-filled spaces. Consider an interface of air and water; the density and Z of the water are greater than those of the air. Thus, most of the sound waves get reflected back to the transducer as an echo and only a few propagate through water and are transmitted. There is also a differential in the Z of air and skin that provides a challenge when attempting to use US to produce images of the body because is necessary to have a small gap between the face of the transducer and the skin surface. This means that, when a sound wave is emitted from the crystals and directed towards the skin, most of the waves would be reflected back to the transducer without entering the body. To counter this effect, a medium that is of similar Z to the crystal and the skin has to be introduced in order to 'bridge' the air gap. This is termed the 'coupling medium' which usually consists of a gel-like substance that is applied on the skin over the area that is to be scanned (Figure 6.33). Once this is applied to the skin, a continuous, more homogeneous medium (crystal > gel > skin) is created through which the US wave can move.

6.6.2.8 US Echo and Creation of the Image

Different tissues reflect signals to different degrees, so strong signals denote one tissue type and weak signals another. The US image is an electronic map of the data generated from a series of returning echoes. These are displayed as different grey levels on the monitor, and thus the contrast is built up. The US wave travels at a known speed, so the time that it takes for an echo to be detected must indicate the distance that it has travelled (speed × time = distance). Therefore, the depth of the interface causing the beam to reflect back can be calculated. It is half the total distance because the pulse travels there and back, and its image is displayed in the correct spatial position. Thus far, the spatial information is only in one dimension. The beam can detect the anterior and posterior boundaries of, for example, the kidney, so its thickness can be determined and the depth of the kidney/liver boundary recognised. Spatial information in the second dimension is achieved in one of two ways:

1. A row of stationary crystals is used and the information from each crystal is processed to provide an image;
2. The crystal is moved so that it scans a section of the patient.

The resolution of the generated image is a measure of image sharpness and this can be affected if two reflectors produce overlapping echoes and these appear as one on the image. The frequency applied can also impact on resolution.

6.6.2.9 Types of US Transducer Probe

The *transducer probe* (probe) converts pulses of electrical energy into US. It then receives US echoes and changes them back into electrical signals, which are then processed and form anatomical images. The bidirectional design of the transducer is very similar to that of a microphone. The probe is hand-held and its position is controlled by the practitioner, who performs the scan. The front side of the transducer which comes into direct contact with the patient is covered in an electrical insulating material. A backing block which quickly absorbs US returning to the probe (stopping the oscillations of the crystal after pulsation) is positioned behind the crystals.

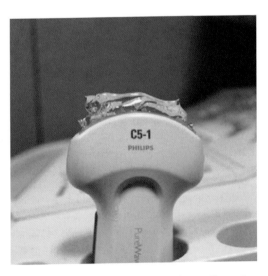

FIGURE 6.33 Ultrasound probe with coupling gel. (Source: courtesy of Philips and Monash University.)

There are two types of transducer probe: the *linear array probe* (linear sequenced array) and the *mechanical movement probe*. The linear array is an example of the static type of probe. It has several hundred tiny crystals which are rectangular in shape and arranged in a straight line. Each crystal has its own electrical connection for the detection and measurement of the echo. The information from each crystal can be updated many times per second to create multiple images (frames) in a rapid sequential format to give the appearance of movement. This is termed 'real-time' scanning and appears as a movie on the screen. The crystal array may be a straight line such as in the probe depicted in Figure 6.34 or arranged in a curved/convex array (Figure 6.35) to afford a wider FOV as the US waves diverge. The internal composition of linear and curvilinear array probes is depicted in Figure 6.36a and b.

The mechanical movement transducer has a motor drive that causes the crystal either to oscillate (Figure 6.36c) or to rotate (Figure 6.36d). The returning echoes are processed in conjunction with information indicating the direction of the transducer at that instant, so the image is displayed in the correct spatial orientation.

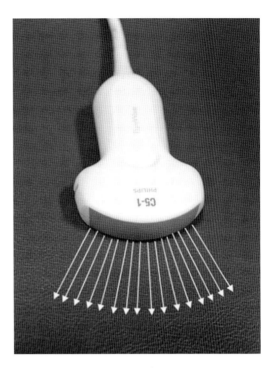

FIGURE 6.35 Convex curvilinear array transducer probe (arrows indicate divergence of initial US pulses). (Source: courtesy of Philips and Monash University.)

6.6.3 Doppler US

Doppler US uses the same principles as the pulse-echo technique, but the interface causing the reflection of the wave is moving, for example in the case of red blood cells. The pulses are generated at a known frequency, but if the blood cell is moving away from the transducer, the returned frequency is lower than the frequency originally generated. The difference between them represents the *Doppler shift*. If, however, the blood cell is moving towards the transducer, the frequency of the returning echoes is higher. In either case, the change in frequency provides information about the speed of movement of the blood cells. This can be displayed in the following ways:

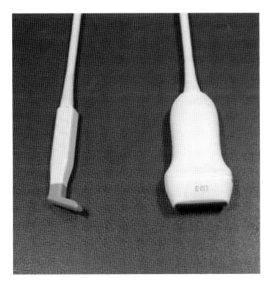

FIGURE 6.34 Ultrasound linear array transducer probes. (Source: courtesy of Philips and Monash University.)

- As a colour image, in which, for example, blood flowing towards the transducer is demonstrated in shades of red and blood flowing away from the transducer in

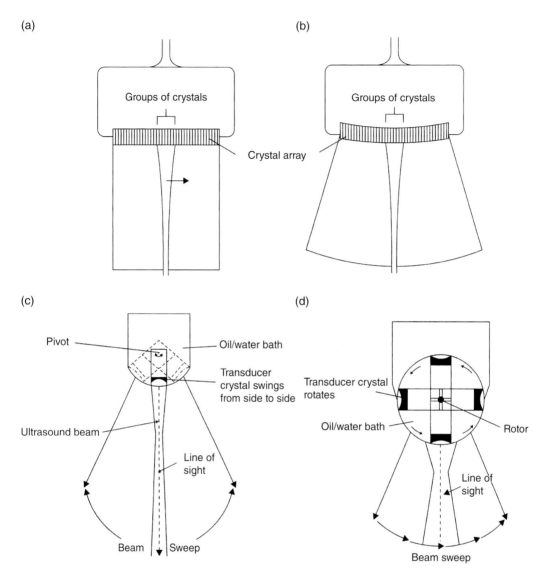

FIGURE 6.36 Ultrasound probes: (a) Linear array probe; (b) curvilinear array probe; (c) oscillating probe; and (d) rotating probe.

shades of blue. The density of the colour indicates the speed of flow. This has the appearance of an angiogram but has the advantage of being non-invasive and does not require the administration of a contrast medium.

- As a spectral graph, in which the range of velocities of blood cells in a given area is displayed over a given period of time. The appearance of the graph will vary with the type of blood vessel imaged,

e.g. the blood in an artery will experience short bursts of high velocity as the heart contracts, whereas the blood in a vein will move at a more constant speed (Figure 6.37).

6.6.4 Safety

US is generally safe when used with low diagnostic frequencies, however it is only recommended for medical use when application of

(a)

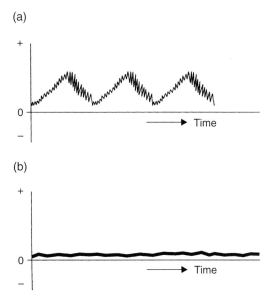

(b)

FIGURE 6.37 Spectral Doppler for: (a) arterial blood, velocity changing with heart beat; (b) venous blood, constant velocity.

the ALARA (as low as reasonably achievable) principle should be employed (minimal output and exposure time). Very high-intensity US has been found to produce bioeffects including physical effects in tissue through which it passes. This higher intensity that is sometimes used for therapeutic purposes causes effects such as a temperature rise (thermal) in the tissues and mechanical (nonthermal) stress, for example formation of tiny gas bubbles (cavitation), so complete safety cannot be assumed (the mechanical and thermal effects are known as biohazards). However, the intensities and pressure levels employed in diagnostic US are constantly monitored for safety and these effects have not been observed at these power levels.

6.7 PET

6.7.1 Introduction

PET is the most frequently used nuclear medicine imaging modality in RT. Rather than allowing visualisation of anatomical detail, PET is a form of functional imaging. As such, PET demonstrates information about the physiological activity of tissues and organs at a molecular level, as opposed to acquisition of anatomical information as is the case with CT, MRI, and US. Thus, PET combines the sciences of physics, chemistry, and physiology. During a PET scan, the patient will initially have an IV injection of a radiopharmaceutical (radioactive isotope/tracer). This radiopharmaceutical is combined with a metabolically active molecule (e.g. glucose) which is readily consumed by living cells and distributes within the body according to a functional pathway. Positrons are emitted from these radioactive isotopes (see Chapter 13). The *in vivo* distribution of the resultant X-rays or gamma rays produced by the positron-emitting radionuclide is then received by external detectors. The dynamics of the radiopharmaceutical reflect the physiological activity of each tissue, and these have different appearances on the visual image display of a PET scan. Tumours can be discerned from healthy tissues in PET due to the unregulated growth of malignant cells and their higher glucose consumption, which appear as areas of more 'concentrated' activity (hot spots) on a PET image.

PET is used in the diagnosis, staging, treatment planning, on-treatment monitoring, and post RT follow up of patients with many different cancers. Before we look at the equipment and physical principles of PET we will briefly discuss its use in RT and oncology.

Cancer diagnosis: PET offers the potential for earlier diagnosis of a variety of cancers, for example in patients with oral cavity tumours [23] and in the diagnosis of recurrences such as in prostate cancer [24]. The advantage of employing PET in the diagnosis of cancer is that greater detail on the stage of the disease can be ascertained. This aids in treatment management decisions. In RT, the use of PET has been seen to impact decisions about treatment intent and also the size of RT target volumes (particularly the inclusion of lymph nodes in the GTV) [25].

Cancer staging, monitoring of response to treatment, and prognosis: The staging of cancers is where PET comes into its own; it has improved staging of primary disease at a molecular level, nodal involvement, and the identification of distant metastases. Thus, the visualisation of active malignant tissues, often before any visible evidence of structural anatomical change, is possible. PET-CT and PET-MR are now both used in the staging of cancers, for example colorectal cancer [26] and oesophageal cancer [27]. These forms of hybrid imaging are covered later in this chapter. PET is also effective in monitoring the response of tumours post-treatment, particularly bony metastases [28], and in predicting prognosis for example in oesophageal cancer [29].

Pre-treatment imaging: In order to be of clinical use in RT planning, because of the inability of PET to demonstrate anatomic detail, PET images are combined with CT images. This amalgamation of images allows for individualised, anatomical, and functional data, providing spatial detection and localisation of the pathophysiological process involved in tumour metastasis. This resultant image represents the location, size, and microscopic spread of disease. In order to acquire anatomical and functional data, the patient will usually be required to have a PET and CT scan undertaken independently of each other. In order to optimise the subsequent combined image, as many parameters as possible are kept consistent. However, it is difficult to achieve the same conditions when the scans are taken at different times. The two independent scans are then combined in a process termed fusion and coregistration (see Section 6.8). This process proves challenging because it is difficult to confirm that both images are aligned accurately, because of the lack of anatomical detail in the PET scan (for example, the detail of bony anatomy which would usually be used on a CT scan to ensure accuracy of overlay of images is just not visible on a PET scan). In recent years, the advent of the PET-CT scanner has alleviated these issues, with this modality allowing for a PET and CT scan to be taken simultaneously.

Monitoring of tumour size and proliferation during RT: There has been an increase in research into the value PET to assess tumour proliferation during RT, for example in lung cancer studies, taking advantage of the ability of PET to generate three-dimensional tumour images with the benefit of being able to image multiple tumour sites simultaneously and repeatedly [30, 31].

6.7.2 Physical Principles of PET

6.7.2.1 Positron Emission

As the radiopharmaceutical undergoes decay, it emits a positron (see Chapter 13). The emitted positron will travel a short distance, often in the submillimetre range, before interacting with a negatively charged electron to produce two 511-keV annihilation photons that travel in opposite directions. It is these annihilation photon pairs that are detected by scintillation crystals housed within ring detectors of the PET scanner. As the two photons travel at almost 180° to each other, a photon pair is identified when two photons hit opposing detectors within the same time frame. It is then possible to identify the origin of the two photons, and thus the location of the emitted positron, by tracing a straight line of coincidence, often referred to as the line of response.

6.7.2.2 Image Reconstruction

Photon pairs recorded by the ring detectors can each be considered to represent a line in space, connecting two detectors along which the positron emission occurred (Figure 6.38). From each photon pair that is recorded, a map of metabolic activity may be generated. This process is similar to the method used in CT scanners, where scintillation crystals absorb the emitted photons and convert them to light. Each crystalline detector is connected to either a photomultiplier tube (PMT) or silicon avalanche photodiode (Si-APD), which creates and amplifies electrical signals in response to the light pulse received from the crystals. The amplitude of the electrical signal is proportional to the intensity of light detected, which in turn is proportional to the radiation absorbed by the crystal.

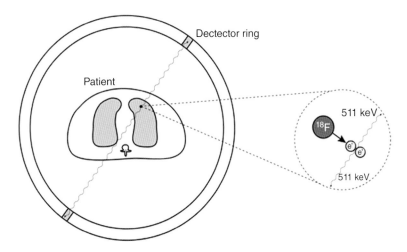

Patient

Dectector ring

511 keV

^{18}F

511 keV

FIGURE 6.38 Registration of annihilation photon pairs from positron emission by a ring of scintillation detectors.

It should be noted that this technique is dependent upon the simultaneous or coincident detection of a photon pair, i.e. photons that are detected more than a few nanoseconds apart are assumed not to form a pair and are therefore disregarded. Image processing algorithms are then used to convert the electrical signals into tomographic images. This description has greatly simplified the image reconstruction process for ease of understanding. However, it should be understood that in practice considerable data processing is necessary to distinguish and correct for a variety of factors such as random photon detection, scatter, differences in tissue attenuation, and detector dead time.

6.7.3 Radiopharmaceuticals Used in PET

The radiopharmaceutical selected for a PET scan depends on the function of the tissue being investigated. The most commonly used radiopharmaceutical in RT planning, which has application across a wide range of cancers, is *^{18}F fluorodeoxyglucose* (FDG), a sugar that is readily taken up by metabolising cells [32]. High FDG uptake measured with PET indicates a high level of metabolic activity within the cells of the tissues being imaged. Differing

regions of metabolic activity will be displayed in the PET image by discrete regions of varying intensity, i.e. highly active regions will have a greater intensity compared with regions of low metabolic activity. Hypoxia markers (e.g. ^{18}F-FAZA-*^{18}F-fluoroazomycin arabinoside,*^{18}F-FMISO-*^{18}F-Fluoromisonidazole*, and ^{64}Cu-ATSM-*N4-methylthiosemicarbazone*) which are tracers that accumulate in areas of low oxygenation have been shown to be advantageous particularly in head and neck cancer and lung cancer. ^{68}G labelled-Prostate-specific membrane antigen (PSMA) and ^{18}F DCFPyl are used in PET imaging for RT planning of prostate cancer [32].

6.7.4 Hybrid Imaging Using PET

It has already been highlighted that one disadvantage of PET is the lack of anatomical detail provided, making it difficult to correlate functional data to structural anatomy. However, this disadvantage has been addressed with the emergence of *hybrid imaging*, in which independent imaging modalities are combined into one unit assembly such as in the case of PET-CT, where a CT scanner is merged with a PET scanner. In these hybrid units the coordinate system is shared between both modalities and image acquisition can be undertaken in direct sequence. As the PET images correspond to the CT images, they can be reconstructed together to provide accurate coregistration of structural and functional data.

At the treatment planning stage, definition of the tumour and healthy tissue is based on CT and frequently supplemented with other imaging modalities such as MRI and/or PET. These other imaging modalities can be registered to the planning CT scan to enhance tumour definition and facilitate accurate and appropriate tumour delineation/contouring.

Accurate image registration is an important requirement for treatment planning; hence image-registration methods that align multimodality images are an inherent feature of most TPSs. In most cases, multimodality image registration is challenging due to the varying patient position at each individual imaging stage, as well as differences in internal organ position due to organ motion. Hybrid PET-CT scanners minimise this inconsistency by acquiring imaging data in the same session, facilitating image fusion without any differences in patient position. In some circumstances it is possible to use the CT data from the hybrid unit instead of an additional planning scan. Considerations such as modification to the couch, installation of a laser alignment system, and commissioning of the TPS to accommodate the CT data may be required.

6.8 Image Registration, Image Fusion, and Multimodality Imaging

As discussed in proceeding sections of this chapter, a variety of imaging modalities have a role to play in the pretreatment process, with each providing supplementary information regarding disease stage, anatomical location and size, cell pathology, and tissue function. These studies can be imported into the TPS (via DICOM) and fused with the planning CT to facilitate definition of the tumour target, as well as surrounding normal tissues. The ability to integrate multimodality imaging studies in the treatment planning process has been pivotal to the introduction of modern RT treatment techniques. Intensity modulated radiation therapy (IMRT), volumetric modulated arc therapy (VMAT), and stereotactic ablative radiotherapy (SABR) are examples of advanced techniques which seek to create a high dose gradient between the treatment target and organs at risk. Therefore, the ability to accurately define the target and avoidance structures through the unification of various imaging information is increasingly more paramount.

6.8.1 Image Registration and Fusion

To use any additional imaging data in the treatment planning process, the dataset(s) first need to be overlaid with one another so that they provide geometrically accurate, clinically relevant information. The process of geometrically overlaying images with one another is known *as image registration*; it describes the method of finding the spatial correspondence between two or more image datasets.

The term is often used interchangeably with image fusion, although strictly speaking *image fusion* refers to the display of different imaging data in a single combined view, after they have been registered with one another. There are several different methods of image registration, ranging from an entirely manual process, where adjustment of the images is performed by the end user until visual alignment of anatomy is obtained, through to highly complex automatic registration algorithms. In the pretreatment setting, automatic registration algorithms are typically used, due to their speed and accuracy.

Irrespective of whether image registration is performed manually or automatically, the process is either extrinsic or intrinsic in nature. *Extrinsic registration* is the use of artificial markers or objects attached to or inserted into the patient that guide the image registration process. An example is the use of fiducials markers placed on the patient's skin or a stereotactic head frame. This method of registration is based solely on external information and does not consider any patient anatomy.

In contrast, *intrinsic registration* utilises patient-based information such as landmarks, surfaces, or voxel intensity to guide the image registration. Intrinsic registration can be subdivided into either rigid or non-rigid methods.

The overall process of image registration can be simplified into four principal steps listed below [33]. However, it should be noted that the process is significantly more complex than this, with further reading suggested at the end of this chapter.

1. Feature detection;
2. Feature matching;
3. Transform Model Estimation;
4. Image resampling and transformation.

6.8.1.1 Feature Detection and Matching

In order to register two or more images, specific features within each image need to be identified that will be used to guide the image registration process.

   a. Landmarks/point based

In this method image registration is based upon a limited number of anatomical landmarks/features or points that are used for alignment. The landmarks/points from each image are compared with one another by pattern matching, so that they resemble each other. The benefit of this method is that registration is based on the underlying patient anatomy or physiology.

   b. Segmentation

In this two-step method, the features of both images are first partitioned (segmented) and then registration is based on minimising the distance between the same anatomical features.

   c. Voxel intensity

This method aligns images by mathematically or statistically matching the grey values/intensity pattern of voxels in each image. The method assumes that when the images are correctly aligned there will be strong similarity between the intensity of the voxels of each image. Intensity-based registration methods work well in simple scenarios but can be ineffective when registering images from different modalities, due to the variation in voxel intensity generated by different imaging techniques.

6.8.1.2 Transformation Model Estimation and Resampling

A transformation model is essentially a mathematical formula that adjusts a number of parameters in order to align or overlay images with one another. An example is applying a translational vector or rotation to an image so that the key features identified between both images have strong correspondence. The degree of corresponding features between the images is determined through a process of resampling the images and a registration metric is then calculated.

6.8.1.3 Registration Metrics

The accuracy of rigid image registration is measured through *similarity metrics*. These metrics essentially assign a numerical value to how similar two images are to each other, with the smaller the numerical value indicating the greater the similarity between the two images. In rigid registration processes, such as those performed in RT TPSs, the accuracy of registration is most commonly measured by the similarity metric known as *mutual information*. This metric is reliable when registering datasets from different imaging modalities, where there may be inherently large differences in voxel intensities. Other similarity metrics include: *cross-correlation*, *sum of squared differences*, and *Dice's coefficient*.

6.8.1.4 Rigid Transformation Algorithms

Rigid transformation algorithms, as their name suggests, are inflexible. They do not compensate for any differences in patient

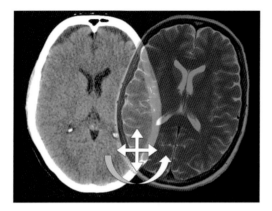

FIGURE 6.39 Example of a rigid image registration process between axial computed tomography (CT) and MR images. The images are aligned through translational and rotational adjustments. The image scale is pre-determined through equipment calibration.

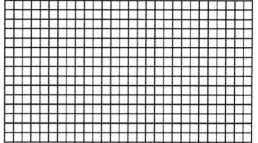

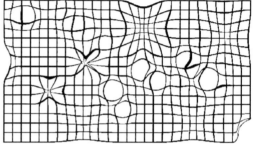

FIGURE 6.40 Deformation of pixel to pixel relationship used by non-rigid registration algorithms.

anatomy or patient position that may exist between images. The pixels within each image are matched with one another through a combination of translation, rotation, and scaling adjustments to achieve the 'best fit'. In this way, the relationship between the pixels within each image remains unchanged. Provided there are no changes in internal or external patient anatomy, a rigid image registration process is relatively simple and efficient. Most TPSs with image registration and fusion software employ this method (Figure 6.39).

6.8.1.5 Non-rigid Transformation Algorithms

Non-rigid transformation algorithms are often referred to as *deformable* or *elastic* algorithms. In contrast to rigid algorithms, they can compensate for differences that exist between images, either due to patient position, patient movement, or organ motion. The pixel to pixel relationship within one image is modified to align it with another. This is known as *deformation, distortion*, or *warping* (Figure 6.40). These algorithms are highly complex due to the degree of freedom allowed in the registration process. Consequently, they can be highly error prone. The use of

deformable registration algorithms is useful when used to remove geometrical distortion in MR images, for example when used in CNS treatment planning. Their role in image guided and adaptive RT is predicted to be significant, as they will enable changes in organ motion and patient anatomy over the treatment course to be accounted for [34].

6.8.1.6 Clinical Context and Quality Assurance

At present, CT is the principal modality used for calculating RT dose distributions. Because CT is the principal dataset on which dose calculations are based, it is referred to as the *primary* or *reference dataset*. Consequently, any other dataset(s) registered with the planning CT, such as an MRI or PET-CT scan, is referred to as a *secondary dataset*.

Verifying the accuracy of any image registration and fusion process is important to ensure that the resultant image is representative of the tumour size, physical location and metabolic function. Errors in alignment can have significant consequences on the accuracy of treatment and the overall clinical outcome for the patient. Therefore, careful inspection of the fused dataset(s) should be performed to validate the registration prior to treatment planning use. In practice, this often involves some degree of compromise; for example prioritising the image registration around the area of intended treatment.

6.9 Hybrid and Functional Imaging

Hybrid imaging is defined as the fusion of two or more imaging technologies into a single platform. The advantage of hybrid imaging systems is their ability to combine molecular imaging information simultaneously with structural anatomical data. In this way, improving the accuracy of imaging information than if this data was acquired independently at a different point in time and likely with a different patient position. Examples of hybrid systems currently available include (but are not limited to); US-MR imaging, PET-CT, and SPECT-CT, as well as the most recent hybrid system, PET-MR.

Functional/molecular imaging has a vital role in the staging of oncologic disease as well as being highly beneficial in the RT treatment planning context. When used in combination with CT and MRI, functional studies can supplement the anatomical information, together providing a powerful collection of imaging information to help define the treatment target, as well as identify areas of higher metabolic activity that could potentially be considered for dose escalation or boost dose. The following sections will briefly introduce some functional imaging techniques and their application to RT and should be read in conjunction with Chapter 13.

6.9.1.1 Functional Imaging
As discussed in Section 6.5.4, fMRI studies can offer functional information regarding blood oxygen level dependence, with BOLD imaging studies having potential use in identifying regions of tumour hypoxia. In the context of pretreatment imaging, this can be valuable in tailoring the radiation dose distribution (dose sculpting). In addition, research has indicated the potential for this imaging technique in identifying patients that may benefit from carbogen sensitisation at the time of RT.

Dynamic Contrast Enhanced CT (DCE-CT) and Dynamic Contrast Enhanced MR (DCE-MR) studies offer useful information regarding blood perfusion. These studies may be considered as an indirect marker for tumour hypoxia; where tumours with low blood perfusion have greater levels of hypoxia and therefore, are likely to be more radio-resistant. An example of use is in pretreatment imaging for prostate cancer, where early research indicates their potential application in locating dominant tumour lesions within the prostate gland as well as predicting treatment response [35].

6.9.1.2 MR Spectroscopy
Early studies of MR spectroscopy (MRS) indicate the potential of this imaging technique regarding cell metabolism, with the potential to differentiate benign tumours from malignant tumours. It may also have a role in identifying radio-resistant tumours that could benefit from dose escalation.

6.9.1.3 Functional PET
Tumour growth relies on a strong demand for glucose, and as such molecular imaging techniques using the radio-tracer FDG have played an increasingly important role in the pretreatment imaging process, for the purposes of disease staging as well as target delineation [36]. Because FDG is more readily taken up by tumour cells than it is by normal tissues, this imaging technique can provide information regarding the metabolic activity of a tumour. An example is the application of FDG-PET in the staging and treatment of lung cancer [37]. Other PET tracers with potential use for biological targeting of RT

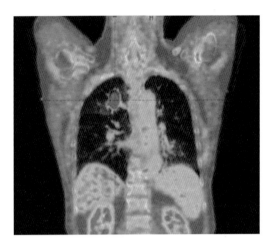

FIGURE 6.41 Coronal view of fused computed tomography (CT) and $^{18}F\ fluorodeoxyglucose$ (FDG) positron emission tomography (PET) in lung cancer. (Source: reproduced with permission Wiley & Sons [34].)

include ^{18}F-misonidazole (FMISO), ^{18}F-thymide (FLT), and ^{11}C-Choline (Figure 6.41).

6.9.1.4 PET-MR

The recent advent of PET-MR imaging systems offers the capability to acquire functional imaging data at the same time as high-contrast soft tissue MR information. Because the PET component of these systems is integrated with MR rather than CT, it offers the further benefit of being non-invasive, with lower radiation exposure to the patient compared to PET-CT.

An example of its clinical application in RT is in head and neck tumours where high sensitivity and specificity imaging information may be obtained to guide the treatment planning process [38].

DICOM transfer of image data between different systems ensures the conformance of internationally accepted standards. However, image transfer errors can still exist. Transfer tests that ensure the correct patient orientation, pixel size, slice thickness and index, and voxel value, etc., form part of the equipment commissioning process, however image datasets from external sources, as is often the case in RT treatment planning, should be performed on an individual patient basis.

6.10 Future Perspectives of Pre-treatment Imaging

As the field of RT continues to evolve in conjunction with technological advancement, the application of functional and biological imaging information in the treatment planning process is set to increase. This offers the opportunity to sculpt the RT dose distribution (known as *dose painting*) based on collective imaging information.

It is anticipated that ongoing developments in the realm of pre-treatment imaging will further allow personalisation of radiation dose to the individual patient, with a growing focus on the prescribing and targeting of dose relative to biological function. Regions identified as radio-resistant may be considered for dose escalation, whilst tissues with microscopic disease may be irradiated to a lower dose. The practical challenges around differences in patient position between modalities and the need for standardised functional imaging methods require consideration, however the extent of clinical application is particularly promising. This is an exciting area of research and development with the potential to maximise the therapeutic ratio between tumour and normal tissue further, potentially increasing tumour control probability (TCP), whilst minimising normal tissue complication probability (NTCP).

References

1. Holmes, K., Elkington, M., and Harris, P. (2013). *Clark's Essential Physics in Imaging for Radiographers*. CRC Press.
2. Carter, C. and Veale, B. (2014). *Digital Radiography and PACS*, 2e. Elsevier.
3. Keall, P. (2004). 4-dimensional computed tomography imaging and treatment planning. *Semin. Radiat. Oncol.* 14 (1): 81–90.

4. Rietzel, E., Pan, T., and Chen, G.T. (2005). Four-dimensional computed tomography: image formation and clinical protocol. *Med. Phys.* 32 (4): 874–889.

5. Li, R., Lewis, J.H., Cervino, L.I., and Jiang, S.B. (2009). 4D CT sorting based on patient internal anatomy. *Phys. Med. Biol.* 54 (15): 4821–4833.

6. Olsen, J.R., Lu, W., Hubenschmidt, J.P. et al. (2008). Effect of novel amplitude/phase binning algorithm on commercial for-dimensional computed tomography quality. *Int. J. Radiat. Oncol. Biol. Phys.* 70 (1): 243–252.

7. Li, H., Noel, C., Garcia-Ramirez, J. et al. (2012). Clinical evaluations of an amplitude-based binning algorithm for 4DCT reconstruction in radiation therapy. *Med. Phys.* 39 (2): 922–932.

8. Yamamoto, T., Langer, U., Loo, B.W. et al. (2008). Retrospective analysis of artifacts in four-dimensional CT images of 50 abdominal and thoracic radiotherapy patients. *Int J Radiat Oncol Biol Phys* 72 (4): 1250–1258.

9. Rai, R., Kumar, S., Batumalai, V. et al. (2017). The integration of MRI in radiation therapy: collaboration of radiographers and radiation therapists. *J. Med. Radiat. Sci.* 64 (1): 61–68.

10. Salerno, J., Finelli, A., Morash, C. et al. (2016). Multiparametric magnetic resonance imaging for pre-treatment local staging of prostate cancer: a Cancer Care Ontario clinical practice guideline. *Can. Urol. Assoc. J.* 10 (9–10): E332.

11. Krishna, S., Lim, C.S., McInnes, M.D. et al. (2018). Evaluation of MRI for diagnosis of extraprostatic extension in prostate cancer. *J. Magn. Reson. Imaging* 47 (1): 176–185.

12. Balleyguier, C., Sala, E., Da Cunha, T. et al. (2011). Staging of uterine cervical cancer with MRI: guidelines of the European Society of Urogenital Radiology. *Eur. Radiol.* 21 (5): 1102–1110.

13. Upadhyay, N. and Waldman, A.D. (2011). Conventional MRI evaluation of gliomas. *Br. J. Res.* 84 (special issue 2): S107–S111.

14. Grady, I., Chanisheva, N., and Vasquez, T. (2017). The addition of automated breast ultrasound to mammography in breast cancer screening decreases stage at diagnosis. *Acad. Radiol.* 24 (12): 1570–1574.

15. Ren, Y., Ye, J., Wang, Y. et al. (2018). The optimal application of transrectal ultrasound in staging of rectal cancer following neoadjuvant therapy: a pragmatic study for accuracy investigation. *J. Cancer* 9 (5): 784–791.

16. Ayuso, C., Rimola, J., Vilana, R. et al. (2018). Diagnosis and staging of hepatocellular carcinoma (HCC): current guidelines. *Eur. J. Radiol.* 101: 72–81.

17. Navani, N., Nankivell, M., Lawrence, D.R. et al. (2015). Lung cancer diagnosis and staging with endobronchial ultrasound-guided transbronchial needle aspiration compared with conventional approaches: an open-label, pragmatic, randomised controlled trial. *Lancet Respir. Med.* 3 (4): 282–289.

18. Merkow, R.P., Herrera, G., Goldman, D.A. et al. (2017). Endoscopic ultrasound as a pretreatment clinical staging tool for gastric cancer: association with pathology and outcome. *Ann. Surg. Oncol.* 24 (12): 3658–3666.

19. Okafor, P.N., Swanson, K., Shah, N., and Talwalkar, J.A. (2018). Endoscopic ultrasound for rectal cancer staging: a population-based study of utilization, impact on treatment patterns, and survival. *J. Gastroenterol. Hepatol.* 33 (8): 1467–1476.

20. Nathoo, D., Loblaw, A., Davidson, M. et al. (2018). A feasibility study on the role of ultrasound imaging of bladder volume as a method to improve concordance of bladder filling status on treatment with simulation. *J. Med. Imaging Radiat. Sci.* 49 (3): 277–285.

21. Claxton, K. and Appleyard, R. (2017). Implementation of ultrasound bladder volume scanning for patients receiving intensity-modulated radiotherapy to the cervix or endometrium: clinical experiences from a United Kingdom radiotherapy department. *J. Radiother. Pract.* 16 (3): 232–244.

22. Han, B., Najafi, M., Cooper, D.T. et al. (2018). Evaluation of transperineal ultrasound imaging as a potential solution for target tracking during hypofractionated radiotherapy for prostate cancer. *Radiat. Oncol.* 13 (1): 151.

23. Keshavarzi, M., Darijani, M., Momeni, F. et al. (2017). Molecular imaging and oral cancer diagnosis and therapy. *J. Cell. Biochem.* 118 (10): 3055–3060.

24. Han, S., Woo, S., Kim, Y.J., and Suh, C.H. (2018). Impact of 68 Ga-PSMA PET on the management of patients with prostate cancer: a systematic review and meta-analysis. *Eur. Urol.* 74: 179–190.

25. Birk Christensen, C., Loft-Jakobsen, A., Munck af Rosenschöld, P. et al. (2018). 18F-FDG PET/CT for planning external beam radiotherapy alters therapy in 11% of 581 patients. *Clin. Physiol. Funct. Imaging* 38 (2): 278–284.

26. Catalano, O.A., Coutinho, A.M., Sahani, D.V. et al. (2017). Colorectal cancer staging:

comparison of whole-body PET/CT and PET/MR. *Abdom. Radiol. (NY)* 42 (4): 1141–1151.

27. Van Rossum, P.S., van Lier, A.L., Lips, I.M. et al. (2015). Imaging of oesophageal cancer with FDG-PET/CT and MRI. *Clin. Radiol.* 70 (1): 81–95.

28. Lecouvet, F.E., Talbot, J.N., Messiou, C. et al. (2014). Monitoring the response of bone metastases to treatment with Magnetic Resonance Imaging and nuclear medicine techniques: a review and position statement by the European Organisation for Research and Treatment of Cancer imaging group. *Eur. J. Cancer* 50 (15): 2519–2531.

29. Chen, H., Li, Y., Wu, H. et al. (2015). 3'-Deoxy-3'-[18 F]-fluorothymidine PET/CT in early determination of prognosis in patients with esophageal squamous cell cancer. *Strahlenther. Onkol.* 191 (2): 141–152.

30. Everitt, S.J., Ball, D.L., Hicks, R.J. et al. (2014). Differential 18F-FDG and 18F-FLT uptake on serial PET/CT imaging before and during definitive chemoradiation for non-small cell lung cancer. *J. Nucl. Med.* 55 (7): 1069–1074.

31. Konert, T., van de Kamer, J.B., Sonke, J.J., and Vogel, W.V. (2018). The developing role of FDG PET imaging for prognostication and radiotherapy target volume delineation in non-small cell lung cancer. *J. Thorac. Dis.* 10 (Suppl 21): S2508.

32. McKay, M.J., Taubman, K.L., Foroudi, F. et al. (2018). Molecular imaging using PET/CT for radiotherapy planning of adult cancers: current status and expanding applications. *Int. J. Radiat. Oncol. Biol. Phys.* 120 (4): 783–791.

33. Bisht, S.S., Gupta, B., and Rahi, P. (2014). Image registration concept and techniques: a review. *J. Eng. Res. Appl.* 4: 30–35.

34. Brock, K.K., Mutic, S., McNutt, T.R. et al. (2017). Use of image registration and fusion algorithms and techniques in radiotherapy: report of the AAPM Radiation Therapy Committee Task group no. 132. *Med. Phys.* 44 (7): e43–e76.

35. Alexander, E.J., DeSouza, N.M., Murray, J. et al. (2015). The accuracy of T2-and Diffusion-weighted Magnetic Resonance (T2W/DWI-MR)

in the detection of intra-prostatic tumour as target volume for focal dose-escalation using Intensity-modulated Radiotherapy (IMRT). *Clin. Oncol.* 27 (3): e3.

36. Iglesias, M.M., Nunez, D.A., del Olmo Claudio, J.L. et al. (2015). Multimodality functional imaging in radiation therapy planning: relationships between dynamic contrast-enhanced MRI, diffusion-weighted MRI, and ¹⁸F-FDG PET. *Comput. Math. Methods Med.* 2015: 103843.

37. Konert, T., Vogel, W., MacManus, M.P. et al. (2015). PET/CT imaging for target volume delineation in curative intent radiotherapy of non-small cell lung cancer: IAEA consensus report 2014. *Radiother. Oncol.* 116 (1): 27–34.

38. Lee, Y.Z., Ramalho, J., and Kessler, B. (2017). PET–MR imaging in head and neck. *Magn. Reson. Imaging Clin. N. Am.* 25 (2): 315–324.

Further Reading

Brock, K.K., Mutic, S., McNutt, T.R. et al. (2017). Use of image registration and fusion algorithms and techniques in radiotherapy: report of the AAPM Radiation Therapy Committee Task Group No. 132. *Med. Phys.* 44: e43–e76.

Bushberg, J.T., Seibert, J.A., Leidholdt, E.M., and Boone, J.M. (2012). *The Essential Physics of Medical Imaging*, 3e. Philadelphia: Lippincott Williams & Wilkins.

Carter, C. and Veale, B. (2018). *Digital Radiography and PACS*, 3e. Elsevier Health Sciences.

Dale, B.M., Brown, M.A., and Semelka, R.C. (2015). *MRI Basic Principles and Applications*, 5e. Wiley Blackwell.

Holmes, K., Elkington, M., and Harris, P. (2013). *Clark's Essential Physics in Imaging for Radiographers*. CRC Press.

Wolbarst, A.B., Capasso, P., and Wyant, A.R. (2013). *Medical Imaging: Essentials for Physicians*. Wiley.

CHAPTER 7

Principles of Treatment Accuracy and Reproducibility

Nick White and Helen P. White

Aim

The aim of this chapter is to overview the range of treatment procedures and immobilisation techniques that can be used to achieve the accurate and reproducible delivery of external beam radiotherapy treatment.

7.1 Introduction

A primary aim of radiotherapy treatment is to optimise the radiation dose to the target volume whilst reducing the dose to the adjacent normal tissues. By conforming the dose distribution to the target volume and limiting normal tissue doses, there is a potential to achieve dose escalation without excessive normal tissue morbidity. Key to this process is the use of effective patient *immobilisation* and assessment of treatment accuracy throughout the delivery process. Positioning inaccuracies may be reduced via the use of dedicated immobilisation devices which allow for accurate reproduction of patient position from fraction to fraction. In addition, it is important to position radiotherapy patients in ways that ensure comfort and stability. By doing so, the incidence of random positioning errors caused by patient movement may be reduced.

Adoption of precision techniques such as *intensity-modulated radiotherapy* (IMRT) and *three-dimensional conformal radiotherapy* (3DCRT) are achievable only if immobilisation techniques are adequate to ensure the elimination of positioning variability. Current radiotherapy practices may also account for variability in the position of internal anatomical structures, and a treatment aim is to attain delivery of a homogeneous tumour dose whilst sparing normal tissue and adjacent organs at risk (OARs). In doing so normal *tissue complication probability* (NTCP) may be limited whilst increasing *tumour control probability* (TCP), thus gaining the best therapeutic ratio for the patient (Figure 7.1).

The patient must be positioned in a stable and comfortable position that minimises movement during treatment delivery and is reproducible at each subsequent visit. There is little value in using advanced treatment techniques and sophisticated dose delivery unless the recipient is positioned with as much care and accuracy as is taken in the

Practical Radiotherapy: Physics and Equipment, Third Edition. Edited by Pam Cherry and Angela M. Duxbury.
© 2020 John Wiley & Sons Ltd. Published 2020 by John Wiley & Sons Ltd.

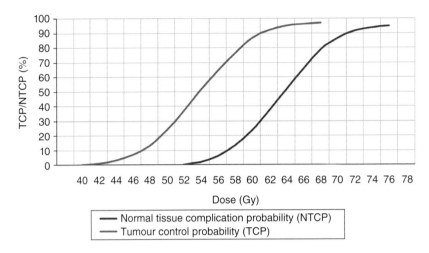

FIGURE 7.1 Radiation dose and probability of effect on normal tissue and tumour control.

planning and delivery of the treatment that he or she is to receive.

The following are the more common standard positions:

- **Supine**: this is probably the most common patient position and also the most comfortable for patients. The patient is positioned on their back, usually with their head towards the treatment machine gantry.

- **Prone**: this position is best adopted when treating more posterior structures such as the spine or the rectum. The patient is positioned on their front, usually with their head towards the treatment machine gantry.

The use of suitable immobilisation devices is usually down to individual department choice, and a number of commercially available devices and materials are available. When deciding the patient position and therefore the immobilisation technique that is to be used, a number of factors need to be taken into consideration, such as:

- Accessibility to the anatomical site for treatment;
- General fitness and mobility of the patient;
- Treatment intent (radical versus palliative);
- The proposed technique/beam arrangement;
- Cost and availability of materials.

It is essential that any positioning or fixation devices are compatible with both the treatment planning equipment (usually a CT [computed tomography] scanner) and the treatment machine, and that they do not create a significant amount of image degradation due to the presence of image artefacts, for example. Special consideration may be given to the pretreatment imaging modality required such as MRI (magnetic resonance imaging) scanners (in which there are limitations allowable with respect to equipment design). Routine use of CT pretreatment planning is also allowable given that most radiotherapy departments use dedicated radiotherapy scanners with a wide field of view (FOV) which allows a range of immobilisation devices to be accommodated during scan procedures.

7.2 Scanner Aperture Size

Historically, scanners designed for diagnostic operation were employed, often located within radiology departments and temporarily adapted to the radiotherapy process through addition of flat couch overlays, immobilisation devices, and an external laser for marking of reference points.

The traditional 70 cm scanner aperture with a 50 cm FOV is too limiting for many radiotherapy techniques, so most manufacturers now produce 'large-bore' versions of their popular multi-slice scanners providing apertures up to 85 cm which enable most radiotherapy patients to be scanned in an optimal position. Reconstruction algorithms may also provide a FOV as large as the physical size of the aperture itself, although quality of image data and CT number accuracy within these extended regions means it may be of limited clinical use. Use of wide-bore scanners inevitably results in a slight reduction in high-contrast resolution and will increase image noise and dose in comparison to standard scanners, although in the radiotherapy context these factors are not usually considered significant in comparison to the benefits provided.

7.3 Reference Points and Anatomical Landmarks

Treatment accuracy is dependent on the correctly reproduced alignment of the patient in accordance with their planned position and as per the pretreatment planning scan. Correct patient positioning permits accurate location of the treatment isocentre(s) with the result that the administered dose can be given confidently in the knowledge that the dose distribution or dose-wash is administered as per the intended treatment plan.

When the patient is initially positioned for treatment, external reference points (usually permanent skin marks such as tattoos) act as fixed points for patient alignment. The patient's surface anatomy (static structures) may also be used to aid accurate positioning both in locating the associated tattoo or to act as a positioning reference point in their own right. Alignment of the external reference tattoos against the in-room laser lights ensures reproducibility in terms of correspondence with the reference CT scan and also fraction-to-fraction reproducibility.

7.4 Treatment Tattoos Versus Semipermanent Skin Marks

Whilst permanent skin tattoos offer a simple and affordable solution to provision of reliable landmarks it may be that for some patients their use is no longer needed. New technologies, including surface tracking, permit real-time analysis of the patient's surface anatomy which also extends to account for dynamic changes in patient anatomy (e.g. as a result of respiratory motion). This coupled with a greater reliance of the analysis of position of internal anatomical structures to guide treatment (e.g. via cone beam image guidance) has led to debate as to the continued worth of permanent (i.e. tattoo) skin marks. Research [1] has suggested that even if it is preferred that an external skin mark is to be used there is no significant difference in systematic and random set up error where semipermanent (e.g. ink marks or henna) are employed compared to tattoos. The option for tattoo-less treatment is appealing given that the cosmetic appearance of radiotherapy tattoos may result in damaging psychological effects associated with poor body image or the tattoo acting as a permanent reminder of treatment [2]. In addition, tattoo-less skin marking may be preferred by some patients due to their cultural or religious beliefs.

However, the decision to use alternatives such as semipermanent skin marks requires a greater degree of care by the patient when washing in order to avoid loss of marks whilst undertaking their radiotherapy and the potential need for treatment replanning. Alternative skin-marking techniques are available, including tattoos only visible under ultraviolet light or the use of semipermanent micropigmentation techniques [3]. Some argue it may be preferable to retain the use of a permanent skin mark as a reference point, for example at patient follow-up or in the case of tumour recurrence, though listening to patient preference might preclude this.

7.5 Lasers and Treatment Setup

Patient setup during treatment planning and radiotherapy delivery requires the use of wall-mounted lasers. These aid in the accurate, reproducible positioning of the patient by being positioned at strategic points within the treatment and planning rooms – usually projecting along the sagittal, transverse, and coronal anatomical planes. Lasers used in radiotherapy positioning are grade two lasers with less than 1 mW output per beam. To aid alignment accuracy the line thickness is approximately 2 mm. The lasers are produced by a plasma tube with a particularly narrow beam profile. Lasers are projected around the room from the tube by a system of small lenses, within the laser mechanism housing, which refract the beam along the required

path. Lasers can be red, green, or blue; these have the same accuracy and usability and are little different in cost, but green lasers are more visible on darker skins. Particular attention must be taken during machine and equipment quality assurance procedures as misalignment of the lasers may result in inadvertent misalignment of the patient during setup.

The use of lasers is twofold; firstly to ensure reference marks are aligned along coincident anatomical planes, and also to notionally locate the treatment isocentre within the patient (defined at the point of the intersection point of the lasers) (Figure 7.2).

This is achieved through the use of defined couch movements (if required) from the setup reference point (usually tattoo intersection point) in the three anatomical planes. Couch shifts during isocentre location can be made automatically via the use of pre-determined shift coordinates calculated from the treatment plan. Daily adjustments are also made if necessary and according to daily image acquisition for image guided radiotherapy (IGRT) protocols.

Final verification checks include the use of the linear accelerator's (LinAc's) optical range finder system. This is a straightforward way of determining that the isocentre is positioned at the intended depth within the

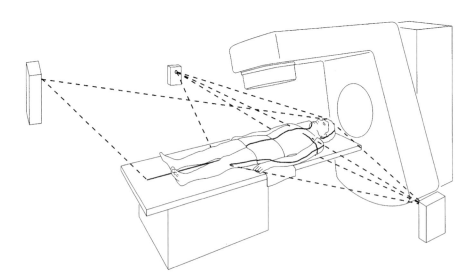

FIGURE 7.2 Laser position in treatment rooms.

patient at the set treatment angle (the isocentre always being located at 100 cm along the central axis of the treatment beam). Deviations from the anticipated focus-skin distance (FSD) reading may indicate an error in the patient setup (e.g. incorrect couch height) but are also an indication in a change in patient anatomy, for example due to treatment-related oedema or conversely, patient weight loss. This is an important manual cue as to whether treatment accuracy can be achieved.

7.6 Volume Definitions and Target Defining Concepts

Achieving treatment accuracy requires radiotherapy practice to adopt recognised convention and accepted nomenclature in the descriptions of treatment volumes as determined initially by the ICRU [4, 5] reports 50 and 62. These volumes consist of a number of defined anatomical limits according to defined parameters as follows.

7.6.1 Gross Tumour Volume (GTV)

The GTV is the extent of the tumour as demonstrated by clinical examination and/or via medical imaging. Treatment accuracy depends in part on the analysis of the morphological extent of the GTV as optimal dose administration to the GTV is essential to obtain local control of the tumour.

7.6.2 Clinical Target Volume (CTV)

Whilst the GTV (i.e. demonstrable disease on examination or via imaging) may appear to define the tumour extent, it is frequently the case that disease extends beyond the tumour margin in a way that cannot be easily detected (it is 'subclinical'). Modern imaging techniques including PET (positron emission tomography) imaging and functional MRI (fMRI) have aided in assessment of such margins, however the extent of the subclinical spread is still a recognisable area of uncertainty and therefore it is necessary to account for this when demarcating treatment volumes, i.e. the CTV must comprise the GTV plus a margin that encompasses areas of suspected subclinical extension. The CTV must receive adequate dose to achieve the therapeutic aim.

7.6.3 Planning Target Volume (PTV)

Radiotherapy delivery may be associated with a degree of uncertainty with respect to positioning of the patient and their internal anatomy. Variability stemming from patient positioning, for example, may lead to a translation of the intended target resulting in underdosage of the CTV and unintended irradiation of healthy tissue. The consequence of this is a risk of treatment-associated morbidity and the failure to achieve optimal tumoricidal dose administration.

Hence the consequences of treatment miss falls into two main categories [6]:

1. Missing the target during the RT course will underdose the tumour and potentially compromise tumour control;
2. Potentially increasing the dose to surrounding normal tissues which in turn potentially increases acute and late side effects.

To overcome variations associated with patient tissue locations and random errors during positioning, a notional PTV is used which includes a margin of tissue which accounts for both physiological displacement of tissues and patient positioning variability. The patient's CTV may be subject to changes in shape, size, and position either within individual treatment sessions (e.g. as a result of breathing, peristaltic bowel movement, or heartbeat), or between separate sessions whereby normal anatomical processes (such as bowel filling) can lead to organ position variability. Such differences (termed *intrafraction* and *interfraction* variability) may be considered via the use of an internal margin (IM).

An additional setup margin (SM) is also required to account for uncertainty relating specifically to beam geometry including:

- Variations in patient positioning;
- Mechanical uncertainties – e.g. gantry, collimators, and couch;
- Dosimetric uncertainty;
- Transfer errors from CT to treatment unit;
- Human factors.

Clearly elimination of such variability is advantageous as this may enable reduction in margins with attendant reduction of dose to the healthy tissues surrounding the CTV. Key to this is the routine use of treatment verification via imaging which permits intervention and treatment correction, for example where setup error or unacceptable gross organ displacement is detected. These imaging techniques coupled with accurate immobilisation strategies may reduce the SM. Strategies to specifically reduce the IM are also employed, such as respiratory gating techniques to account for organ motion or true IGRT techniques whereby tumour movement is accounted for. For example, via the use of cone-beam CT (CBCT), or via the use of implanted fiducials, which may act as a surrogate for target position.

The increased information gleaned from the submillimetre accuracy of pixels of information derived from CT (and PET) scanning has permitted implementation of intensity modulation of radiotherapy treatment involving treatment-planning optimisation algorithms coupled with dose administration via multiple small beamlets of radiation. Adoption of IMRT requires a reassessment of treatment margins and uncertainties associated with their use, particularly since IMRT can result in steeper gradients of

dose between the target volume and adjacent OARs. IMRT therefore requires the additional consideration of patient positioning and management of patient motion (such as gating). Whilst the aforementioned GTV and CTV remain anatomical or oncological concepts, IMRT presents a new assessment of PTVs used to account for organ variability over time in order to achieve optimisation of dose to the CTV whilst limiting doses to OARs [7].

7.7 Treatment Bolus and 3D Bolus Printing

During radiotherapy treatments, delivery of dose to the tumour site as per the preplanned distributions is essential. There are instances where the irregularities in the patient's surface may result in an inhomogeneous dose being received, for example where the patient has a complex body contour resulting from surgery. The addition of an artificial 'bolus' material (*tissue equivalent material*) may be advantageous in such cases as this acts to compensate for the variation in the patient's contour. During electron beam radiotherapy, bolus may also be used to modify depth dose distribution in combination with beam energy selection.

A number of commercially available bolus materials are available such as Superflab. The use of such bolus, whilst acting to smooth contour irregularity, necessarily results in a loss of the skin-sparing effect of megavoltage radiotherapy (whereby the dose maximum point for a beam of radiation lies beneath the patient's skin). The use of bolus may result in an increased surface skin dose and therefore result in an increase in patient treatment reactions. For some patients this form of modification of dose distribution is in fact desirable, particularly where the intended treatment volume sits superficially as in the case of electron therapy, or where a surgical resection scar potentially harbours tumour cells that may otherwise lie within the dose 'buildup' zone. It is essential that such boluses possess the same dosimetric characteristics as human tissues since tissue equivalence ensures suitable tissue defect compensation.

In such cases it may be preferable to use a bolus material that is customised for each patient since uniform flat-surfaced materials covering a wide area may result in a loss of contact with the patient's skin across irregularly contoured anatomical sites, particularly over the nose, ear, and scalp [8]. Where air gaps result there may be an unintended modulation effect on the intended maximum and skin doses administered to the patient. Avoidance of such gaps can be achieved by carefully positioning bolus materials such as paraffin gauze or wax, however it can be difficult to achieve uniformity of bolus thickness in doing so.

Recent developments in 3D printing technologies have led to the development of bespoke bolus materials that are patient-specific and allow for boluses that are closely matched to the patient's anatomy, as their manufacture permits generation of a bolus that has a complex functional shape and uniform thickness. During bolus manufacture, the patient's computer-generated treatment plan (including bolus outline) acts as the template for production of the printed bolus, and this allows for a high degree of outline conformity. 3D printers work by serially printing material layer by layer from a digital template (in this case derived from the patient's CT treatment plan or via the use of a 3D optical scanner). This template acts to 'slice' the printed material into individual layers which are then added sequentially during the printing process. Printing itself utilises a dedicated 3D printer. It is important to ensure that the fabrication materials employed during the printing process are as closely tissue-equivalent as possible, and full analysis of their dosimetric parameters is necessary before their use is adopted. Evidence [8] suggests such individualised 3D printed boluses have the potential to increase setup reproducibility and overcome the disadvantages that commercially available flat boluses may provide due to avoidance of unwanted air gaps.

It may also be possible to manufacture 3D printed boluses which themselves are malleable rather than constructed of hard materials [9]. This further aids patient comfort and increases adaption of the bolus material to the patient's surface.

7.8 Immobilisation Shells

Immobilisation shells are devices that enable the fixation of patients into their treatment position in an effort to limit movement and to obtain treatment reproducibility. Shells are required to be used often for several weeks of treatment, and so must be durable and hard wearing. To be effective they should accurately follow the patient's contour and restrict movement through each of the anatomical axes. For most anatomical sites the immobilisation shell should be semi-rigid, whilst being smooth against the patient's skin surface to ensure patient comfort. In addition, the practical use of patient shells requires that they accommodate the use of surface markers for treatment setup such as the position of the isocentre, beam entry points, or field edges. Suitable materials for radiotherapy treatment shells should ideally be thin enough to ensure minimal beam attenuation, whilst retaining enough strength to maintain patient position and withstand recurrent use over several days or weeks of treatment.

7.9 Immobilisation Equipment for Head and Neck Treatment

The need for accurate immobilisation in the head and neck region is paramount due to the need to treat target volumes that are often small and located adjacent to radiosensitive structures. The use of highly conformal treatment dose distributions means that patient movement is potentially catastrophic and may result in a geographical miss of the target volume and overdose of critical structures. In practical terms this is minimised by using small setup tolerances of the order of 1–2 mm in an effort to reduce systematic errors and ensuring a high degree of accuracy; this may be quality assured by the regular use of treatment verification imaging. IMRT and 3DCRT techniques in the head and neck can be attempted only in the knowledge that the proposed immobilisation strategy eliminates unacceptable patient movement. For most radical treatments to the head and neck a comfortable rigid external fixation shell is usually indicated in order to ensure precise positioning. The adoption of 'universal' systems to prevent patient motion is also important where a patient is to undergo a variety of differing imaging procedures, and these facilitate attempts at image fusion.

7.9.1 Head Supports

Before a patient's immobilisation shell is constructed attention should be paid to the choice of headrest. A suitable headrest allows the patient to adopt the required treatment position comfortably at a designated height above the treatment couch. Most radiotherapy departments employ a system that allows a choice from a number of standard headrests, which follow the contour of the patient's head and neck and offer a choice of positioning options to accommodate a range of anatomical variation. For example, during positioning it may be necessary to eliminate excessive neck flexion and reduce curvature of the spinal cord in the anterior direction. Headrests should also ideally limit rotational and lateral movements of the head. This can be ensured by using a headrest that is slightly higher at its edges. A reasonable choice of headrest is important because the head position selected for treatment is dictated by the site and type of the lesion to be treated.

Certain treatments may require elevation of the patient's chin and extension of the neck (e.g. during treatment of parotid gland tumours). This can be facilitated by the use of a headrest with a pronounced neck curve and deeper 'head bowl'.

Most headrests are manufactured using materials such as *polyurethane foam* or *thin plastic composites*, although *carbon fibre* options are available. These materials need to be durable because they are for reuse and should therefore be washable for infection control purposes. Materials used should exhibit minimal beam attenuation properties because it may be necessary to employ treatment beam arrangements that treat through the cushion support (e.g. when treating from a posterior-oblique direction). A number of manufacturers now offer custom supports providing individualised head moulds that employ vacuum-cushion technologies or water-activated resins.

7.9.2 Baseplate Systems

For accurate treatment it is necessary to fasten the head immobilisation devices to the scanner and treatment couch top via a dedicated baseplate. The baseplate system should allow easy attachment to the couch and may be indexed such that the patient can be positioned along the longitudinal plane. Most systems also allow for the lateral movement of the headrest so that the patient can be positioned in an offset position towards the edge of the treatment couch. This position may be necessary for the treatment of lateralised volumes and the use of posterior oblique gantry angles without the risk of gantry–couch collisions. The fixation system used should permit a variety of treatment positions, e.g. prone head and neck treatments or supine treatments in the extended, neutral, or flexed position. Provision should be made for the angulation of the baseplate in order to ensure the option to select a tilted position as required in flexed 'chin-down' positioning, e.g. for use during the treatment of pituitary disease.

7.9.3 Facial Masks

For the purpose of irradiation of head and neck tumours, facial masks are most frequently used. It is important that the masks used provide suitable immobilisation and retain a degree of rigidity to prevent patient motion. A good shell should closely follow the contours of the patient and should have the following characteristics [10]:

- Permit localisation of the lesion to be accurately determined from surface markers attached to the shell;
- Enable an accurate position of the patient to be reproduced from fraction to fraction;
- Guarantee an accurate and constant patient contour;
- Can be labelled and marked clearly and remove the need to draw marks on the patient;
- Offer accurate beam entry and exit points;
- Provide a base for the addition of buildup material.

Initial patient positioning is made according to local protocol and this usually coincides with the planning CT scan. In the UK these procedures are usually led by therapeutic radiographers although many departments employ specialist mould room technicians.

Before mask construction it is critical that a suitable amount of attention be paid to the proposed patient position with respect to the position of the head, neck, and shoulders. A decision needs to be made as to whether the immobilisation shell is required to encompass just the head (e.g. from skull vertex to chin), or whether a 'full' shell (including shoulder fixation) is necessary, for example where lateral fields extending inferiorly are intended.

Patient preparation for mask construction usually commences with the patient removing all clothing from the upper body. When positioning the patient it is usual to employ identifiable reference points on the patient's surface such as the nose, chin, and forehead. Shoulder and arm position may influence the reproducibility and stability of a patient setup. Many departments rely on patients maintaining the treatment position themselves, but it may be necessary to employ an additional positioning device to effectively retract the patient's shoulders downwards. This may be particularly useful in patients receiving larynx or pharynx irradiation using lateral treatment beams and who may have a short neck or high shoulders. Such devices usually consist of an elastic strap system with grab handles or wrist straps for the patient to hold on to, which manoeuvres the shoulders inferiorly during treatment setup. The length of the strap is adjusted for each patient in order to bring the shoulders inferiorly and away from the radiotherapy beams. Research [11] suggests that use of such shoulder retraction may effectively lengthen the neck region and permit irradiation of the paravertebral region and cervical soft tissues and increase the range of beam angles that are deployed during techniques such as IMRT.

There are two principal types of shell in use: clear plastic (*polyethylene terephthalate glycol*) (PETG) and *thermoplastics*. In the UK PETG plastic shells are now used only rarely although their use has been retained in other countries.

PETG plastics are relatively cost-effective and combine both strength and durability. In addition they offer the advantage of good optical properties in that the patient's anatomy can be viewed through the shell. It is important that an assessment is made as to the suitability of fit on a day-to-day basis due to the risk of problems resulting from patient weight loss, or conversely tissue swelling as a result of treatment side effects. Construction of PETG plastic shells can be an involved process requiring the use of full mould room facilities. The immobilisation material is heated until soft, and then vacuum formed over a positive impression of the patient's anatomy (usually constructed via the use of a plaster of Paris mould). Repeat visits of the patient for the purpose of shell construction and fitting may also be necessary. A full description of the process of shell construction can be found elsewhere [10].

More commonly employed materials include *perforated thermoplastics*. During construction it is necessary to select a suitable length of the immobilisation material according to need, e.g. a full shell may be required that extends over the shoulders and upper thorax – a consideration for those patients for whom supraclavicular nodal or anterior lower neck irradiation is indicated (Figure 7.3).

Mask construction requires the material first to be softened (usually via the use of a hot water bath) and subsequently draped over the patient's face. Whilst soft, it is necessary to mould the plastic across the patient's contours, ensuring that the material follows the outline of the bony prominences in the head and neck. During subsequent use of the mask it can be accurately sited on these landmarks.

When cooled the material becomes stiff and serves as rigid immobilisation. Slight shrinkage of the material usually ensues, although this does not usually compromise patient fit. One advantage of such materials is that they are relatively easy to adjust should a patient gain or lose weight, requiring shell modification to ensure acceptable fit. When reheated the material has a tendency to flatten and return to its original shape – so-called 'plastic memory'. By local heating of the material (e.g. via the use of a heat gun) the mask can be reformed to accommodate changes to the patient contour.

A reliable fixation mechanism must also be used to attach the shell to the dedicated

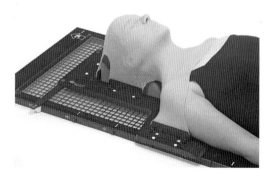

FIGURE 7.3 Thermoplastic immobilisation shell extending over shoulders. (Source: image courtesy of Oncology Systems Ltd., Shrewsbury, UK, and CIVCO Medical Solutions, Iowa, USA.)

baseplate system, which allows secure attachment whilst allowing for easy release of the patient from the device. Attachment of the mask to the baseplate system usually involves three, four, or five points of attachment dependent on the system employed and the anatomical extent of the shell employed. The baseplate system may also permit for insertion or removal of a dedicated plastic spacer (or 'shim') between the shell and the baseplate, and in some departments this is done to account for a degree of shell shrinkage after forming, or to compensate for patient swelling or weight loss during treatment. This however may introduce uncertainty with respect to isocentre positioning and careful assessment of patient anatomy is necessary via imaging.

7.9.4 Bite Blocks

For some treatments it may be necessary to treat the patient with the mouth open or to move the tongue away from the target volume during treatment. Despite the external fixation methods outlined previously, there is still scope for treatment position uncertainty due to jaw movements and movement of the tongue. A bite block (or mouth 'gag') provides a means of maintaining the mouth in the open position and ensuring that the tongue remains depressed. Many radiotherapy departments opt to manufacture in-house devices that employ materials used for dental impressions such as specialised *dental wax* or *dental compound*. When used, this material is heat softened and shaped around a suitable plastic tube, which ensures that the patient's airway is not compromised during use. The patient then bites down onto the wax and in doing so an impression of the teeth is obtained. The material is left to harden, and on subsequent use when inserted into the mouth the patient is able to relocate the block into the desired position. The resultant position of the bite block and tongue depressor is illustrated in Figure 7.4.

It is important that the construction of the bite block be undertaken after any remedial

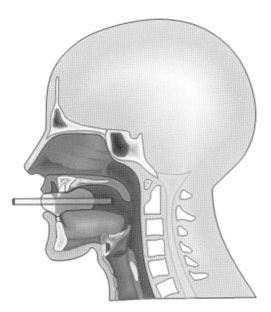

FIGURE 7.4 Position of mouth bite *in situ*.

dental work has been carried out (e.g. dental extraction), and that it is ready for use before the construction of a facial mask. The use of bite blocks may present some problems for edentulous patients or patients experiencing severe oral mucositis, and for all patients it is usual to disinfect the bite block after each use.

Commercially there are bite blocks available that can also aid head stability, where the bite block attaches to the overlying thermoplastic cast. Rotation and flexion movements may be reduced in addition to suitable tongue displacement.

7.10 Immobilisation Techniques and Proton Beam Radiotherapy

One of the most important factors that determines treatment accuracy during proton beam radiotherapy is effective patient immobilisation. Proton radiotherapy allows for a dose distribution to a defined depth point within the patient. Via modulation this dose may be spread out at the location of the intended target with minimal doses proximal and distal to this location due to the effect of the Bragg peak. Consequently, changes to the patient position and the movement of the target volume itself may be associated with significant dosimetric errors since movement of the target beyond the location of the (spread-out) Bragg peak can lead to the tumour lying in a zone of steep dose fall-off. This is much more of a critical consideration than that seen in photon radiotherapy where there is a gradual fall-off in depth dose distribution [12]. In addition immobilisation devices may influence the lateral dose gradient of the administered beam which may lead to a loss of dose sparing in OARs that are lateral to the beam.

As with photon beam radiotherapy, consideration should be given so that any immobilisation device employed should not limit the treatment angles selected. This is particularly important in proton radiotherapy where the patient may be in close proximity to the treatment aperture. Careful analysis of immobilisation devices is required to identify the proton range pullback caused by the materials used, and a comparison made between measured range and the range predicted by the treatment planning system. It is also important to consider the proton stopping power of materials used within custom supports (e.g. for head and neck support) as this may vary due to a change in their chemical and physical characteristics during the process of manufacture itself. Immobilisation devices such as thermoplastic masks may be employed as with photon radiotherapy, however it is important to ensure these are attached and indexed in a manner that is compatible with the proton treatment couch (which may be a robotic couch for example). The physical presence of the mask frame or table edge may also add to proton range uncertainty. In addition, it may be important to carefully assess the thickness of material employed during shell construction since differing gradients in thickness may influence proton range. Previous experience in construction of immobilisation devices specific for proton therapy has included the use of devices using carbon composites as they may be constructed with a uniform thickness [13]. Proton radiotherapy is indicated for some paediatric tumours and as such it is important to be mindful of the comfort, ease of setup, and tolerance to immobilisation amongst these patients.

Organ motion is a particular concern during proton radiotherapy and it is likely that treatment delivery will routinely address this phenomenon via approaches such as respiratory motion control and image guidance, perhaps via the use of implanted fiducials to facilitate organ tracking.

7.11 Immobilisation Equipment for Breast Treatment

A significant proportion of work within a radiotherapy department is breast irradiation and this is a challenge due to the complexities of breast planning, given the range of anatomical variation present amongst this patient group. The breast itself has a complex shape and has an irregular contour and changing tissue separation along the length of the intended treatment volume [14]. In addition, breast techniques are required to adequately treat the chest wall and overlying tissues whilst reducing excessive doses to the lung and heart. Rotation of the patient's torso coupled with respiratory motion can compromise treatment accuracy. Patients may also be required to adopt treatment positions that permit supraclavicular and axillary nodal irradiation. For these patients, treatment position is a crucial factor in the determination of accurate field matching with breast tangents, and stability and reproducibility of the patient's position can determine whether there will be overdosing at the match line. The demand for positional accuracy can be a challenge in patients who have limited mobility in the upper limb, e.g. after partial mastectomy or axillary lymph node clearance.

7.11.1 Positioning

Radiotherapy to the breast or chest wall conventionally requires the patient to be irradiated via the use of glancing tangential fields across the patient's thorax, although IMRT techniques are becomingly more widely adopted. These can be achieved only if the patient is positioned in a manner such that the arm on the affected side of the body is placed into an abducted position away from the chest wall. It may be appropriate for both arms to be elevated for treatment and positioning may be more reproducible in this position. Additionally, the use of the bi-arm (both arms up) technique may realise reduction of irradiated lung volume within the treatment field, however, machine restrictions may permit the elevation and support only of the ipsilateral arm.

For many patients it is also appropriate to elevate the upper thorax in order to ensure that the sternum is lying horizontally. By doing so the need for collimator angulation when using static tangential fields is removed, and the irradiated lung volume can be reduced in the caudocephalic direction. To achieve this treatment position, a positioning device is required to maintain thoracic elevation and arm abduction. The device must allow for adjustment of patient position required during the planning process whilst permitting the adoption of a comfortable treatment position to suit each individual patient. Most frequently radiotherapy departments will make use of a dedicated *breast board*. Modern breast boards employ an ergonomic design that permits the patient to be placed in a suitable position for treatment that is comfortable and stable. It is also necessary for such devices to be compatible with both the CT scanner and the treatment couch. Earlier CT planning techniques were limited to those patients whose position could be accommodated by the width of the CT aperture; however, recently the wider availability and increased use of dedicated radiotherapy 'wide-bore' scanners (i.e. bore width of 80–90 cm) allows the use of CT planning for most breast patients positioned on a breast board.

7.11.2 Breast Board Design

A number of breast board designs are commercially available. Earlier wooden devices have been superseded by the use of acrylic materials and many modern devices are now constructed from low-density foam within a carbon fibre outer shell. This ensures minimum attenuation of the treatment beam should treatment beams encroach onto the breast board itself. The practical use of such equipment is relatively straightforward and each patient's individual position can be readily reproduced by reliance on an indexing system, allowing the relocation of the arm, elbow, hand, and wrist (Figure 7.5).

Patient position may vary along the caudocephalic plane; however, this can be addressed by an indexed 'hip-stop' and knee immobilisation to prevent the patient from sliding down the board during treatment. Additional use of vacuum mould immobilisation systems with breast boards may be of use in a few patients for whom comfort is difficult to achieve, although their routine use may not translate as significant elimination of setup error [15].

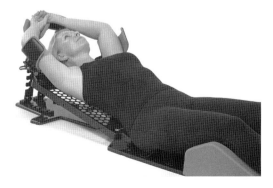

FIGURE 7.5 Carbon fibre breast board. (Source: image courtesy of Oncology Systems Ltd., Shrewsbury, UK, and CIVCO Medical Solutions, Iowa, USA.)

The patient's head position is maintained by a dedicated headrest system that itself can be relocated according to the comfort and anatomy of the patient, whilst permitting the extension of the chin away from the radiation beams. The headrest system should ideally permit lateral rotation of the head if required, for example during irradiation of the supraclavicular region.

7.11.3 Immobilisation for Larger Breast Size

Patients with larger breast size present some particular challenges with respect to immobilisation of the target organ and achieving optimal dosimetry. For these patients the supine position can result in the movement of breast tissue superiorly and laterally, requiring the adjustment of posterior field borders laterally, which can lead to a considerable increase in the volume of irradiated lung. As a consequence, it may be appropriate to select a method of immobilising the whole breast and/or selecting the use of a nonstandard treatment position.

Most frequently used breast immobilisation devices are constructed in house and usually include the manufacture of a custommade 'treatment brassière' made from thermoplastic or polyurethane-based plastics. Preformed shells may also be available. Their use maintains the position of large or flaccid breasts in a reproducible position whilst moving the contralateral breast away from the treatment position. They may also be effective at eliminating excessive skinfolds, which can help reduce the likelihood of skin toxicity. However, the use of immobilisation shells for breast immobilisation necessarily reduces the phenomenon of skin sparing. One solution to this is to cut out areas of the immobilisation device, but this can lead to uncertainties in the reliability of the breast position. Modified devices such as a *microshell* have undergone trials, which may go some way to achieving breast support with minimal increases in skin-surface dose [16].

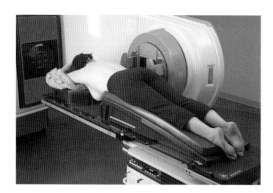

FIGURE 7.6 Prone breast board. (Source: image courtesy of Oncology Systems Ltd., Shrewsbury, UK, and CIVCO Medical Solutions, Iowa, USA.)

Alternative positioning strategies for this patient group have also been suggested and include the use of decubitus or prone positions. Use of the prone position for patients with pendulous breasts potentially improves dosimetry, reduces normal tissue irradiation, and improves setup reliability [17]. A number of positioning aids are available that permit customised prone patient positioning, such as *prone breast boards* (Figure 7.6).

An important consideration for this treatment position is the location of the contralateral breast, which should ideally be rotated away from the treatment beam. A suitable aperture should be present in the prone breast board on the ipsilateral side, which allows the breast to fall under gravity into the required treatment position through an open treatment couch panel. The resultant position of the affected breast permits the use of lateral treatment fields during treatment delivery.

Whilst this prone technique may be effective for some large-breasted patients, one important consideration is the position of the presenting primary lesion within the breast. Where the original lesion is in proximity to the chest wall, the prone position may be inappropriate as suitable coverage of the target volume may not be achievable because the lateral treatment fields would collide with the treatment couch. In addition, such techniques may be inappropriate or unfeasible for some patients, for example in the immobile

or very elderly patient, or where positioning is difficult due to morbid obesity [18].

Adoption of IMRT and 3DCRT for breast irradiation has introduced a new focus on positioning and immobilisation for these patients, given that historically breast patients were positioned primarily via the focus on immobilisation of their thorax rather than the breast tissue itself (unless the patient is larger breasted and requires a bespoke immobilisation intervention as described previously). More recently interest has developed in larger-breasted patients being immobilised in support bras that are more akin to the patient's own underwear in an effort to overcome the attendant loss of skin sparing seen with plastic shells for example. Keller et al. [19] investigated the use of a fabric strapless custom-fit bra with plastic stays in larger-breasted patients. In this trial an increase in radiation dermatitis was seen in those patients fitted with the bra compared to those who were not, although gains were seen in reduction of the amount of irradiated lung and heart where the bra was used. A limitation of this study however remains that the immobilisation bra, whilst *custom-fit*, is not *custom-made* and the bra itself as a form of immobilisation in its own right should arguably be subject to rigorous testing including assessment of reproducibility and dosimetric assessment. More recently consideration has been given to the feasibility for the use of a novel radiotherapy-specific support bra that facilitates accuracy of breast positioning, with concomitant reduction in doses to OARs (namely heart and lungs) particularly, although not exclusively, amongst women with larger breasts [20]. Development of such a device has included preclinical assessment of design materials via phantom studies and suitability assessment using healthy volunteers. Importantly codesign of equipment with healthcare professionals is necessary in order to maintain ease of setup and allow radiotherapy procedures to continue unhindered, including assessment of patient skin reactions and patient alignment. Such devices potentially result in the reduction of the use of permanent tattoos and also maintain the dignity of the patient, who historically has been positioned with her body undressed from the waist upward – often for several minutes at a time and in the presence of two or more therapeutic radiographers. For many patients this loss of modesty has the result of causing an increase in anxiety or distress which itself can prejudice treatment accuracy where this anxiety results in additional patient movement or tensing of body posture.

7.12 Respiratory Movements

Movement due to respiration can be a significant influence in altering the anatomical position of the target volume and may constitute a major cause of intrafraction variability. Chest wall movements may also reduce the reliability of surface reference marks, which can lead to setup errors. The effects of these movements are obviously important when considering the treatment of intrathoracic or breast disease but may also exert an influence on organ position at more remote anatomical locations such as the pelvis. Dedicated breathing control systems such as the *active breathing control* (ABC) system [21] provide for regulation of patient breathing via the use of a modified ventilator system that aims to minimise the margins for breathing motion. At a predetermined tidal lung volume inspiratory and expiratory airflow is temporarily blocked, thus immobilising the chest momentarily (nasal air flow is prevented due to the use of an occlusive nasal clip) (Figure 7.7).

The system is usually employed in conjunction with thorax immobilisation devices such as vacuum bags or immobilisation frames. This in effect restrains the patient within a breath-held position which has the potential to produce a reproducible position for planning and for use in gated radiotherapy techniques.

ABC devices operate via the use of control valves that close and dictate flow direction

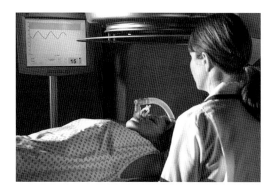

FIGURE 7.7   Active breathing coordinator. (Source: image courtesy of Elekta Ltd.)

at specific points in the breathing cycle. Lung volume detection is critical in the process in order to achieve the predetermined chest position. *Pneumotachograph spirometry* or motion detection imaging may be used together with the use of dedicated computer software to accomplish this. Importantly, ABC systems should also include an abort button that restores airflow in the event of patient distress.

The value of breath-hold techniques (either with ABC devices or via free breathing) is that they reliably hold the patient's thorax at predetermined points in the breathing cycle. For lung cancer patients this potentially provides defined positional information of the clinical target volume throughout the breathing cycle and may also eliminate breathing artefacts during CT imaging procedures. Breath-hold techniques are also shown to be particularly useful amongst patients receiving radiotherapy for left-sided breast cancer [22]. Amongst these patients there may be an appreciable reduction in cardiac dose received where the patient is treated in the breath-hold position. This is due to the fact that in the breath-hold position the patient's heart is moved away from the irradiated field as a consequence of lung inflation and associated expansion to the dimensions of the thorax. Despite these potential benefits it seems likely that the efficacy of breath-hold techniques is heavily reliant upon the use of patient training before their use; a lack of patient cooperation or poor patient compliance may be problematic, particularly where patients present with concurrent respiratory disease, which makes breath-holds problematic. The therapeutic radiographer has a crucial role to play in the communication of information to such patients in order that the technique is achievable. These techniques by their very nature may increase treatment times and necessitate additional staff training however.

7.12.1 Surface Tracking

Strategies for tracking and analysing the patient's surface during the breathing cycle permit an assessment of dynamic changes in the position of the thorax. An adaptive and dynamic assessment of anatomy may therefore in one sense move the focus of treatment accuracy away from one purely based on immobilisation alone. In the case of radiotherapy to the thorax, an assessment of the patient's position is automatically made and compared against an ideal (preplanned) position, and if the patient moves out of tolerance during treatment delivery, the treatment is temporarily stopped via a beam hold command sent to the LinAc's control unit. Technologies that have been employed include the use of external surrogates such as reflective skin markers, or the use of an external belt worn by the patient which allows for analysis of breathing amplitude via the use of pressure sensors.

Video-based patient motion tracking systems are available such as the real-time position management (RPM) system (Varian Medical Systems, Palo Alto, CA). This system involves motion tracking of the patient's breathing cycle via the use of infrared cameras trained onto a reflective surface marker on the patient's skin which will act as a surrogate for thorax expansion. The patient is required to undertake a voluntary deep inspiration manoeuvre and may be assisted by the aid of a visualised trace on a computer screen. The camera video system will detect the position of the surface marker and analyses breathing motion and expansion of the thorax. The RPM system is linked with the LinAc such that if the patient's position deviates away from the preplanned breath-hold

position the beam will switch off. Hence the system ensures the breath-hold position is reproducible and does not fall outside of predetermined limits of breathing motion.

Marker-free systems are also employed whereby 3D stereo cameras are used to create a 3D rendered model of the patient's surface anatomy. This may be used to track the patient's treatment position and make a comparison against the 'ideal' position. Again it is necessary to define acceptable error range for patient setup, and thereby only administer treatment when the patient reaches a position that is acceptable in comparison to the planned reference position.

Respiratory motion may also be an important factor that needs to be controlled for example during stereotactic radiotherapy treatments such as stereotactic ablative radiotherapy (SABR). For ablative radiotherapy to liver lesions there may be considerable variation in the location of the target volume during the breathing cycle due the close proximity of the liver to the right dome of the diaphragm. Techniques that have been employed to help reduce organ motion at this site include voluntary deep inspiration breath-hold (DIBH) or deep exhalation breath-hold (DEBH) manoeuvres. Abdominal compression via the use of a dedicated abdominal compression plate may also prove to be useful, however this technique is unsuitable for patients who have previously undergone abdominal surgery or for those who are morbidly obese.

Analysis of tumour motion in the case of lung SABR may be possible via the use of 4D-CT treatment planning whereby the excursion of the tumour during respiration may be analysed during free breathing. This may result in the use of an IM that is slightly larger to account for translation of the tumour during the breathing cycle. Alternatively respiratory gating may be used but this brings with it additional technical challenges. As with other techniques involving analysis of respiratory motion, a degree of patient training or coaching may be necessary such as provision of dedicated written information prior to pretreatment planning or the use of a dedicated 'practice' or 'day 0' set up appointment (without treatment). Real-time feedback to the patient may also be provided via the use of patient goggles linked to a video display to assist rhythmic breathing or the use of audible patient cues such as a tonal metronome.

7.12.2 Technical Issues Relating to the Use of 4D-CT

Within the CT scanner fast tube rotation times of 0.5–1 second, allowing rapid acquisition of large volumes of data, although advantageous from a diagnostic perspective could be considered undesirable in some therapy scenarios because they generate image data at a rate unrepresentative of the period of radiotherapy delivery. Techniques may be required that acquire scan data over timescales comparable with the breathing cycle (Figure 7.8), through use of low pitch (slowing couch movement) or combining slow tube rotation with thin reconstruction slices.

If *4D-CT* is to be employed, scanner control software should provide the means whereby the breathing cycle demonstrated during scan acquisition can be related to the images reconstructed. Using low pitch and thin slice thickness (around 1 mm) it is possible to divide the study into a number of sub-studies, each relating to an identifiable segment of the respiratory cycle. This data can then be used to either 'gate' treatment delivery on the LinAc (exposure only occurring within predefined ranges), or alternatively it can used to identify extremes of organ and tumour movement, enabling a composite PTV to be produced.

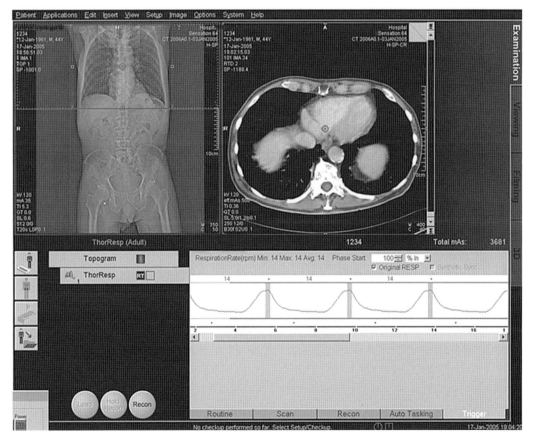

FIGURE 7.8 Four-dimensional computed tomography (4D-CT): demonstration of respiratory cycle during image acquisition.

7.13 Thorax Immobilisation

For simple techniques in the thorax it is not necessary to use complex immobilisation devices. For parallel pair techniques to the chest it may be necessary only to select a reproducible position that ensures patient comfort by the use of a standard range of foam wedges and cushions.

For planned volume techniques it is usual to position the patient in an arms-up position in order to accommodate obliquely placed treatment fields whilst avoiding the patient's arms. This can be achieved by using a *chest board* which, like breast boards, allows for a range of upper-limb positions to be selected but without the use of a thoracic incline. In these patients it is important that the arm receives adequate support and many of these devices feature a dedicated elbow support or characteristic 'wing'. *Vacuum bag systems* or positioning moulds may also be used (Figure 7.9).

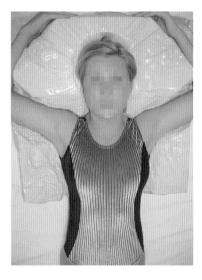

FIGURE 7.9 Thoracic positioning mould. (Source: image courtesy of Smithers Medical Products Inc.)

7.14 Immobilisation Equipment for Pelvic Treatment

Reproducible positioning of the patient is crucial when treating the pelvis, due to the juxtaposition of critical structures and the high-dose treatment zone. In addition, interfractional differences in anatomical position of soft-tissue structures within the pelvis should be considered, and these themselves can be affected to varying degrees by the positioning of the patient.

For many pelvic treatments the use of simple leg and/or ankle immobilisation is considered appropriate and there is evidence that the use of immobilisation can reduce the incidence of positional errors > 5 mm to between 4 and 8% of displacements detected on portal imaging [23].

For supine treatment positions a variety of foam rubber supports are available that help maintain stability and aid reproducibility, not least due to the fact that the supports offer additional comfort in the region of the lumbosacral spine for patients lying on a hard treatment couch. There are a number of commercially available devices, and many aim to raise the knees whilst achieving a suitable treatment position. Ankle-positioning devices may also be used where a consistent foot position is desirable during treatment; such devices often take the form of so-called 'ankle stocks' and may extend as far superiorly as the knee joint as 'leg stocks'. These devices have the beneficial feature that they act to separate the feet whilst limiting external or internal rotation of the lower limb, which in turn can govern the accuracy of pelvic position.

Alternative methods of pelvis immobilisation can be employed that aim to provide individualised bespoke positioning tailored to the contours of each patient. These can take the form of half-body positioning systems that may extend from hip to ankle. Vacuum bag systems may be used which comprise a reinforced bag containing polystyrene beads positioned beneath the patient. Using a vacuum pump air is extracted and the bag moulds to the contours of the patient. This mould is retained as long as the access port is sealed. This is a relatively easy process and the bags can be reused once treatment is complete. Care is required to prevent puncturing of the device because any leakage may result in a loss of the rigid patient outline.

Alternatively, body moulds can be formed via the use of foaming chemicals within a bag that provides rigid immobilisation. Such systems (e.g. Alpha Cradle, Smithers Medical Products, Inc.) employ expanded polyurethane foam that is moulded to the contours of the patient. This foam expands and hardens after the mixing of constituent chemicals, and the expansion process takes place with the patient lying on the device within a supporting 'cradle'. During the construction process care is required to eliminate excess air from the bag, and to ensure that the foam is distributed equally across the region of the patient's back, legs, and hips. A decision needs to be made whether to use hip-to-ankle or a shorter hip-to-knee mould. Such systems are non-reusable and may constitute some additional storage requirements compared with more simple techniques. In addition, one report describes the possibility of difficulties with placing elderly and obese patients into and out of their cast [24].

Prone treatments present further positioning challenges. For patients undergoing irradiation of a rectal carcinoma a prone position is favoured, due to the need to irradiate posteriorly located treatment volumes, using posterior beams to encompass the buttocks. Treating in the prone position enables a degree of separation of the natal cleft, which can help maintain the skin-sparing effect. Immobilisation of prone patients can be inherently problematic, and there are marked difficulties, particularly with elderly patients. The discomfort experienced by patients arises as they attempt to 'balance' their bony pelvis on a hard couch top. Simple immobilisation devices such as ankle pads afford a degree of comfort by allowing slight flexion of the knee joint, avoiding contact of the dorsum of the foot with the couch top. Patients are ordinarily positioned with their arms above their heads; however, care needs to be taken to ensure that the patient's arms and head are comfortable because variation can introduce variability of pelvic skin markings. This can be facilitated via the use of a dedicated positioning aid such as a modified prone pillow. Other confounding factors such as the presence of an abdominal ileostomy pouch can lead to uncertainties as to the accuracy of patient positioning. Prone treatments may also be indicated for other pelvic malignancies such as carcinoma of the prostate gland, although daily setup variability appears less accurate than supine setups, particularly in the absence of immobilisation devices [25].

In obese patients prone positioning presents additional problems due to the uncertainty and variability of skin marks and patient comfort issues, and that the prone position itself may increase the risk of irradiation of small bowel. Invasive surgical techniques to immobilise the bowel have been attempted such as the use of *omentoplasty* or *intrapelvic prostheses* [26]; however, the need for surgical immobilisation is rare due to significant developments in imaging and treatment planning. Positioning and immobilisation devices may be used that address the position of abdominal and bowel variability. The use of a 'belly board' or open-couch device may increase comfort and has been highlighted as one method of reducing gastrointestinal toxicities [27]. These devices may be constructed from a variety of materials such as polystyrene, although the use of carbon fibre devices is indicated if the device occludes treatment beams. Each device requires the patient to be supported in a manner in which the abdominal region can be comfortably accommodated whilst lying in the prone treatment position (Figure 7.10). Adequate support for the upper legs and symphysis pubis is necessary, as is adequate support for the patient's arms and head. Reproducibility is aided by the use of an indexing system on the device, which enables the isocentre to be located in the longitudinal direction.

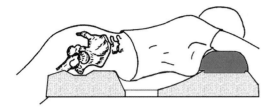

FIGURE 7.10   Patient position during use of prone 'belly board'. (Source: image courtesy of Oncology Systems Ltd., Shrewsbury, UK, and CIVCO Medical Solutions, Iowa, USA.)

Whether supine or prone, consideration should be given as to the use of rigid external immobilisation devices for pelvic irradiation. The use of thermoplastic immobilisation shells may be appropriate for patients with mobile skin marks; however, previously reported potential gains in the accuracy of positioning [28] may be countered by additional costs and increased setup complexity. In addition, it should be ensured that such external fixation devices are compatible with CT scanners.

7.14.1 Organ Position Due to Differential Filling

Current approaches to pelvic treatment delivery require day-to-day reduction in setup variability in patient position. Translational and rotational movements may be reduced via the use of external fixation devices or the use of patient supports that aid comfort and stability. However, there is a new focus on the notion that the variable position of individual organs themselves should be considered. Uncertainty in the position of the target volume potentially negates improvements in planning accuracy and the use of highly conformal techniques. One of the frustrations of treatment accuracy is that, although it is quite possible to achieve a level of immobilisation of bony elements of the pelvis, there may be a large variability in internal anatomy between successive fractions (*interfraction variability*) or during each treatment fraction (*intrafraction variability*). Potential methods that decrease

the volume of normal tissue in the high-dose region should lead to decreased morbidity, providing scope for dose escalation [29].

Irradiation of the prostate gland presents some significant challenges due to the often pronounced effect that differential rectal filling and flatus distension have on the position of the prostate gland itself, and the motion of the rectal wall relative to the high-dose region. Reproducibility of the rectal position can be achieved by encouraging the patient to void the rectum before treatment. This relatively simple solution may be unreliable however, not least due to difficulties in compliance for patients who are required to empty their rectum 'at will', and subjective perceptions of what constitutes an 'empty' bowel by the patient. In addition, the rectum position may still be variable when empty [30].

With the adoption of image guided techniques many radiotherapy departments have developed their own protocols for preparing patients prior to their treatment. These are determined mindful of the fact that bladder filling and rectal distension may have a significant effect on the position of the prostate and local anatomy and may affect the success of dose conformity. A number of strategies exist in preparing the patient such as drinking of a predetermined volume of water to ensure adequate bladder filling, and the use of microenemas or suppositories to ensure rectal emptying – both at predetermined times prior to acquisition of the pretreatment CBCT image. Careful analysis of the pretreatment image should also be made to determine rectum and bladder status – in the eventuality that the bladder is too empty for example, the patient may be asked to consume further water. More generally patients may be provided with treatment advice that may aid in achieving reproducible organ position on a daily advice – this includes maintaining a good level of hydration, and adoption of a diet that may reduce production of bowel gas (which can cause unintended rectal distention and associated prostate shift).

Patient preparation is obviously also important in the administration of radiotherapy to other anatomical loci. Research [31] suggests that radiotherapy for cervical cancer is subject to variability in position of the pelvic organs, and that even with strict fluid drinking protocols patients may struggle to obtain optimal bladder capacity, which may be related to radiation-induced cystitis for example. Patient preparation protocols allow for a reduction in organ position variability however this is entirely as successful as the patient is compliant – that is, nonadherence to advice may lead to treatment delay or potential inaccuracies. Invasive approaches to organ immobilisation have been trialled as a possible solution.

One method in which these variables are reduced is the use of internal immobilisation methods such as the use of an inflated rectal balloon catheter. The catheter is tested for leaks and subsequently covered by a protective sheath before being inserted into the patient's rectum. Depression of the syringe plunger introduces between 50 and 100 cm^3 of air into the balloon (according to patient comfort), which once inflated acts to immobilise the prostate and displace rectal tissue in the posterolateral direction. The procedure is undertaken during planning CT scans and then for each subsequent treatment fraction. Despite this being a potentially distressing invasive procedure, which might be thought to decrease patient comfort, the use of the rectal balloon is reported as being tolerated well by patients.

In addition there may be a dosimetric precedent for the use of an air-filled balloon catheter, since at the interface between the air and tissue there is a slight reduction in dose. This phenomenon appears to affect only a small region of the anterior rectal wall in the region of the interface without compromising dose coverage to the target volume. Research [32] indicates that dose at this point is reduced to approximately 15% less than where a balloon catheter is not used. Potentially this may result in a dose reduction to the anterior rectal wall, resulting in reduced acute rectal toxicities.

The use of an intrarectal balloon significantly reduces prostate motion. An increased degree of immobilisation of soft-tissue structures potentially makes PTV delineation more

reliable and may permit smaller treatment margins to be used. Such precise targeting is essential for 3DCRT and in particular in the use of IMRT. The use of a rectal balloon catheter presents an additional treatment procedure that may add to the workload of the radiographer, although routine use and patient compliance would hopefully facilitate the procedure.

7.14.2 Prostate Spacers

An alternative approach to limit rectal toxicity during prostate radiation is via the use of a dedicated rectal spacer. Rectal spacers involve the introduction of a biodegradable material into the space between the prostate and rectum which expands and provides a space between the prostate and the rectal wall. Various spacer materials have been trialled including the use of collagen, hyaluronic acid, expandable biodegradable balloons, or polyethylene glycol (PEG) hydrogels. It is important that the material used is nontoxic and biocompatible, and to this end materials used elsewhere, such as in the field of medical implants, are favoured. In the case of hydrogels they may be cost effective spacers as well as having a superior distribution within the perirectal space.

The spacer itself is surgically implanted into the patient via a transperineal approach under local, regional, or general anaesthesia whilst the patient is positioned in the lithotomy position. This procedure is ultrasound guided and accurate positioning of the implant may be facilitated by first introducing saline liquid via a needle inserted into the space between the rectal wall and the fascia overlying the prostate (Denonvilliers' fascia) occupied by perirectal fat (a procedure known as hydrodissection). In the case of the use of hydrogels (such as the SpaceOar system in Figure 7.11) the spacer is then deposited via the same in-dwelling needle into the desired location via the introduction of two precursors where it polymerises and solidifies *in situ* within 10 seconds. Solidification typically lasts about three months and is eventually

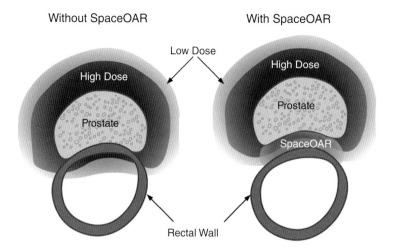

FIGURE 7.11 Hydrogel prostate spacer *in situ*. (Source: used with permission by Augmenix Inc., Bedford MA.)

biodegraded and reabsorbed into the patient's body after about six months and is eventually eliminated from the patient's body via renal clearance. Injection or insertion of the spacer typically achieves a separation of the prostate and rectum of between 1.0–1.5 cm dependent on the system employed and is well tolerated by the patient.

Without the use of spacers the anterior rectal wall ordinarily encroaches into the high-dose region, however spatial separation of these adjacent anatomical structures can significantly reduce the volume of rectal wall irradiated. In one study [33] the volume of rectum receiving 70 Gy (the V70) was reduced by 56%.

The potential gains for the use of such spacers are fourfold:

1. They result in a reduction of rectal dose and therefore a reduction in treatment toxicity and improved quality of life;

2. Reduction of dose to the organ at risk realises the potential to escalate prescribed dose;

3. Their use may facilitate hypofractionated treatment regimes resulting in a shorter treatment schedule for the patient;

4. They may permit retreatment with radiotherapy in the event of tumour recurrence.

Complications from spacer implantation are reportedly rare and late toxicity rates have been shown to be reduced via their use [33]. Consideration must be given to the additional time and resources required for implantation of spacers and whether their use is more generally acceptable to patients. Additional associated costs of their use may be justified given the potential gains made due to reduced incidence of acute and chronic toxicities, meaning prostate IMRT including the use of the implanted spacer may be cost effective [34]. Whilst there is evidence for the use of spacers as a means of spatial separation and sparing of rectal wall, their use does not eliminate prostate motion, and additional strategies such as the use of fiducial markers may be necessary.

7.14.3 The Use of Implanted Fiducial Markers

The issue of organ motion remains a complex one as organ motion can be uncertain, complex, and patient-specific with a significant range of random error in organ positioning. Assessment and analysis of the patient's position is possible via strategies such as surface tracking and using bony landmarks as stable reference points for image matching procedures.

However, it can be difficult to accurately locate soft-tissue structures without the use of a radiopaque fiducial marker introduced as a surrogate for tumour location. A good example of this is the accurate localisation of the prostate gland in radiotherapy for which the PTV may be small and subject to a large degree of variability in its position due to the influence of dynamic changes to surrounding anatomical structures. This prostate motion is greatest in the superior–inferior and anterior–posterior axes, compared to left to right. Awareness of such movement is particularly important in the delivery of radiotherapy techniques in which there is a high degree of conformity to the prostate and the use of tighter safety margins such as *volumetric modulated arc therapy* (VMAT).

It is important that fiducials are biologically inert and are readily visible on imaging including megavoltage portal imaging. A number of commercial seed designs are available including those with a characteristic cross-cut or 'knurled' surface which improve the seed's grip once implanted and reduces the possibility of seed migration (Figure 7.12). Materials employed most frequently involve the use of 24-carat gold seeds although polymer-based fiducial markers are available that are specially optimised for proton radiotherapy. These are also suitable for imaging via MRI (via modified MRI sequencing) and CT and have the benefit that they are associated with minimal imaging artefacts.

Responsibility for insertion of fiducials is assumed by a suitably trained healthcare professional. In the UK practice varies but implantation may be undertaken by senior urology medical staff, urology clinical nurse specialists, oncologists, or advanced clinical practitioner (ACP) therapeutic radiographers. The process of fiducial implantation usually takes place via the use of general or local anaesthesia, although anaesthetic-free insertion is reported as being well tolerated by the patient and helps reduce the procedure time [35]. *Trans*-rectal ultrasound (TRUS) is used to visualise the prostate gland and seeds are introduced via the rectal wall. At least three fiducials are introduced into the prostate gland (base and apex of the gland on one side and in the middle of the gland on the contralateral side) (Figure 7.13).

Additional fiducials are usually unnecessary since the migration and loss of implanted seeds is reportedly rare, although it is important to avoid implantation low down in the base of the prostate in proximity to the urethra to mitigate this risk of loss. Alternatively, a transperineal insertion may be undertaken and is favoured in some centres as this may potentially reduce the risk of post-implantation infections. Prophylactic antibiotic cover is usually administered irrespective of the method of insertion.

Once implanted, fiducial markers act as stable markers. Treatment planning CT is then employed to image the patient using the fiducial implants, although a short delay is often implemented between implantation and CT scanning. This is to allow resolution of post-implantation prostate swelling, permits time for the fiducials to lock into position, and allows the patient to recover from any side effects. Fiducial use is beneficial as it permits alignment of the prostate itself and extends

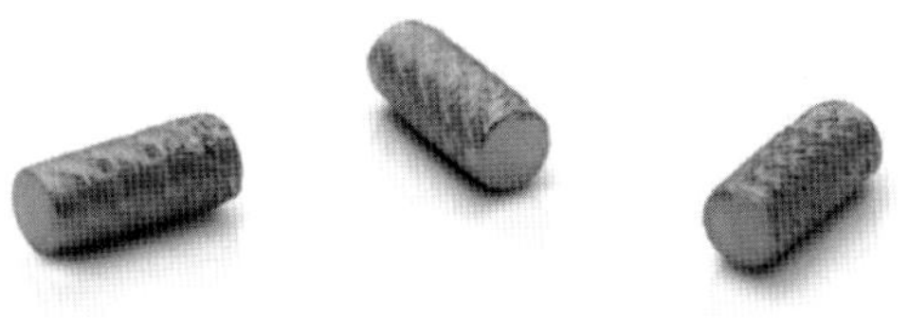

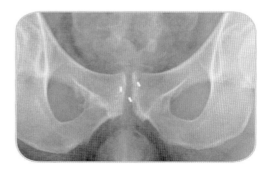

FIGURE 7.12 Gold fiducials. (Source: image courtesy of CIVCO Radiotherapy.)

FIGURE 7.13 Radiograph of gold fiducials *in situ*. (Source: image courtesy of CIVCO Radiotherapy).

the accuracy of image-matching techniques by assessing both bony landmarks (e.g. pelvic bones) and soft tissues which otherwise would be difficult to visualise via portal imaging or CBCT techniques.

7.14.4 The Use of Ultrasound Imaging for Treatment Verification

As described, differential bladder filling may affect prostate position, and may also be an influence on the likelihood of bowel and urinary treatment toxicities (although this is uncertain). The degree of success of bladder filling depends on patient compliance, and there may also be a wide range of individual bladder filling rates amongst men receiving radiotherapy for prostate treatment. As a consequence, a set patient preparation protocol based on defined water consumption may not realise adequate bladder filling in some patients. A solution to this is to assess the degree of bladder filling before daily treatment administration via the use of ultrasound scanning. Many radiotherapy departments now routinely employ ultrasound imaging to improve treatment accuracy by assessing bladder volumes prior to treatment administration. In doing so, assurance is gained that the daily bladder volume aligns with the degree of bladder filling at the point that the planning CT was undertaken. Non-invasive transabdominal bladder scanning via the use of a handheld scanner is reported as being effective and well tolerated by patients and does not impact on overall treatment times [36]. In addition this procedure allows for an assessment of bladder status during patient set up without associated radiation dose, i.e. a decision may be made regarding patient status prior to the use of CBCT (see also Chapter 6).

Ultrasound devices may also be used for assessment of positional accuracy of the prostate itself and this extends to its use to assess intrafraction variability of the prostate. It is recognised that prostate displacement *within* treatment administration is likely to be a common occurrence. If this motion can be tracked, treatment accuracy can be assured by suspending the treatment should the degree of prostate movement exceed a predefined threshold. Systems such as the Clarity® Auto-scan TPUS (Elekta) employ a non-invasive transperineal ultrasound scanner. During patient setup the ultrasound probe is placed against the patient's perineum. The probe is locked into a motorised housing which permits an automatic sweeping motion that replaces a manual sweep of the probe. Automated sweeping of the probe during scanning permits image reconstruction of the prostate in 3D and informs the need for adjustment of patient position to account for interfraction variability. In addition the use of the Autoscan probe may also allow for 4D real-time intrafraction motion monitoring. Assessment of prostate motion in this manner is well tolerated by patients and maintains treatment accuracy. Dynamic radiotherapy that includes motion correction may thus allow for maintenance of target coverage and reduction of radiation exposure of OARs. Ultrasound guided techniques in particular also preclude the need for implanted fiducials.

7.15 Superficial Radiotherapy

Patient immobilisation for the treatment of superficial lesions tends to be simplistic with patient comfort and stability achievable via the use of foam pads, cushions, and immobilisation blocks. Whether using electrons or superficial X-ray photon beams, the aim is to position the patient in a manner in which the affected site is accessible to enable close contact with machine applicators, whilst being comfortable for the patient.

For superficial skin lesions in the head region the stability of the patient's head position can be maintained by the use of a securing headband or surgical tape, coupled with laterally placed sandbags, which can

(a)

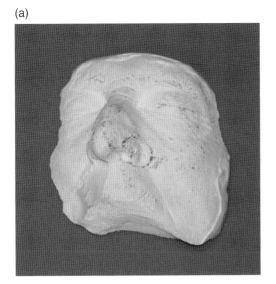

(b)

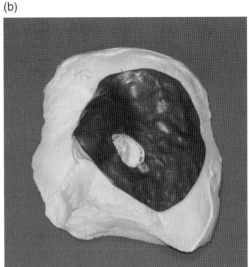

FIGURE 7.14 (a) Impression of patient's face constructed from stone plaster; (b) custom-made lead cutout in position surrounding lesion.

effectively act to 'chock' the patient's head in position. The treatment technique may also require the use of a custom-made lead cutout that defines the radiation field and provides shielding to adjacent structures. The lead cutout is formed so that it follows the contours of the patient's face such that accurate repositioning is achievable. Construction of the lead cutout requires it to be hammered into shape over a positive preformed cast of the patient's face (Figure 7.14).

For treatment, the cutout is positioned over the treatment site so that the treatment field encloses the lesion plus its treatment margin. A suitable applicator size is chosen to cover the treatment site. Very slight movements in the patient's head position should not therefore result in a geographical miss because the lead cutout may move with the patient's head and the target remains within the treatment beam. For some treatments there is the risk of dosing the radiosensitive mucous membrane lining the nose or inside the lip. In such cases it is possible to use a lead strip inserted into the nasal vestibule or the buccal cavity as additional protection. If treatment involves electron therapy there is a need to line this additional lead shielding, as a means of absorbing any secondary electrons

liberated by interaction of the primary beam and the lead.

For superficial treatments elsewhere in the body it may not be necessary to immobilise patients in ways other than to achieve patient comfort with a degree of reproducibility. However, in the use of electrons for phased treatments it is usual to administer these fields with the patient in their associated photon treatment position to prevent an inaccurate junction at any photon–electron match line.

7.16 Position Reproducibility in Emergency or Palliative Radiotherapy

Emergency and palliative radiotherapy techniques usually require a greater focus on patient comfort rather than strict immobilisation as the affected patient may be in discomfort or pain. Complex immobilisation procedures such as use of multi-point fixation head shells and bespoke headrest systems may not be used as these involve additional procedures that may delay treatment delivery and may not be needed for simple radiotherapy techniques (such as opposed radiation fields). Treatment accuracy and reproducibility are still paramount even across short-course radiotherapy regimens. A careful assessment of the patient's individual and holistic needs should always be made prior to consideration of radiotherapy administration not least since disease treated with palliative intent may not always be associated with an attendant likelihood of poor tolerance of radiotherapy. Even for patients with metastatic disease there may be a case for more complex and involved high-dose treatments particularly in the case of oligometastases which may be amenable to high-dose stereotactic treatment [37].

For some patients with advanced disease and with a poor prognosis it is necessary to attempt radiotherapy with the minimum of distress to the patient and reduce their treatment burden. To this end patient comfort is achievable by the addition of a soft mattress for positioning on the treatment couch since patient sag and its effect on reproducibility is unlikely to be a concern. Likewise, a degree of comfort is achieved via the use of foam rubber supports and treatment pillows.

7.17 Immobilisation for Less Common Techniques

There are a number of treatment scenarios for which a conventional supine or prone treatment position is unachievable, or where the patient's position needs to be adapted to facilitate access to the treatments site, e.g. where an electron field is to be employed.

7.17.1 Seated Treatments

For emergency cases (e.g. superior vena cava obstruction) or where a patient's immobility prevents the patient from being able to lie down, it may be necessary to administer treatment with the patient in a seated position. For this purpose a dedicated *treatment chair* can be used. A number of commercially available chairs are available which are either secured on the couch top or can be used as freestanding devices within the treatment room. Once transferred into the treatment chair, the treatment position is maintained by the use of arm supports and a Velcro head strap. Some systems may also use a baseplate system that additionally enables the use of thermoplastic immobilisation masks.

For patients for whom thoracic fields are indicated and for whom a horizontal position is unobtainable, it may be necessary to administer a parallel pair technique with the patient in the treatment chair. This is achieved by administering an unobstructed posterior treatment field via a mesh 'treatment window' in the back support panel. In addition the provision of arm supports permits the use of 'arms-up' or 'arms-down' positions with such devices. Accurate field positioning can be achieved in such systems as the full range of couch and tabletop movements is permissible.

A recent feasibility study [38] has explored the deployment of a novel seated position for head and neck patients treated with radical intent. The rationale for an upright or seated treatment stems from the fact that these patients may struggle to cope with the demands of their planned treatment in the conventional supine position, particularly where treatment side effects (such as dyspnoea or dysphagia) make lying flat difficult or even impossible. Contingency for treating head and neck cancers whilst the patient is seated includes the use of a dedicated treatment chair that allows fixation of a thermoplastic shell and adapted upright baseplate system. Since few departments retain the capacity for 2D imaging (e.g. via the use of a treatment simulator) treatment planning would necessarily need to employ the imaging capacity of modern LinAcs located within the treatment room. Initial trials suggest the possibility for a reproducible patient positioning that is well tolerated, and that it may be possible to translate these initial 2D imaging studies into the acquisition of workable LinAc-situated CBCT imaging for the purpose of treatment planning.

7.17.2 Unconventional Positions

For certain techniques it is necessary for the patient to adopt an unconventional position, e.g. where the anatomical area for treatment is difficult to access. For disease involving the anal margin or perineum it may be necessary to immobilise the patient in a lateral position with the knees drawn upwards. Positioning and immobilisation are facilitated by the use of supports between the patient's knees and under the ankles. An alternative approach is to position the patient hunched over a supporting pillow in order that the treatment site may be accessed. A relative degree of comfort may be difficult to achieve and it may be necessary for treatment centres to improvise using a combination of pillows and foam rubber immobilisation supports or to develop in-house immobilisation devices.

7.17.3 Total Body Irradiation

Individual total body irradiation (TBI) techniques have evolved over time and vary between individual departments. Patient immobilisation and positioning present a number of challenges, not least due to the need to undertake extensive *in vivo* dosimetry at a number of anatomical loci on these patients. TBI techniques ordinarily require treatments at extended treatment distances, and it is not usually practical to achieve such treatments on the usual treatment couch. Many departments utilise a dedicated TBI couch that allows the patient to adopt a semi-recumbent position for treatment and can be moved easily to the required treatment position and rotated for lateral exposures. For treatment the patient may adopt a position with the arms across the chest to act as compensators, and additional supporting straps may provide the additional support for this purpose. An alternative would be to position the patient such that he or she is lying on their side. Immobilisation can be achieved in this position via the use of an immobilising vacuum bag or bespoke foam support.

Alternatives to the use of a TBI couch may include use of a chair or devices that support the patient in the standing position.

7.17.4 Total Skin Electron Irradiation

Total skin electron (TSE) irradiation is indicated for patients with diffuse skin lesions such as mycosis fungoides (a form of cutaneous T-cell lymphoma). Treatment may be technically demanding as an aim of therapy is to achieve a uniform dose distribution to the whole of the surface dermal and epidermal layers of the patient's body, whilst ensuring comfort and stability during positioning. A number of treatment techniques are employed. In the case of administration of large electron fields the patient is placed in a standing position at an extended treatment distance, e.g. 700 cm source to skin distance (SSD). The patient position is changed up to six times within each individual fraction of electron therapy by repositioning the patient via a series of rotations including raising the patient's hand to ensure suitable coverage of the patient's surface with the incident electron field. For these techniques it may be possible to deliver the treatment via the use of two (i.e. dual) overlapped treatment fields, particularly where room dimensions do not permit longer SSDs. However the need to reposition the patient up to six times plus the use of two fields of radiation results in a longer procedure for the patient. Alternatively, a rotational technique may be employed using one field and the patient is automatically rotated in the standing position with the treatment beam switched on. To accomplish this, a dedicated motorised TBE (total body electron) therapy turntable is employed which automatically rotates the patient at a constant speed to ensure good dose homogeneity throughout each fraction of treatment. Such techniques have the advantage that beam matching is unnecessary and treatment times may be reduced. Alternative patient positioning strategies have also been employed such as the use of a six dual field technique with the patient placed in dedicated supine and prone positions rather than standing. For all patients receiving TBE treatment it may be necessary for the patient to wear external eye shields to prevent corneal ulceration, however this is necessarily excluded for patients with disease involved in their eyelids (see Chapter 8 for further details of this technique).

7.17.5 Radiotherapy Treatment of the Penis

Irradiation of patients with carcinoma of the penis requires an immobilisation strategy that may also provide a means of achieving a homogeneous dose distribution and ensuring the necessary use of buildup. This is achieved by the use of a two part Perspex or wax block containing a cylindrical cavity, within which the penis is supported. Perspex blocks have the advantage that they are transparent and permit suitable visualisation of the immobilised penis to permit treatment verification. The position of the penis relative to the block can be maintained by packing the cylinder with paraffin gauze or by the use of a Tubigrip to hold it in position. The use of tissue-equivalent packing material also helps to ensure uniform dose coverage. The treatment block itself is positioned on top of a lead scrotal shield, and it is usually necessary to secure the immobilisation device in place by the simple use of surgical tape or securing straps. For patients who have undergone extensive surgery such as partial penectomy

the use of the block is unsuitable as the penile remnant is too short to be accommodated. In such cases bespoke immobilisation is employed, such as the use of a custom wax buildup.

7.18 Immobilisation Equipment for Treatment of Extremities

The irradiation of the extremities requires precise limb positioning, a task that is affected by a high degree of mobility in the arm and leg. The lower limb position, for example, requires alignment with respect to the normal anatomical range of motion, including rotation, flexion, extension, abduction, and adduction. For the limbs, there are also exacerbating considerations such as the need to irradiate long muscle compartments whilst ensuring the sparing of a strip of tissue in order to reduce the likelihood of oedema. It is usual to consider the immobilisation of the entire affected limb because relatively small deviations in the position of the proximal limb can result in large translational and rotational displacement of the distal structures. Practical immobilisation of the limb also requires consideration as to whether the proposed treatment position permits treatment through a range of gantry and couch angles. In addition, the patient position must ensure avoidance of critical structures and adjacent anatomy. In the case of the leg this means avoidance of the contralateral limb, whilst immobilisation devices for the upper limb must allow for the arm to be positioned away from the torso. Tumours located in the distal lower limb are often treated with the patient in a 'feet to gantry' position in order for the treatment site to be brought into range of the clinical beam, whilst permitting the full range of couch movements to be used during setup.

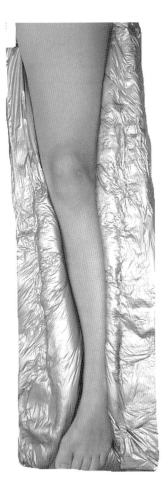

FIGURE 7.15 Leg immobilisation using positioning mould. (Source: Image courtesy of Smithers Medical Products Inc.)

Limb immobilisation can be achieved in a variety of ways including the use of vacuum bag systems or positioning moulds (Figure 7.15).

Alternatively, thermoplastic materials can be employed that can completely immobilise the treated limb. For lesions of the lower limb it is possible to construct an immobilisation 'boot' which anchors the ankle joint and prevents rotational movements. Where used with sagittal skin tattoos a high degree of reproducibility can be afforded. However, it is important to consider immobilising the entire affected limb using an immobilisation shell to prevent movement. In the upper limb similar positioning strategies are used, although it is favourable to choose immobilisation devices that permit the affected limb to be positioned in the abducted position so as not to inadvertently include the normal tissues of the trunk or axilla. CT planning of limbs can prove to be technically difficult, particularly when there is a need for the elevation of the unaffected limb. In this case there is a need to adapt the position of the contralateral limb during the scanning procedure so that the patient will be clear of the CT aperture.

7.19 Immobilisation of the Paediatric Radiotherapy Patient

Whilst they form a small proportion of patients referred for radiotherapy, there may be significant difficulties and challenges in the treatment of children with radiotherapy. For these patients, anaesthesia or sedation may be a necessary strategy to ensure the elimination of excessive movement, particularly as in many cases there are tight constraints with respect to the proximity of the location of OARs and the high-dose volume. Irradiation of the central nervous system in particular may prove to be challenging, as usual approaches to patient immobilisation (i.e. the use of an immobilisation head shell) may be distressing to the very young. The use of general anaesthesia or sedation is usually indicated in the youngest of patients who may lack the understanding of the need for remaining still during treatment. In addition, increased complexity of the technique of radiotherapy procedures is accompanied by protracted treatment times. Paediatric general anaesthesia brings with it a number of additional technical and practical challenges with many radiotherapy departments requiring suitable spaces allocated for anaesthetic induction and patient recovery. The emergence of the specialist paediatric therapeutic radiographer has aided in the management of the administration of paediatric radiotherapy, and their role as a treatment coordinator is invaluable. Special consideration is needed for management of aspects of concurrent treatment such as careful management of chemotherapy central lines and other aspects of patient care. In addition, it is important to coordinate the process of anaesthesia itself to include management of anaesthetic-associated patient fasting and the impact of this on patient nutrition [39].

7.19.1 The Role of Play Therapies During Paediatric Radiotherapy

Play therapy or play preparation refers to the use of a specialist healthcare professional responsible for the psychological preparation of the patient via interactive play. Fundamentally play therapy ensures that the youngest radiotherapy patients may have their radiotherapy procedures explained via the use of language and communication techniques particular to their individual stage of development [40]. This allows for a greater degree of cooperation, and for some children play therapy may reduce the need for sedation or anaesthesia (although this also likely to be dependent on the age of the patient). Play as a specific intervention may be employed throughout the radiotherapy planning and delivery process including pretreatment planning and treatment administration. This also extends to the inclusion of immobilisation devices themselves within play therapy. Thermoplastic masks may be safely decorated according to the wishes of the patient and may serve to reduce apprehension or fear of the process of immobilisation itself by affording the patient a degree of control and choice over an otherwise difficult situation for them. Achieving anaesthesia-free treatment delivery may also be achieved via play strategies whilst the patient is secured into the treatment position. This may include use of toys or audiovisual tools (such as DVDs [digital versatile discs]) as a distraction technique.

7.20 Stereotactic Radiotherapy

Stereotactic radiotherapy involves the use of multiple small conformal beams of radiation that are precisely administered to the patient. This is usually achieved via the use of a three-dimensional external coordinate system that is used to localise the intended treatment site within the patient. Adequate immobilisation is a necessary prerequisite to ensure treatment accuracy, and for treatment sites in the head region the positioning strategy requires elimination of all head motion such that the head is completely restrained: usually achieved via the use of a dedicated head frame that incorporates a three-dimensional referencing system permitting positioning accuracy in the order of 1 mm.

Invasive immobilisation devices were originally used for such purposes, whereby a *stereotactic head frame* such as the Brown–Roberts–Wells device was attached directly to the head via self-tapping cranial screws secured under anaesthesia. This head ring or 'halo' device thus served to fix the patient's head whilst presenting a reliable set of external stereotactic coordinate points. These are of use in single fraction treatments (stereotactic radiosurgery), e.g. in the delivery of treatment of an arteriovenous malformation (AVM); however, they are generally considered too uncomfortable for protracted radiotherapy treatments over a number of days (stereotactic radiotherapy).

Non-invasive, relocatable, head immobilisation devices are available for use in fractionated techniques. Many of these utilise a custom-made bite-block system in which the patient bites down on an integral bespoke bite plate constructed from dental impression material (Figure 7.16).

A vacuum cushion may also be used in an effort to reduce lateral deviation and rotation of the head. Additional head support may be offered via the use of head fixation straps, individualised occipital pads, or an external fixation device such as a thermoplastic shell.

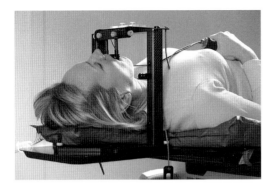

FIGURE 7.16 Immobilisation system for stereotactic radiotherapy using bite block and vacuum bag cushion. (Source: Image courtesy of Elekta Ltd.)

Stereotactic radiotherapy techniques may also be undertaken at other extracranial locations, e.g. within the thorax, abdomen, or pelvis. This is usually achieved using a suitable immobilisation device such as a vacuum bag coupled with an external *stereotactic body frame*, which provides a referencing system for accurate definition of the coordinates of an internal target during CT or MRI planning procedures. Organ motion can compromise the accuracy of target localisation at these sites however, and it may be necessary to adopt the use of organ stabilisation strategies (e.g. ABC) in tandem with stereotactic body immobilisation. SABR involves the precise irradiation of a lesion and is associated with the use of a high radiation dose delivered in a small number of fractions, and a highly conformal dose distribution with very tight margins is favoured. Given that the daily dose administered for such patients is much greater than in conventional radiotherapy (e.g. 11 Gy per fraction with lung SABR) it is clear that inaccurate or imprecise treatment delivery would have a significant impact on the patient.

7.21 Conclusion

In this chapter we have explored a variety of techniques by which patients may be immobilised to assure treatment reproducibility. It has been shown that current notions of treatment accuracy extend to the consideration of the physiological and anatomical translocation of organs between and during treatments. Strategies to manage these phenomena include a close analysis of anatomy and organ motion via routine patient imaging, management of normal anatomical motion (such as breathing motion), and adaptive techniques. Development of new technologies including MRI linear accelerators and routine use of new modalities such as proton radiotherapy require accuracy and reproducibility to be considered as the cornerstone of effective radiotherapy administration.

Acknowledgements

The authors of this chapter would like to acknowledge the information provided by the various manufacturers mentioned in the text.

References

1. Probst, H., Dodwell, D., Gray, J.C., and Holmes, M. (2006). An evaluation of the accuracy of semi-permanent skin marks for breast cancer irradiation. *Radiography* 12: 186–188.
2. Clow, B. and Allen, J. (2010). Psychosocial impacts of radiation tattooing for breast cancer patients. *Canadian Woman Studies* 28: 46–52.
3. O'Neill, A., McAleer, S., McCarty, H. et al. (2018). Semi-permanent tattoos in breast radiotherapy (STaBRad) study: a randomised-controlled clinical trial comparing the 'Precision Plus Micropigmentation System' to permanent skin tattoos in radical breast radiotherapy patients. *Journal of Radiotherapy in Practice* 17: 12–19.
4. International Commission on Radiation Units and Measurements (1994). *Prescribing, Recording, and Reporting Photon Beam Therapy ICRU Report 50*. Bethesda, MD: ICRU Publications.
5. International Commission on Radiation Units and Measurements (1999). *Prescribing, Recording, and Reporting Photon Beam Therapy (Supplement to ICRU Report 50). ICRU Report 62*. Bethesda, MD: ICRU Publications.

6. National Cancer Action Team (2012). *National Radiotherapy Implementation Group Report Image Guided Radiotherapy (IGRT) – Guidance for Implementation and Use*. London: NCAT.

7. International Commission on Radiation Units and Measurements (2010). *Prescribing, Recording, and Reporting Intensity-Modulated Photon-Beam Therapy (IMRT) ICRU Report 83*. Bethesda, MD: ICRU Publications.

8. Kim, S.W., Shin, H.J., Kay, C.S., and Son, S.H. (2014). A customized bolus produced using a 3-dimensional printer for radiotherapy. *PLoS One* 9 (10): e110746.

9. Park, J.W., Oh, S.A., Yea, J.W., and Kang, M.K. (2017). Fabrication of malleable three-dimensional-printed customized bolus using three-dimensional scanner. *PLoS One* 12: e0177562.

10. Bomford, C.K. and Kunkler, I.H. (2003). *Walter and Miller's Textbook of Radiotherapy*, 6e. Edinburgh: Churchill Livingstone.

11. Newbold, K.L., Bhide, S., Convery, H. et al. (2012). Prospective intra-patient evaluation of a shoulder retraction device for radiotherapy in head and neck cancer. *Medical Dosimetry* 37 (3): 293–295.

12. Wroe, A.J., Bush, D.A., Schulte, R.W., and Slater, J.D. (2015). Clinical immobilization techniques for proton therapy. *Technology in Cancer Research and Treament* 14 (1): 71–79.

13. Bussière, M.R. and Adams, J.A. (2003). Treatment planning for conformal proton radiation therapy. *Technology in Cancer Research and Treament* 2 (5): 389–399.

14. Winfield, E.A., Deighton, A., Venables, K. et al. (2003). Survey of tangential field planning and dose distribution in the UK: background to the introduction of the quality assurance programme for the START trial in early breast cancer. *British Journal of Radiology* 76: 254–259.

15. Nalder, C.A., Bidmead, A.M., Mubata, C.D., and Beardmore, C. (2001). Influence of a vac-fix immobilization device on the accuracy of patient positioning during routine breast radiotherapy. *British Journal of Radiology* 74: 249–254.

16. Latimer, J.G., Beckham, W., West, M. et al. (2005). Support of large breast during tangential irradiation using a micro-shell and minimizing the skin dose – a pilot study. *Medical Dosimetry* 30: 31–35.

17. Algan, Ö., Fowble, B., McNeeley, S., and Fein, D. (1998). Use of the prone position in radiation treatment for women with early stage breast cancer. *International Journal of Radiation Oncology, Biology, Physics* 40: 1137–1140.

18. Stegman, L.D., Beal, K.P., Hunt, M.A. et al. (2007). Long-term clinical outcomes of whole-breast irradiation delivered in the prone position. *International Journal of Radiation Oncology, Biology, Physics* 68 (1): 73–81.

19. Keller, L.M.M., Cohen, R., Sopka, D.M. et al. (2013). Effect of bra use during radiation therapy for large-breasted women: acute toxicity and treated heart and lung volumes. *Practical Radiation Oncology* 3 (1): 9–15.

20. Cancer Research UK. 2018. *A study about the S4A support bra for women having radiotherapy for breast cancer*. https://www.cancerresearchuk.org/about-cancer/find-a-clinical-trial/a-study-about-the-s4a-support-bra-for-women-having-radiotherapy-for-breast-cancer (Accessed 25.10.18).

21. Wong, J.W., Sharpe, M.B., Jaffray, D.A. et al. (1999). The use of active breathing control (ABC) to reduce margin for breathing motion. *International Journal of Radiation Oncology, Biology, Physics* 44: 911–919.

22. Ledsom, D., Reilly, A.J., and Probst, H. (2018). Assessment of deep inspiration breath hold (DIBH) amplitude and reduction in cardiac dose in left breast cancer patients. *Radiography* 24: 98–103.

23. Langmack, K. and Routsis, D. (2001). Towards an evidence based treatment technique in prostate radiotherapy. *Journal of Radiotherapy in Practice* 2: 91–100.

24. Mitine, C., Hoornaert, M., Dutreix, A., and Beauduin, M. (1999). Radiotherapy of pelvic malignancies: impact of two types of rigid immobilisation devices on localisation errors. *Radiotherapy and Oncology* 52: 19–27.

25. Weber, D., Nouet, P., Rouzaud, M., and Miralbell, R. (2000). Patient positioning in prostate radiotherapy: is prone better than supine? *International Journal of Radiation Oncology, Biology, Physics* 47: 365–371.

26. Logmans, A., Trimbon, J.B., and van Lent, M. (1995). The omentoplasty: a neglected ally in gynaecologic surgery. *European Journal of Obstetrics and Gynaecology* 58: 167–171.

27. Allal, A.S., Bischof, S., and Nouet, P. (2002). Impact of the 'belly board' device on treatment reproducibility in preoperative radiotherapy for rectal cancer. *Strahlentherapie und Onkologie* 5: 259–262.

28. Malone, S., Szanto, J., Perry, G. et al. (2000). A prospective comparison of three systems of patient immobilisation for prostate radiotherapy. *International Journal of Radiation Oncology, Biology, Physics* 48: 657–665.

29. Patel, R., Orton, N., Tomé, W.A. et al. (2003). Rectal dose sparing with a balloon catheter and ultrasound localization in conformal radiation therapy for prostate cancer. *Radiotherapy and Oncology* 67: 285–294.

30. Bridge, P. (2004). A critical evaluation of internal organ immobilisation techniques. *Journal of Radiotherapy in Practice* 4: 118–125.

31. Jadon, R., Pembroke, C.A., Hanna, C.L. et al. (2014). A systematic review of organ motion and image-guided strategies in external beam radiotherapy for cervical cancer. *Clinical Oncology* 26 (4): 185–196.

32. Teh, B.S., McGary, J.E., Dong, L. et al. (2002). The use of rectal balloon during the delivery of intensity modulated radiotherapy (IMRT) for prostate cancer: more than just a prostate gland immobilization device? *The Cancer Journal* 8: 476–483.

33. Pinkawa, M., Corral, N.E., Caffaro, M. et al. (2011). Application of a spacer gel to optimize three-dimensional conformal and intensity modulated radiotherapy for prostate cancer. *Radiotherapy and Oncology* 100: 436–441.

34. Vanneste, B.G., Pijls-Johannesma, M., Van De Voorde, L. et al. (2015). Spacers in radiotherapy treatment of prostate cancer: is reduction of toxicity cost-effective? *Radiotherapy and Oncology* 114 (2): 276–281.

35. Alexander, S.E., Kinsella, J., McNair, H.A., and Tree, A.C. (2018). National survey of fiducial marker insertion for prostate image guided radiotherapy. *Radiography* 24 (4): 275–282.

36. Hynds, S., McGarry, C.K., Mitchell, D.M. et al. (2011). Assessing the daily consistency of bladder filling using an ultrasonic Bladder-scan device in men receiving radical conformal radiotherapy for prostate cancer. *British Journal of Radiology* 84: 813–818.

37. Spencer, K., Parrish, R., Barton, R., and Henry, A. (2018). Palliative radiotherapy. *British Medical Journal* 360: k821.

38. McCarroll, R.E., Beadle, B.M., Fullen, D. et al. (2017). Reproducibility of patient setup in the seated treatment position: a novel treatment chair design. *Journal of Applied Clinical Medical Physics* 18: 223–229.

39. Stackhouse, C. (2013). The use of general anaesthesia in paediatric radiotherapy. *Radiography* 19: 302–330.

40. Scott, L., Langton, F., and O'Donoghue, J. (2002). Minimising the use of sedation/anaesthesia in young children receiving radiotherapy through an effective play preparation programme. *European Journal of Oncology Nursing* 6 (1): 15–22.

Further Reading

Bentel, G. (1999). *Patient Positioning and Immobilization in Radiation Oncology*. London: McGraw-Hill.

Marcu, L., Bezak, E., and Allen, B. (2012). *Biomedical Physics in Radiotherapy for Cancer*. Collingwood: CSIRO Publishing.

CHAPTER 8

Radiotherapy Beam Production

David Flinton

Aim

The aim of this chapter is to describe the equipment used to deliver radiotherapy, including kilovoltage, linear accelerators, cyclotrons, gamma knife, and intraoperative radiotherapy. To complete this chapter there is a section on the current treatment techniques used to deliver radiotherapy.

8.1 Introduction

Most of the equipment used to deliver radiotherapy is detailed within this chapter, the exclusion being brachytherapy systems (see Chapter 14). The chapter is divided into various sections, each dealing with a different type of equipment.

8.2 Kilovoltage Equipment

Kilovoltage units once dominated the provision of external beam radiotherapy, until *cobalt-60 units* and then *linear accelerators* were introduced, both of which could offer

improved delivery of dose at depth and, in the case of linear accelerators, *superficial therapy* with electrons. Despite this, kilovoltage units remain useful in the treatment of superficial conditions, especially small tumours or conditions near the eye where they have advantages over electron therapy. The current Department of Health recommendation [1] is that a superficial unit be part of the minimum complement of treatment units present in a radiotherapy department. Currently there are approximately 58 units in the UK, treating about 6000 patients a year [2].

8.2.1 Range of Kilovoltage Energies

X-ray therapy of kilovoltage beams can be divided into the three areas described below, arranged according to their degree of beam penetration [3]. Despite this classification of beams, treatment units will not necessarily fall into just one category because they usually offer a range of energies that may cross these boundaries:

- **Very low energy:** X-rays with a half-value layer (HVL) between 0.0035 mm and 1 mm of aluminium (Al). X-rays

Practical Radiotherapy: Physics and Equipment, Third Edition. Edited by Pam Cherry and Angela M. Duxbury.
© 2020 John Wiley & Sons Ltd. Published 2020 by John Wiley & Sons Ltd.

generated at an accelerating potential of <50 kV. Sometimes beams in this energy range, particularly those with a generating voltage below 30 kV are referred to as *Grenz rays*. This type of beam is not commonly used in the UK, but it is used with more frequency in both Germany and the USA. This energy is used primarily in the treatment of inflammatory skin conditions such as eczema and psoriasis, which have other safer methods of treatment available including topical use of emollients and steroid creams, non-topical treatments such as retinoids, and immunosuppressant light therapy. As a result of these 'safer' options in the UK it is recommended [4] that very low energy X-rays are used only on inflammatory skin conditions that are either unresponsive to these other treatments or under research conditions.

- **Low energy:** X-rays with an HVL between 1 and 8 mm of Al. The X-rays are generated at a potential difference between 50 and 160 kV. Treatment is usually reserved for small superficial lesions on the skin. In the past beams using a generating voltage between 50 and 150 kV were referred to as *superficial*.

- **Medium energy:** X-rays with an HVL >8 mm Al, covering the X-rays generated at a potential of between 160 and 500 kV. Beams of these energies are primarily used in the treatment of skin tumours, but the higher-energy units can have a role to play in the palliative treatment of metastases. Beams generated using a potential of between 150 and 500 kV were referred to as *orthovoltage* or *deep X-ray*.

Contact therapy is a specialised form of kilovoltage treatment that is predominantly used in the treatment of rectal carcinomas using a technique that is sometimes referred to as a Papillon treatment, after the doctor who developed it in the 1950s, or endocavity irradiation. Surgery is the main treatment method for rectal cancer and the Papillon method is usually reserved for patients who decline surgery or are not fit enough for the standard treatment, although it can also be used before or after surgery to reduce the risk of local recurrence [5]. The treatment utilises an X-ray unit operating at a generating voltage of between 40 and 50 kV. The patient can be treated on an outpatient basis with a local anaesthetic that allows a proctoscope to be inserted and positioned over the tumour. The X-ray tube applicator then fits into the proctoscope and comes into contact with the tumour.

The main reason for this type of treatment is the physical property of an extremely rapid fall-off of dose in tissue rather than a radiobiological advantage. The depth dose falls from a surface dose of 100% to 60% at 5 mm depth, so allowing a high local dose to the tumour whilst sparing normal tissue. Typical total doses are 90 or 110 Gy in three or four fractions delivered every two weeks.

8.3 Superficial and Orthovoltage Equipment

The main components for this type of equipment are a generator, control console, tube mounting, X-ray tube, cooling system and collimators; an optional patient information system can also be used.

8.3.1 Generator

A generator serves to increase the main voltage to the voltages required for X-ray production through the use of transformers, and then rectifies and smooths the waveform (see Chapter 3). These actions increase the efficacy of X-ray production and increase the stability of the beam output, the electrons being accelerated by an almost constant potential difference across the tube.

At higher energies it is necessary to use two balanced generators operating together: one to supply the negative potential to the cathode, and the second the positive potential to the anode. Tubes that have this arrangement are called 'bipolar tubes'; the anode has a positive potential and the cathode a negative potential with respect to the ground potential (earth). This is a safer arrangement at higher voltages because this effectively halves the maximum voltage that any one component may have. The lower-energy tubes working off one generator are termed 'unipolar', the cathode having a selectable negative potential and the anode always being at ground potential.

8.3.2 Control Console

Modern control consoles contain a microprocessor to monitor and manage the exposure and in some cases, a dual microprocessor that allows an independent backup timer for safety.

All operating parameters that affect or could affect dose delivery and radiation quality must be displayed on the console, which can be interlocked with numerous tube components, and a select and confirm system ensures correct choice of treatment parameters, such as energy, filter, and collimator. Certain units are interlocked in such a way that inserting the filter automatically defines beam energy selection.

The control panel is switched on via a key that should be kept safe when the unit is not in operation. Typical data inputted/confirmed by the operator are: dose/time set, time limit (usually 5% greater than the expected duration of treatment), filter, applicator, kV, and mA. (Most modern units contain an ionisation chamber in the sub-tube assembly which allows treatment to be performed by setting dose [monitor units, MU] as opposed to treatment time, which is used in the older X-ray units.) Other information available before and during treatment are: a light signifying whether X-rays are on; the dose rate; and the dose administered/time treated. Pausing the treatment is possible via an interrupt key, or the treatment may be terminated via the stop button. In the case of power failure an internal battery will maintain details of the treatment up to the point of power failure which can be recorded. A separate operating mode also exists that is accessible by either password or a separate key that allows physicists/engineers to calibrate the unit and configure parameters.

8.3.3 Tube Mounting

The mounting for kilovoltage units, unlike linear accelerators, is not *isocentric* (Figure 8.1). Units are usually either supported by the use of a ceiling support or have a floor-mounted stand and require manual force for any movement to occur. Movement can usually occur in three axes – longitudinal, transverse, and vertical – as well as the tube being able to rotate as well as tilt. Counterweights and tensator springs help provide a consistent resistance and allow a smooth, even movement of the tube, as well as allow accurate fine positioning movements. Use of electromagnetic brakes helps improve accuracy of setup, locking the movement when desired – an advantage over the mechanical locks used on older units, which often used to give further tube movement when applied. In the case of power failure, the mounting system must maintain the weight of the tube

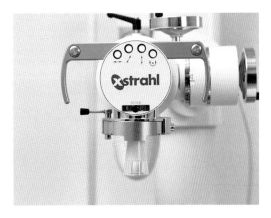

FIGURE 8.1 Kilovoltage unit. (Source: image courtesy of Xstrahl Ltd.)

and allow the patient to be removed; this can be done by freeing all the locks except the vertical movement, so allowing the tube to be removed from the patient with no danger of the tube descending onto them.

8.3.4 Tube Design

The basic tube design is dissimilar to both the tube described in Chapters 3 and 6. The standard design used is that of a stationary anode (Figure 8.2). Recent developments in the design of kilovoltage tubes have seen the gradual replacement of the glass-enveloped X-ray tube, used for over 80 years with metal-ceramic tubes. The use of metal-ceramic tubes has several advantages. Metal-ceramic tubes are smaller and more robust than glass tubes of equivalent energy. They enable more flexibility in the electrical circuitry associated with the tube and have a higher output.

Metal-ceramic tubes consist of a cathode assembly held within an evacuated tube. A ceramic insulator holds the assembly in place and electrically insulates it from the metal tube envelope. The cathode assembly consists of a single *tungsten filament* that is heated by an electrical current passing through it. Tungsten may be doped with another element such as rhenium to lower the work function further, which means that less heat energy is needed to

remove an electron from the material. When hot the filament emits electrons by *thermionic emission*. The filament is set into a *focusing cup* which has a static negative charge on it. The static charge stops the electrons from spreading out, forcing them together, and ensuring that the electron beam moving to the anode has a small cross-sectional area.

The anode structure is either welded directly to the metal tube envelope or isolated from the envelope by *ceramic insulators*. The target is recessed within a copper anode, which provides a hood for the anode. Situated on one side of the hood is a *beryllium* ($Z = 4$, $A = 9$) window. Because of beryllium's low atomic number, mass, and density it is relatively transparent to X-rays, so allowing the desired X-rays to exit whilst the hood removes the unwanted low-energy X-rays produced by electrons hitting the anode outside the target area (extra-focal radiation).

The target is usually made of tungsten due to its high atomic number ($Z = 74$). A high atomic number material is usually used as it is more efficient at producing X-rays.

$$\text{Efficiency of X-ray production} = 9 \times 10^{-10} \, Z \, V$$

$$(8.1)$$

Where Z is the atomic number of the target metal and V the tube voltage.

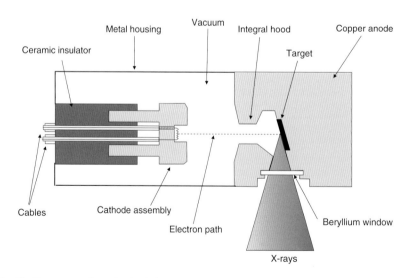

FIGURE 8.2 Stationary anode unipolar tube.

Using this formula Eq. (8.1), for a tube operating at 300 kV the efficiency would be approximately 2%, the other 98% of energy deposited in the target being turned into heat.

The *target angle* is usually in the order of 30° in kilovoltage treatment tubes. This is a lot higher than the 17° used in the simulator tube or 5–17° found in the various diagnostic X-ray tubes. Having a target angle of this magnitude affects the photon beam in a number of ways. Firstly, the larger target angle causes the apparent *focal spot* to be larger, which could have the effect of increasing the geometric penumbra; however, this is negated by collimating at, or close to, the patient's surface. The second effect is to reduce the 'anode heel effect', which is caused by self-attenuation of the beam in the target material. As the amount of material travelled through depends on the exit direction, we get a variation in X-ray intensity (photon fluence) across the anode–cathode axis of the beam (Figure 8.3). This effect cannot be removed completely but is reduced in tubes with large target angles. In tubes operating over a range of energies the anode heel effect is energy dependent: the greater the generating voltage the deeper the electron interaction in the target, and the

greater the degree of attenuation within the target.

All tubes have *inherent filtration* which, together with the added filtration, will give the total filtration of the beam. The inherent filtration consists of the beryllium window of the hood and the tube window, the Xstrahl 150 system having an inherent filtration of 0.8 ± 1 mm of beryllium.

8.3.5 Cooling System

In stationary X-ray tubes most of the heat is removed from the target via conduction. *Thermal conduction* is dependent on four factors: the material, cross-sectional area, temperature difference, and length, the last being an inverse relationship. Copper is used because it is an extremely good thermal conductor, having a thermal conductivity of 385 W/m/K compared to 130 W/m/K for tungsten. There has to be an extremely good thermal link between the tungsten target and copper anode to allow heat to be easily transferred into the copper. The copper block in which the target is set is relatively large, allowing easy passage of the heat energy to

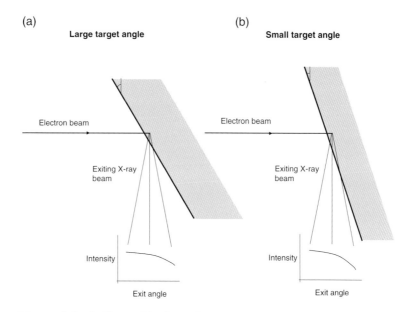

(a) **Large target angle**
(b) **Small target angle**

Electron beam

Exiting X-ray beam

Intensity

Exit angle

FIGURE 8.3 The anode heel effect and its dependence on target angle.

the cooling system. The cooling system maintains a high temperature difference across the anode so ensuring rapid removal of heat away from the target.

At lower energies, because the X-ray tube is unipolar in design (the anode is at earth potential), water can be used to cool the anode. Either the heated water is then replaced with new cool water (lost water system) or the water can be recirculated, having been cooled by a refrigeration unit or fan. For the higher-energy bipolar tubes, because the anode is not at earth potential, water can no longer be used as a cooling agent as it is a conductor of electricity, so oil is used instead as it is an electrical insulator. The heated oil is then cooled using either air or water.

8.3.6 Collimation

The common method of beam collimation for kilovoltage energies is removable applicators. Applicators allow the operator to easily see if the beam direction is perpendicular to the skin's surface (skin apposition) and ensures that stand-off, if present, is even and minimal. This is important because stand-off and stand-in can have major consequences to the dose

received (see inverse square law, Chapter 2). Another function of the applicator is to define the treatment distance. Applicators can be found in a range of different focus skin distances (FSDs), ranging from about 15 to 50 cm, the larger FSDs generally offering larger field sizes.

The applicator assembly (Figure 8.4) consists of a rigid baseplate, which is used to attach the applicator to the unit. Within the baseplate is a layer of lead of sufficient thickness to collimate the beam to less than 1% of the incident intensity. Within the lead is an aperture that collimates the beam to the desired field size. A second layer of lead may be present where the wall of the applicator joins with the plastic end cap. This second lead insert acts to trim the penumbra of the beam, effectively collimating the beam near the skin's surface. A photograph of a selection of applicators can be seen in Figure 8.5. Note the small indentations visible on the base plate of some of the applicators that form part of the interlock system that identifies the applicator when in use.

The walls of the applicator are made from either steel or copper. The walls of the applicator do not receive any primary radiation and their primary function is to attenuate any

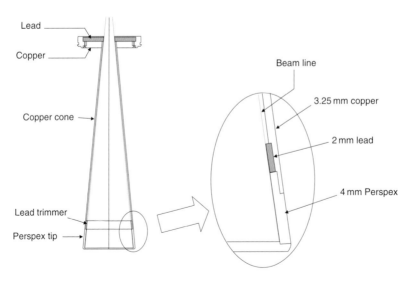

FIGURE 8.4 Typical kilovoltage applicator. (Source: adapted from an image provided by Xstrahl Ltd.)

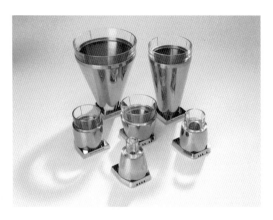

FIGURE 8.5   Open ended kV applicators. (Source: image courtesy of Xstrahl Ltd.)

scattered radiation, which will be of low energy. The plastic end of the applicator can be of either an open or a closed design. With closed-end applicators it is possible to add a little compression when treating, which can allow the smoothing out of uneven surfaces, so reducing variation of stand-off. Compression should be avoided with open-ended tube designs because this can lead to stand-in of tissue, the soft tissue 'bulging' into the applicator, leading to a higher dose being received than expected. The plastic end cap also has lines etched onto the plastic of visual reference marks that can aid with the correct placement of the applicator.

Applicators are only available in set sizes and shapes, and further beam shaping might be needed to limit the radiation field to the desired treatment area. This can be achieved by the use of cutouts consisting of sheets of lead or a low melting point alloy (LMPA). Cutouts are shaped to the body contour and sit on the patient, covering the area needing to be shielded with a hole cutout of the lead in the desired shape of the field. The applicator is then positioned over the cutout. The thickness of the material used for the cutout is dependent on the beam energy but should reduce the dose to at least 5% of the incident beam. The cutout effectively reduces the area of the beam, reducing the amount of scatter produced and so affects the dose rate. Because of this change in dose when a cutout is used, a cutout factor needs to be applied.

8.3.7 Beam Quality

The penetrating power of a beam varies with beam energy and it is usual with megavoltage beams to describe quality by stating the generating potential used. For kilovoltage beams this is not sufficient because filters are used that can significantly affect the emerging beam's quality. As a result of this it is more usual at these energies to use both the generating voltage and the HVL of the beam to describe beam quality.

8.3.8 Filtration

The quality of the beam exiting the tube can be improved by the addition of filters into the beam. A filter holder is positioned after the primary collimator and is interlocked so that the machine cannot be switched on without a filter present. Quality filters are usually made of one the following three materials: aluminium, copper, and tin. Composite filters can also be used that are made from two or more of the materials. Composite filters consist of layers of material that are always arranged in order of decreasing atomic number as you move away from the target. Each of the materials has a k absorption edge associated with it: the higher the atomic number of the material, the higher the energy that the absorption edge has. The absorption edge for tin occurs at 29.2 keV and above this energy tin is a good absorber of X-rays, but just below this energy the amount of photoelectric absorption is much smaller. Characteristic radiation will also be created by the interaction with the k-shell electrons at energies between 25 and 29 keV. Copper's absorption edge is smaller occurring at 9 keV, and so will be a good attenuator of X-rays just above this energy, which will include most of the energies below 29.2 keV and the characteristic X-rays from the tin. Aluminium's absorption edge is 1.6 keV so will cause a significant reduction of X-rays above 1.6 keV, and so will significantly reduce the low energy X-rays that the copper has let through as well as its characteristic X-rays (see Chapter 5). A quality filter made of tin, copper, and aluminium is sometimes referred to as a *Thoraeus filter*.

As the unit cannot work without a filter the units are provided with warm-up filters. Warm-up filters are usually made of lead, to absorb most of the primary beam, but some low-energy warm-up filters can be made from brass. Warming up the unit is very important as it allows heat to build up slowly in the tube through a series of short exposures of increasing energy so preventing uneven expansion in the tube due to thermal stress and prolonging the life of the tube. Some units have automatic warm-up sequences; in the Xstrahl Medical consoles these are automatically stored and displayed on power-up ready to be run before clinical use. Depending on the idle time of the unit this may have to be repeated during the day.

8.3.9 Kilovoltage Beam Characteristics

At kilovoltage energy the interaction effect is a mixture of the photoelectric effect and Compton scattering. Both interactions give rise to electrons that will be absorbed close to their site of production. Compton also gives rise to scattered photons which may travel a significant distance in tissue before depositing their energy. A significant amount of scatter is sideways and backwards (*backscatter*). The sideways scatter explains one of the characteristics of isodose curves for kilovoltage beams (see Chapter 5). The sharp edge to the beam is caused by the collimation at or near the skin's surface. Beyond this sharp edge are small amounts of radiation caused by scattered radiation moving outside the exposed area.

The amount of backscatter depends on the field size, tissue, and beam quality (Figure 8.6)

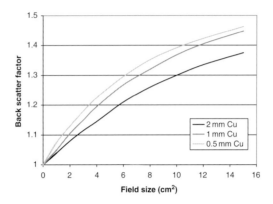

FIGURE 8.6 Effect of field size and energy on backscatter.

used as well as the thickness of underlying tissue but is independent of the treatment distance. The *backscatter factor* (BSF) can be calculated using Eq. (8.2), where $K_{air,s}$ is the air kerma rate at the surface of a water phantom, $K_{air,f}$ is the air kerma rate at the same point with the phantom removed, $(\mu_{en}/\rho)_{w,air}$ is the ratio of the mass energy absorption coefficients for water and air in the presence of the scattering medium or free space. According to Klevenhagen and Thwaites [6] only small differences in beam quality occur on going from free space to surface irradiation, so although not strictly true we can assume that the (μ_{en}/ρ) terms cancel each other out and BSF can be calculated from the simpler equation – Eq. (8.3).

$$\text{BSF} = \frac{K_{air,s}\left(\left[\mu_{en}/\rho\right]_{w,air}\right)_{s}}{K_{air,f}\left(\left[\mu_{en}/\rho\right]_{w,air}\right)_{f}} \qquad (8.2)$$

$$\text{BSF} = \frac{K_{air,s}}{K_{air,f}} \qquad (8.3)$$

Backscatter can also have a major effect on dose received when lead is used as shielding behind the target volume. The interactions that occur in the lead shielding can cause a significant increase in dose on the beam side of the lead due to the high backscatter component at these energies. This can effectively be removed by coating the lead shielding with a tissue-equivalent material such as wax that will absorb the backscatter before it reaches the patient.

8.4 Inverse Square Law

Application of the inverse square law is especially important at kilovoltage energies due to the short treatment distances used when compared with linear accelerators. Small changes in treatment distance can lead to significant changes in dose. The importance of this variation in treatment distance, 'stand-off and stand-in', is therefore especially important at kilovoltage energy. Figure 8.7 shows how treatment distance can affect the dose received at some commonly used kilovoltage treatment distances compared with a treatment distance of 100 cm FSD.

Where stand-off and stand-in occurs, a factor can be calculated that can be used to modify the dose per MU at the surface of the patient (Eq. 8.4):

$$\text{Stand-off} = \frac{\text{FSD}^2}{\text{FSD} + \text{Stand-off}^2}$$

$$\text{Stand-in} = \frac{\text{FSD}^2}{\text{FSD} - \text{Stand-in}^2} \qquad (8.4)$$

These factors can then be used with the dose rate to calculate the modified dose rate due to the inverse square law. To calculate the dose at the surface, the reference surface dose rate needs to have the following factors

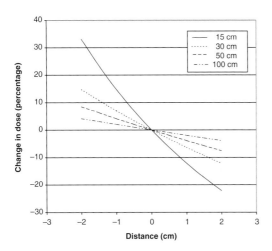

FIGURE 8.7 Effect of changes in treatment distance on the dose received.

applied: applicator factor, BSF and stand-off/in factor, and cutout factor if used.

8.5 Quality Assurance Tests

Daily, monthly, and annual quality assurance tests are usually carried out by physicists or radiographers. Daily functional checks of the treatment unit should include: tube movement in all dimensions and that the locks work; filter interlocks work correctly; beam status indicators work; beam turns off when the key is turned to the off position; emergency off and interrupt buttons all function correctly; the kV and mA are both correctly displayed; and correct operation of backup timer.

Output of the unit should be checked using a Farmer ionisation chamber or other suitable detector at the chosen energy and filter combinations. Other checks that should also be carried out before treatment are: to ensure that the patient monitoring devices work; door interlocks terminate treatment; and that the couch movement and brakes all work correctly.

Table 8.1 shows tests recommended within the IPEM (Institute of Physics and Engineering in Medicine) report and their tolerances. It also shows the recommended frequency of testing and results from a study by Palmer et al. [2] indicating the number performing the tests as recommended within the report.

8.6 Linear Accelerators

8.6.1 Introduction

The production of photon beams using a conventional X-ray tube permits a maximum beam energy only in the kilovoltage region. To produce higher-energy beams a different technology is required: the linear accelerator. The aim of this section is to provide an overview of this technology, and the mechanisms of production of a clinical beam.

TABLE 8.1 Kilovoltage unit quality control tests and frequency of testing in UK radiotherapy centres.

Parameter	IPEM Report 81 recommended	% following recommendation	Tolerance (IPEM Report 81)
Interlocks	Daily	83%	functional
Fixtures	Daily	33%	functional
Filter interlocks	Daily/weekly	49% perform test daily	functional
Output constancy	Daily	93%	±5%
Output	Monthly	64%	±3%
Timer accuracy	Monthly	57%	±2%
Linearity	Monthly	34%	±2%
Backup timer	Monthly	56%	functional
Radiation field size	Monthly	38%	±2 mm
HVL constancy	Monthly	62%	±10%
HVL full check	Annually	62%	±10%
Field uniformity	Annually	49%	±5%
Applicator factors	Annually	60%	±3%
Focal spot	Unspecified	Most check on commissioning only 44%	functional

Source: Adapted from Palmer et al. [2].

8.6.2 C-Arm Linear Accelerators

Three manufacturers – Accuray, Elekta, and Varian – dominate the linear accelerator market. Linear accelerators (LinAcs) are machines that consist of several discrete components (Figure 8.8) functioning together to accelerate electrons to a high energy using radiofrequency (RF) waves before the electrons 'hit' a target to produce X-rays. After this the X-ray profile is flattened, shaped (collimated), and measured before clinical use. Linear accelerators are now also capable of producing X-ray beams of different energy (*multi-energy units*) and/or producing both X-rays and electrons (*multimodal units*).

8.7 Production and Transport of the RF Wave

8.7.1 RF Generators, the Magnetron, and Klystron

To accelerate the electrons to the required energy an RF wave is needed. This can be produced from one of two devices: either a magnetron or a klystron.

The magnetron consists of a cathode situated in the middle of a circular chamber which, when heated, releases electrons by

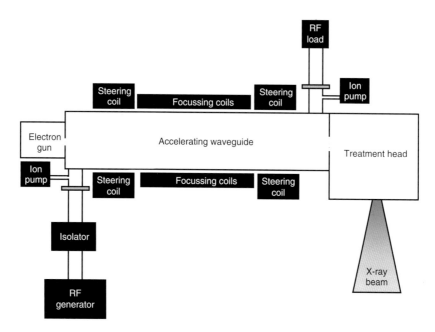

FIGURE 8.8 Major components of the linear accelerator.

thermionic emission. Surrounding the cathode but separated by an open evacuated space (called the interaction space) is the anode which has cavities milled into its structure. Above and below the magnetron as drawn is a permanent magnet that produces an axial magnetic field. The magnetic field is perpendicular to the electron's initial radial motion, which causes the electrons produced by the cathode to spiral outward in a circular path rather than moving directly to the anode (see later section on Lorentz forces).

The cloud of electrons, influenced by both the high voltage and the strong magnetic field, form a rotating pattern called a 'space charge wheel' that resembles the spokes of a spinning wheel (Figure 8.9). Spaced around the rim of the circular chamber are cylindrical resonant cavities. As the electron spokes pass the openings of the cavities, they cause the free electrons in the metal to spiral around the cavity (like charges repel), first one way then the other; this oscillation induces a resonant, high-frequency radio field in the cavity. An aerial then extracts the RF wave.

A klystron is an RF amplifier. The RF wave is produced by an oscillator. The wave then passes into the main body of the device, which consists of a series of resonant cavities. Electrons produced by an electron gun also enter the main body in phase with the RF wave. The oscillating RF field causes the electrons either to slow down (electrons arriving early in the phase) or to speed up (electrons arriving late in the phase), so causing the electrons to bunch together. When the electron bunches pass over the output cavity they excite a voltage on the output cavity, and the electrons will lose kinetic energy. The excitation of the cavity emits an RF wave that, as the electron bunches were arriving at a time interval equal to one cycle of the RF wave, will be in phase and add its power to the existing RF wave. The RF power then exits the klystron and the electrons, which have lost a significant amount of their energy, are then absorbed in an *electron catcher* or *beam dump.*

8.7.2 Feed waveguide

In a linear accelerator electrons are accelerated by the action of RF electromagnetic waves. Relatively low-energy electrons are

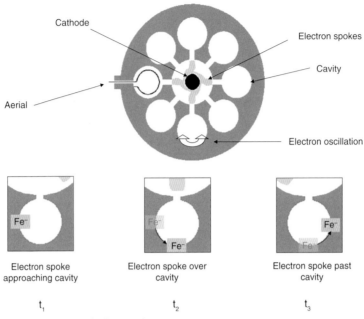

Electron spoke
approaching cavity

Electron spoke over
cavity

Electron spoke past
cavity

t_1

t_2

t_3

Fe⁻ = free electrons in the metal

FIGURE 8.9 Magnetron (cross section).

injected into an accelerating structure and gain energy as they travel down the structure. A waveguide is used to transfer the RF wave to the accelerating structure which consists of a series of hollow tubes. The waveguide contains *sulphur hexafluoride* (SF_6), a synthetic inert nontoxic gas at approximately two times atmospheric pressure. Although the gas itself is inert and nontoxic it does decompose into several toxic products including sulphur tetra-fluoride and hydrogen fluoride. The Intergovernmental Panel of Climate Change recognises it as the most powerful of all greenhouse gases, so disposal of the gas has to be done with care.

A gas is present as the transfer of RF waves is more efficient in a medium; however, due to the high energy of the RF wave electric arcing can take place. Sulphur hexafluoride is excellent at quenching the arcing, so stops excessive loss of power in the transfer of the RF wave to the accelerating structure. At the end of waveguide is an alumina disc (Al_2O_3) in a thin copper sleeve that allows the RF wave to pass but isolates the gas-filled RF waveguide from the vacuum in the accelerating waveguide.

Figure 8.8 shows the waveguide structure as a straight line, but because of the position of the RF generator in relation to accelerating waveguide, the RF waveguide has to change directions a number of times; this may cause some reflection of the wave back towards the RF generator. Reflected RF waves passing back into the RF generator can detune the system. To stop this happening a circulator or isolator is introduced into the RF waveguide which can protect the RF power generator by stopping any returning waves reaching it.

8.7.3 Production and Acceleration of the Electron Beam

8.7.3.1 Electron Gun

Electrons are produced by thermionic emission from a heated cathode of a material such as tungsten or lanthanum hexaboride LaB_6. An electrostatic field produced by the *cathode cup* focuses the electrons to a small area of the anode. The *anode*, unlike that in kilovoltage units, contains a hole where the electrons are focused, so rather than hit the anode they pass through the hole and enter the accelerating structure.

Two basic types of electron gun exist: the *diode* and *triode*, with most LinAcs using a triode design [7] as the triode design is more flexible, allowing independent regulation of gun current and beam energy, and is smaller in design. In the diode gun the voltage applied to the cathode is pulsed, so producing bunches of electrons rather than a continuous stream. The triode gun obtains discrete bunches of electrons by introducing a third component to the structure – a grid positioned just in front of the anode, between the anode and the cathode. The cathode has a constant potential and the voltage to the grid is pulsed. When the voltage applied to the grid is negative the electrons are stopped from reaching the anode. When the voltage from the grid is removed the electrons accelerate towards the anode. The grid can therefore control the frequency of electron pulses entering the accelerating structure. The high voltage pulses to the cathode or grid are produced and controlled by a modulator which is also connected to the RF power generator.

8.7.4 Accelerating Structure

The main function of the accelerating structure is to accelerate the electrons, giving them energy that can then be converted into X-rays.

It is important that the electrons are correctly placed on the wave for maximum acceleration, which occurs in the first part of the accelerating structure, sometimes referred to as the bunching section. If we consider the electron bunches on the RF wave in Figure 8.10, they will all receive energy from the wave, causing them to be accelerated. The electron bunch in position 1 will receive a greater acceleration causing them to catch up with bunch 2. Electron bunch 3 will receive less acceleration and move backwards on the wave in relation to bunches 1 and 2, until finally all the bunches merge together at the same point on the wave.

The energy given to the electrons is in the form of kinetic energy, but as the velocity of the electrons increase a significant proportion of the energy can be in the form of a gain

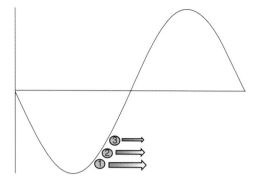

FIGURE 8.10   Electron bunching.

in mass (see relativistic changes and acceleration). This is referred to as a 'relativistic change in mass'. As energy and mass are equivalent and interchangeable, $E = mc^2$; this can still be regarded as an increase in energy.

Equation (8.5) can be used to calculate changes in mass with velocity. Increases in mass equates to an increase in energy, but also an increase in mass will require an increase in the force applied to give the same acceleration ($F = ma$):

$$m = \frac{m_0}{\sqrt{1 - v^2/c^2}} \qquad (8.5)$$

where m = mass, m_0 = resting mass, v = velocity, and c = the speed of light (approximately 3×10^8 m s^{-1}).

When entering the accelerating structure, the electron is travelling at approximately $0.4c$ (1.2×10^8 m s^{-1}) and on exiting the accelerating structure approximately $0.98c$ (2.94×10^8 m s^{-1}). Given the resting mass of an electron (9.10956×10^{-31} kg) it is possible to calculate the mass of the electron when it exits the accelerating structure.

$$m = \frac{9.10956 \times 10^{-31}}{\sqrt{1 - (2.94 \times 10^8)^2 / (3 \times 10^8)^2}}$$

$$\rightarrow m = \frac{9.10956 \times 10^{-31}}{\sqrt{1 - (8.64 \times 10^{16}) / (9 \times 10^{16})}}$$

$$\rightarrow m = \frac{9.10956 \times 10^{-31}}{\sqrt{1 - 0.96}} \rightarrow m = \frac{9.10956 \times 10^{-31}}{\sqrt{0.04}}$$

$$\rightarrow m = \frac{9.10956 \times 10^{-31}}{0.20} \rightarrow m = 4.58 \times 10^{-30} \text{ kg.}$$

The mass is still small but has increased by a factor of 5 and as it gets closer to the speed of light the mass continues to increase rapidly.

Two different types of waveguide may be used, depending on the type of wave present: the travelling or standing wave.

8.7.4.1 Travelling Wave Waveguide

In the travelling wave waveguide the wave enters at the electron gun end of the waveguide, travels the length of the waveguide, rather like a wave travelling towards the beach, and then exits at the opposite end of the accelerating structure. Once the wave has exited it can be either fed back into the input end of the accelerating structure or alternatively absorbed by an RF load.

The waveguide consists of a hollow tube containing discs of copper that resemble washers with a hole in the centre through which the electrons can travel. Copper is used due to its high electrical conductivity, reducing power loss from the structure. The discs also function to reduce the wave's speed of propagation, allowing the wave and the electrons' velocities to be matched at the start of the waveguide. The discs are spaced less frequently as it moves down the waveguide

allowing the speed of the wave's propagation to increase.

As the travelling wave moves down the waveguide its electrical field induces a corresponding region of charge in the tube and the copper discs, as shown in Figure 8.11. Electron bunches entering cavities B and F at time t_1 will experience acceleration; they will then move through to the next cavity in sequence C and G, which at t_2 will have changed polarity due to the wave also moving forward, and again be accelerated. This continues along the length of the accelerating structure until the RF wave is removed.

8.7.4.2 Standing Waveguide

In the standing waveguide, when the travelling wave reaches the end of the waveguide, it is reflected back in the opposite direction by reflective discs. When the original travelling wave and the reflected travelling wave moving in the opposite direction interfere with each other a new wave pattern is formed: a standing wave. The standing wave has fixed points that never undergo any displacement, called nodes, which are the result of destructive interference of the two travelling waves, i.e. they cancel each other out. Midway between every consecutive node there are points that

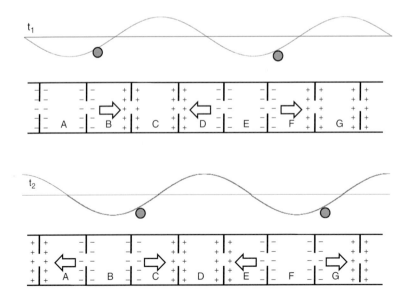

FIGURE 8.11 Travelling wave.

undergo maximum displacement called anti-nodes. Anti-nodes are points that oscillate back and forth between a large positive displacement and a large negative displacement. The anti-nodes are the result of a mixture of constructive interference and destructive interference of the two travelling waves. When the two waves forming the standing wave are completely in phase, the resulting standing wave has twice the amplitude (either positive or negative) of the travelling waves. When completely out of phase the two waves cancel each other out. As it is the standing wave that causes the acceleration of the electrons it is not essential for the wave to enter

the waveguide at the electron gun end of the accelerating structure.

The theory of operation is basically the same as the travelling waveguide, the wave producing regions of positive and negative charge that will attract and repel the electrons. Figure 8.12 shows a typical standing wave oscillation, the lines showing the amplitude of the wave at different points in time. Those electrons entering a cavity at the optimum point in the wave cycle (cavities C and G at time point 1 and cavities A and E at time point 2) will find themselves accelerated (Figure 8.13). As the standing wave is a composite of two travelling waves

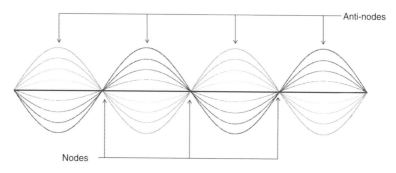

FIGURE 8.12 Standing wave.

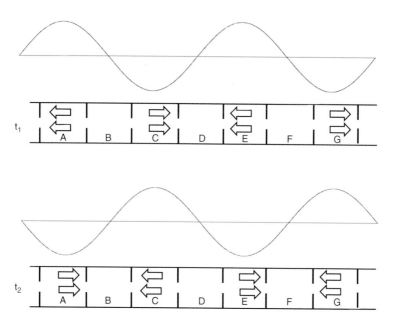

FIGURE 8.13 Standing wave acceleration.

the resultant force on the electrons will be greater. Note that because the nodes are always in a fixed place, every other cavity (cavities B, D, and F) always has a zero field and so can never contribute to the acceleration of the electron bunch. In practice the cavities that contain the nodes can be moved out to the sides of the accelerating structure, making the overall length of the accelerating waveguide much shorter. These cavities are called side-coupled cavities.

8.8 Ancillary Equipment

8.8.1 Cooling System

The accelerating waveguide requires a stable operating temperature as changes in temperature will cause a change in the dimensions of the accelerating waveguide (within about $0.5\,^{\circ}C$), which will affect its efficiency. The RF generator and target also require cooling and a single cooling system usually supplies all these components. A water pump continually circulates water around these structures, which then goes to a heat exchanger.

8.8.2 Loads

Loads are used to absorb microwaves and therefore wasted power without reflection.

8.8.3 Lorentz Forces

The next four components all rely on Lorentz forces to work. When a charged particle moves in either an electrical field or magnetic field it will be subjected to the Lorentz force. In radiotherapy we are mainly concerned with magnetic fields which use the equation $F = qv \times B$. The Force (F) felt by the charged particle is dependent on its charge (q), the velocity it is with (v), and the magnetic field strength (B). There is also a vector component.

There will be no force exerted on the charged particle if the particle is travelling parallel to the magnetic field and is at its strongest when the charged particle is travelling at right angles to the magnetic field.

If a charged particle is travelling at right angles to the direction of the magnetic field a force will be exerted on the charged particle at right angles to both the direction of travel and magnetic field, causing the charged particle to change direction, and so we can make the particles move in the direction we want (Fleming's left hand rule).

8.8.4 Vacuum Pumps

A vacuum of approximately 10^{-7} torr is maintained within the accelerating structure by *ion pumps*. This high vacuum prevents electrons losing energy through collisions with gas molecules as they traverse the waveguide. Ion pumps only work effectively at vacuums below 10^{-3} torr and to get to this pressure a mechanical pump is needed. Ion pumps only work on ions that are attracted by a potential difference between two titanium electrodes. When the positive ions reach the titanium electrode it 'sputters' and forms a 'gettering material' which absorbs the gas molecules, effectively removing the ions from the waveguide. To elongate the track of the electrons the pump is situated within a magnetic field. This causes the electrons to spiral towards the anode, which is important because the chance of an atom entering the ion pump is random and elongating the ion path increases the chance of ionisation of any gas atoms in the waveguide. The larger positive ions, due to their mass being so much greater, tend to travel in a straight line to the cathode of the vacuum pump [8].

8.8.5 Focusing Coils

During acceleration the electrons have a tendency to diverge that is strongest at the gun end of the waveguide. Two factors cause this: the RF wave itself, which has a small radial component, and the electrostatic repulsion of the electrons on each other. Focusing coils surrounding the waveguide produce a magnetic field with the lines of force running lengthways along the waveguide; these stop the electrons from diverging as they are accelerated.

8.8.6 Steering Coils

The accelerating structure may contain minor imperfections that can affect the position of the electrons in the accelerating waveguide. The electrons will also be influenced by any external magnetic fields such as the Earth's magnetic field and, as the position of the waveguide changes in relation to these fields, the electrons may move from their optimum trajectory down the centre of the waveguide. Steering coils exert an electromagnetic force on the electrons, keeping them in the centre of the waveguide. The electromagnets are situated in pairs, two on the x and two on the z axis, to control for any deviation in these planes. A set of steering coils is present at either end of the accelerating waveguide.

8.8.7 Bending Magnets

Linear accelerators with horizontally mounted accelerating structures require the direction in which the electrons are travelling to be changed before they hit the target. When the electrons leave the accelerating structure, they enter the *'flight' or 'drift' tube* which is an evacuated tube where no further acceleration takes place and transfers the electrons to the bending cavity. Bending magnets positioned either side of the cavity can be used to change the electrons' direction of travel. Three bending systems are in common use: the 90° and 270° systems, so called because of the angle the electrons are turned through, and the 112.5° slalom system where the electrons take a zigzag course (Figure 8.14).

The simplest bending system, the 90° system, produces a larger focal spot on the target than the other two systems. Electrons leaving the accelerating waveguide have slightly different energies. Electrons with higher energies will be deflected less by the magnet, whereas low-energy electrons will undergo a larger angle of deflection. The other two systems bend the different electron energies to varying degrees. High-energy electrons will be bent to a greater degree than slower electrons, so allowing the electrons to be focused on a single point on the target 'achromatic'.

The 270° system has the disadvantage of needing the head to be larger to accommodate the electrons orbit. This extra height of the head raises the *isocentre* of the unit because a greater amount of space is needed to allow the

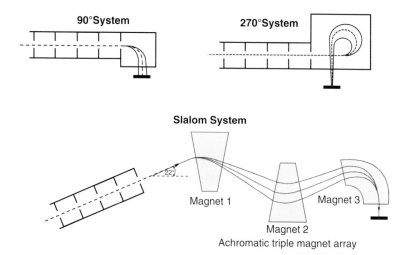

FIGURE 8.14   Bending magnets. (Source: Slalom system diagram courtesy of Elekta Medical Systems.)

head to move under the couch. An alternative to raising the isocentre height that has been utilised is a pit or sinking floor under the couch, which can open/drop when the gantry rotates under the couch. Elekta's answer to this problem was to introduce the slalom system, a variation of the 270° system that again produces the small focal spot, but without the need for a significant increase in head size.

8.9 Treatment Head

The head of the LinAc contains various structures, shown in Figure 8.15. Each component is described in sequence below.

8.9.1 Target

At high energy the photons produced by the *electron target* interaction are mainly created in the forward direction. A *transmission target* allows most of the photons produced to be used and is therefore more efficient than a

reflection target. As with kilovoltage tubes the target is made from a metal with a high atomic number such as tungsten or gold, due to the increased efficiency of X-ray production. The target needs to be thick enough so that all the electrons that are directed onto the target via the bending magnet can interact and produce X-rays, but not too thick because this will start to attenuate the beam as the X-rays have to pass through the target.

The efficiency of X-ray production at megavoltage energy is significantly better than at kilovoltage energies due to the faster moving electrons at approximately 30%, so less heat will be produced than in kilovoltage units. Cooling is relatively simple as less heat is produced and the target is at earth potential, so can be done by water circulating around the edge of the target structure. Some LinAcs contain a second target consisting of a target with low atomic number, as a megavoltage beam created using a low-Z target will have an increased number of low-energy photons present which improves soft-tissue contrast when imaging [9]. The flattening filter is also removed in imaging mode.

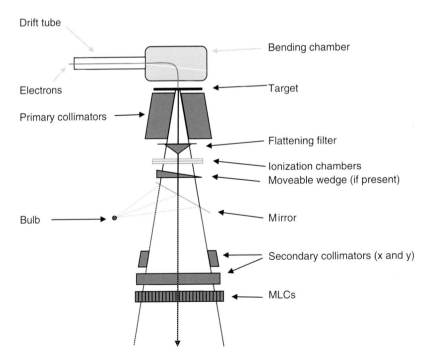

FIGURE 8.15 Components in a linac head.

8.9.1.1 Beam-Flattening Filter

The spatial arrangement of X-rays produced at the target is greatest along the central axis of the beam and decreases in intensity further away from the central axis. This beam would be unsuitable for treatment purposes because it would be impossible to give a uniform dose at any given depth. The beam-flattening filter needs to reduce the intensity of radiation most at the central axis and then decreasingly so as it moves away from the central axis. To do this the filter needs to be thicker in the middle and gradually reduce in thickness from the centre, giving a conical-shaped filter. The filter being positioned close to the point of X-ray production will have relatively small dimensions. Filters are usually made of brass or copper or similar material. Materials with a high atomic number would make the filter smaller but would give greater changes in the beam quality across the beam and reduce beam hardness. Dual-energy machines will have a different flattening filter for each of the beam energies.

Some methods of beam delivery no longer require the use of a beam flattening filter and some of the newer LinAcs do not have one present and can operate in Flattening Filter Free (FFF) mode. The use of FFF mode has recently been growing rapidly as technology and techniques change. Conventionally radiation beams were given using square or rectangular shaped beams, then shaped beams were used. With these beams it was important to keep the beam profile flat to allow the delivery of a homogenous dose to the planned target volume (PTV). However, it flattens the beam profile at the cost of a reduced dose rate, especially on and near the central axis, in addition to causing an increase in scattered radiation, more radiation leakage from the LinAc head, beam hardening, and for very high energy LinAcs, increases neutron contamination [10, 11].

Newer techniques such as IMRT (intensity-modulated radiotherapy), where we want to vary the fluence of the beam during treatment, means that flat beams are unnecessary. Also, for small fields which tend to be used in stereotactic procedures the treatment field is virtually flat over the central few centimetres meaning the filter is not needed [12]. Inverse planning methods detailed in Chapter 9 take into account a non-flat beam profile in the planning algorithm which would be extremely difficult with forward planning.

FFF beams typically replace the flattening filter with a thin copper or brass foil in order to remove any electrons that have passed through the target. Without the flattening filter present to attenuate the beam there will be a much higher dose rate which in turn means a faster treatment time, so reducing the time the patients' have to stay still for treatment.

8.9.1.2 Ionisation Chamber

The ionisation chamber in the head of the linear accelerator is a dual, sealed, parallel plate chamber. The chamber is sealed so that it will give a constant reading at a constant dose rate regardless of the temperature and pressure. The advantage of having a dual system is that the secondary dose monitoring system can terminate the beam when the selected MUs are exceeded by a set limit. The ionisation chamber has a number of sectors that provide feedback to the steering coils and bending magnet, ensuring that the clinical beam is flat and has symmetry. When the change exceeds the tolerance range and automatic adjustment cannot bring it within these parameters, automatic cutouts engage, and the machine will stop.

8.9.1.3 Optical System

As the linear accelerator does not use applicators an optical system is needed to define the FSD and show the beam direction. A light is positioned to one side of the head and a mirror reflects this light through 45° to run along the path the X-rays take. The mirror is made of Mylar®, a thin, strong polyester film with one surface covered in a reflective material such as aluminium that is a few micrometres thick, so as not to reduce the intensity of the radiation beam to any great extent. The geometry of this system is very important; the light beam and X-ray beam must directly superimpose on each other or the radiation beam will not correspond to the visualised field. This check, which can be done with an X-ray film, should be part of the routine QA programme.

8.9.2 Collimators

The linear accelerator has at least two sets of collimators: the *primary collimators* and the *secondary collimators*. The primary collimator is circular and defines the maximum angle of the exiting beam. It is situated close to the target so as to reduce its size. The secondary collimators are situated after the mirror and consist of two pairs of adjustable lead blocks that restrict the radiation emerging from the head to determine square or rectangular field sizes ranging from approximately 4 cm^2 up to 40 cm^2 at 100 cm FSD, although the latter may have slightly rounded corners due to the primary collimator. The secondary collimators are calibrated so that the collimator reading will give the corresponding field size at 100 cm FSD. Due to beam divergence the field size at any other distance will be different and a calculation using similar triangles (see Chapter 2) will need to be done to determine it. Secondary collimators can move either symmetrically around the central axis of the beam or asymmetrically. Where one of the collimators coincides with the central axis that one side of the field has no beam divergence.

A potential issue with the secondary collimators is *transmission penumbra* (Figure 8.16) which is caused by the beam going only through part of the collimator. To reduce this effect the collimators do not slide straight in and out but rather move through an arc so that the edge of the collimator is always parallel to the beam edge. Transmission through the collimators is typically less than 2% of the primary (open) beam, the CLinAc iX having a reported transmission of less than 0.5%.

A further type of collimator called multi-leaf collimators (MLCs) is also usually present. The MLCs consist of a number of leaves of tungsten, each of which can move independently and shape the beam. As they are present on only one axis it is possible to

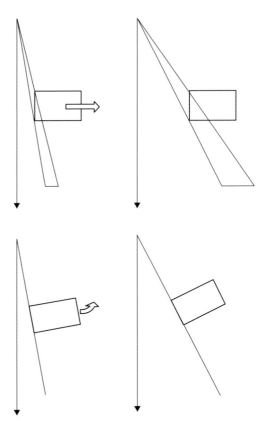

FIGURE 8.16 Transmission penumbra.

have different degrees of tumour conformation depending on the collimator orientation. Figure 8.17 demonstrates this showing MLC conformity in two different directions with the conformity being significantly better in (a) compared to (b).

For standard MLCs each leaf corresponds to a shielded width of around 1 cm at an FSD of 100 cm. Full field 0.5 cm MLCs are now available from Elekta and Siemens. This figure is reduced to values of 3–5 mm for micro- and mini-MLCs, although these systems have limited field sizes. If the leaves were straight blocks of tungsten next to each other, there would be considerable leakage of radiation through the gaps. To reduce inter-leaf radiation leakage the gap is kept as small as possible and the MLCs are shaped so that they have stepped or overlapping sections, the shapes are slightly different for each of the manufacturers as is their position. Figure 8.15 shows them below the secondary collimators

(a) (b)

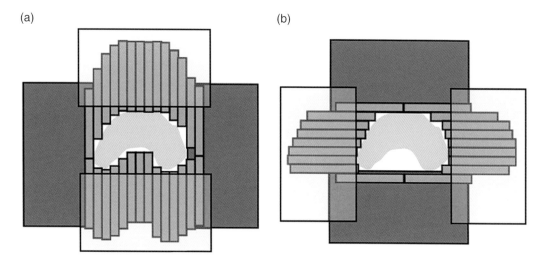

FIGURE 8.17 Multi-leaf collimator arrangement. MLCs positioned on (a) Y axis and (b) X axis.

which tends to be done in the Varian units, although they can also be placed above the secondary collimators which is the preferred method in Elekta units.

The stepped and overlapping sections are not the full thickness of the blade and so cannot reduce the beam intensity by the same value as the blade. Symonds-Tayler and Webb [12] suggest a value of 14% transmission compared with 2% through the leaf. The secondary collimator is also used to reduce interleaf leakage and will be positioned just behind the outermost leaf absorbing most of the leakage before it reaches the patient. Another issue with MLCs is the penumbra. The MLCs are not set up to move in an arc as with the secondary collimators and, to overcome the changing geometry with the beam, they are designed with rounded leaf tips. Although this shape allows some transmission of the beam through the blade tip it is independent of the position of the leaf. The greater the maximum MLC field size the greater the curvature needed.

The function of all the collimators mentioned is to define the beam, which they do by attenuating the part of the beam that is not required. The collimator material needs to have a high density because the major interaction process at these energies is the Compton interaction. The most frequently used materials are lead and tungsten.

8.9.3 Wedges

In older units a number of wedges, typically 15°, 30°, 45°, and 60°, could physically be placed in the treatment head by the radiographer. The wedge, made from a dense material such as lead or steel attached to a backing plate that would fit into a wedge holder, was usually situated between the ionisation chamber and the mirror. The use of manual wedges has largely been superseded, first by *motorized wedges*, which consist of a physical wedge of a large wedge angle, usually around 60°. The wedge is permanently situated in the treatment head (see Figure 8.15 for its position relative to other structures) and can be moved into the beam automatically for part of the treatment to give the desired wedge angle. Another method of obtaining a modified beam profile is through dynamic or *virtual wedges*. As the name suggests there is no physical wedge, but the effect is created by moving one of the collimators across the beam at a precalculated speed during the treatment to give the same effect on the beam profile as a wedge. Any of the four collimator jaws could create this effect, but in practice it is limited to one set of jaws. One advantage of this system of wedging the beam is that the average beam energy remains constant across the full width of the beam. With a physical wedge there will be a degree of beam hardening that will depend on the thickness of filter traversed.

Wedges are needed to improve dose uniformity within the PTV and compensate for missing tissue and beams coming in with different *hinge angles*. The angle does not relate to the wedge itself but rather the angle through which the isodose is turned, the *wedge angle* being defined as 'the complement of the angle between the central axis and a line tangent to the isodose curve at the depth of 10 cm' [13]. Many current techniques such as IMRT and tomotherapy remove the need for a wedge entirely.

8.10 Patient Support System

The patient support system is often overlooked but is a complicated and important part of the treatment equipment. The support system carries the couch, which the patient lies upon during treatment.

The couch top is usually made from carbon fibre which is further strengthened by supporting struts. Carbon fibre is used for two main reasons. Firstly, it has a high rigidity and tensile strength meaning that there will be minimal flexing under load, which we sometimes refer to as couch sag. The flexing of the couch reduces spatial accuracy of radiation dose delivery; the greater the degree of sag the greater the treatment positioning inaccuracy.

Carbon fibre, as well as having a high tensile strength, also has a low attenuation of X-rays which is important for a number of reasons. Different couch designs have different attenuation factors, but it is usually less than 13%, although it will be dependent on various beam parameters such as the gantry angle, beam energy, and field size. Another consideration would be if an Omniboard (see Chapter 7) is being used, as again this would increase the amount of beam attenuation. Low attenuation is important for imaging of the patient, as at certain gantry angles the X-ray beam must be able to pass through the couch to reach the detector and so a low attenuation is essential to allow the beam exiting the patient to reach the detector. Also, it is important that the couch has a homogenous attenuation as any change in attenuation of the couch will affect the image quality.

Having a low attenuation is also important in relation to the dose received by the patient. When using fields that go through the couch before reaching the patient the beam is attenuated by the couch, which will decrease the dose reaching the patient and significantly increase skin dose, the couch acting as a buildup material [14]. This can be accounted for at the treatment planning stage, or alternatively some couches have removable panels that allow replacement of the carbon fibre section with thinner sections such as a 'tennis racket' insert, a section containing mylar over an open nylon string section. Another solution is to offer different couch top modules, some of which will have different sections with reduced attenuation to allow treatments such as an under-couch treatment. Often overlooked is the increase in skin dose on the exit side of the patient if the beam exits through the couch. This is due to the couch creating backscatter as the beam is attenuated so increasing the exit dose. Sheykhoo [15] identified an increase in dose on the exit side of between 14 and 20% for a 6 MV beam when the couch was present.

The couch is flat to aid patient reproducibility and is also indexed, a system of graduated measurements that aid with the precise and repeatable patient positioning. The couch also contains attachment points for a range of inserts that help with patient positioning and reproducibility.

Couch movement is controlled in the room either by buttons on the side of the patient support system or on a pendant. Remote movement is also possible from the control panel outside of the room, which following imaging allows for the correction of any misalignments in the patient setup before treatment begins.

Until recently patient support systems only had four types of movement: vertical (z), longitudinal (x), lateral (y), and rotation (yaw). Recently however, couches have been designed that allow the couch some degree of roll (rotation around the longitudinal x axis) and pitch (rotation around the lateral y axis), this now means that radiographers can easily correct for translational patient positioning errors, movements in the x, y and z directions, as well as rotational errors (roll, pitch, and yaw) on set. Couches that move in these six dimensions are said to have six degrees of freedom. This type of couch improves spatial accuracy, which for some treatments would directly relate to improved clinical outcomes. Couches on LinAcs with a ring gantry such as the Halcyon and Tomotherapy units have no rotation (yaw) movement.

8.11 Imaging Systems

Most modern-day C-arm LinAcs have imaging devices present in the form of an electronic portal imaging device (EPID) and/or an onboard imager (OBI).

EPID devices are flat panel detectors that are positioned opposite the head of the LinAc so that the image is created by the megavoltage X-ray beam being produced by the LinAc. The EPID is usually flush against the LinAc when not in use and can be extended automatically into position when imaging is needed. During use the position of the detector can be manually adjusted in the vertical, longitudinal, and lateral directions.

OBI consists of two robotic arms, one holding an X-ray tube, and the other a flat panel detector. Typically, the tube is an oil-cooled rotating anode X-ray tube with two possible focal spots (4 and 8 mm) and a target angle of approximately 14° [16]. The potential difference across the tube can be varied between approximately 30 and 140 kV [17] which means that image quality will be high, as the resulting X-ray interactions in matter will predominantly be via the photoelectric effect. Two pairs of adjustable collimators can be used to limit the irradiated area. The arms are positioned opposite each other and at 90° to the head of the LinAc, and like the EPID when not in use are retracted towards the gantry. As with the EPID detector, when in use the flat panel detector's position can be adjusted manually in three directions.

The most common form of flat panel detector used is an amorphous silicon (a-Si) detector. The detector consists of a phosphor payer which converts radiation into visible light. Common materials used are caesium iodide that has been doped with thallium (CsITl) or terbium doped gadolinium oxysulfide (Gd2O2S:Tb). Behind the phosphor screen is a matrix of a-Si transistors (photodiodes) on a glass baseplate that converts the light produced in the phosphor layer into electrons. In the EPID system a copper plate is positioned in front of the scintillator [18] which shields the detector from low energy scattered secondary radiation and also acts as a buildup layer converting photons into secondary electrons, increasing efficiency of the system. Both flat panels have an active imaging area of approximately 40×30 cm and are positioned in a protective plastic housing which has touch guards.

Potentially both the EPID and OBI systems can operate in two modes either producing a 2-dimensional image or producing a 3-dimensional cone beam computed tomography (CBCT) image. The OBI system can also operate in fluoroscopy mode that can be used for pretreatment verification of respiratory motion and the validation of the gating thresholds.

CBCT, as the name implies, uses a cone-shaped beam of radiation that is directed onto the flat panel detector rather than a fan beam that is used in CT scanners to produce the image. Because a cone beam is used, only one rotation of the beam is needed to produce the image compared to the multiple slices needed in a CT unit, although the method of creating the image, 'filtered back-projection', is the same (see Chapter 6). A specialised filter is needed when performing CBCT called a 'bowtie' filter. These filters change the flux of the beam reaching the detectors attempting

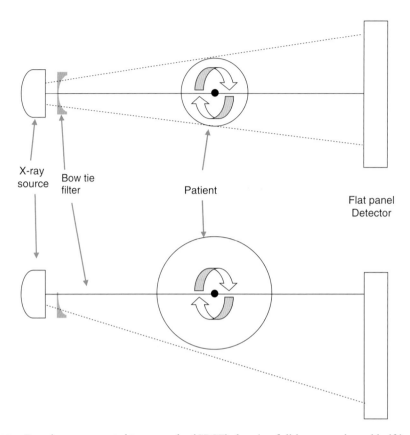

FIGURE 8.18 Cone beam computed tomography (CBCT) showing full-beam mode and half-beam mode.

to balance out the difference in distance the X-rays take, and the patient's shape, as seen in Figure 8.18. This reduces patient dose and also improves the quality of the image by reducing the amount of scatter reaching the detector. CBCT can operate with two different modes, full-fan and half-fan. The full bowtie has a relatively small field of view and so is most suitable for small areas such as the head and neck area. For larger areas a half-beam mode is used which requires a half bowtie filter and the flat panel detector to be moved so that it is no longer centred on the central axis of the beam (see Figure 8.18).

CBCT scan times are equivalent to the time needed for the gantry to rotate around the patient, although additional time will be needed for the digital reconstruction of the image. Additionally, at the end of the rotation the arms need to be retracted and the gantry angle reset as well as allowing time for image matching by the radiographers and application of any corrections needed, meaning that the whole process usually takes between three and five minutes. Far better-quality images can be obtained with kV CBCT with much lower doses [19] than with MV CBCT, however there are some benefits to using MV CBCT, such as the image being less susceptible to imaging artefacts from metallic objects, and when used for planning of treatments MV CBCT images provide more accurate treatment plans compared to kV CBCT-based planning.

8.11.1 Electron Beams

To produce a clinical electron beam a number of changes need to be made to the linear accelerator. The most obvious is the removal of both the target and the beam-flattening filter (Figure 8.19). These structures are made

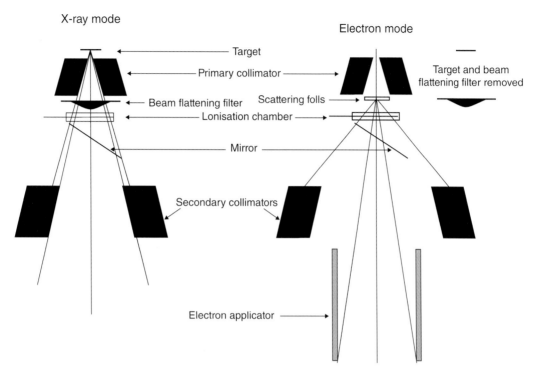

FIGURE 8.19 LinAc treatment head components when treating with X-rays and electrons.

of metal and being in the electron path would effectively remove all the electrons and create X-rays through bremsstrahlung interactions. Similarly, the secondary collimators must be opened as they are not used to collimate the beam, and although not in the direct path of the electrons, electrons hitting the metal would produce X-rays that would contaminate the beam.

The beam-flattening filter is often positioned in a rotating carousel that also contains a number of *electron-scattering foils*. When the electron mode is selected the carousel rotates, removing the flattening filter, and the correct scattering foil for the selected energy is automatically inserted. A scattering foil is needed to spread the thin beam of electrons out over a useful area and a metal such as copper is usually used, which gives the best trade-off between scattering of the beam and bremsstrahlung X-ray production. A single foil produces a dose profile with a high central intensity of electrons, but further scattering in air and from the walls of a solid applicator produce a beam of more uniform intensity.

When open-sided applicators are used the foil usually consists of two thin metal layers. The second sheet creates further scatter of the beam spreading the electrons out over a larger area because the scatter from the air alone within the applicator is not enough to produce a uniform beam. A number of different scattering foils are present for the different electron energies in order to produce a suitable electron beam.

Another less frequently used method to spread out the narrow electron beam is to scan the beam over a large area using electromagnets. As there is no scattering foil in the beam this produces an electron beam with far less X-ray contamination.

Electron beams have to be collimated close to the patient's surface to reduce dose outside the treatment area from electrons that are scattered by the air. The applicators are made of a material with a relatively low atomic number such as aluminium to reduce the amount of bremsstrahlung X-ray production.

It is also important when changing from X-ray to electron mode that the gun current is reduced. X-ray production is inefficient, and this affects the dose rate. Removal of this inefficient process would lead to a significant increase in dose rate with electron beams. For the dose rate to remain the same the gun current is reduced when in electron mode.

8.12 Other Linear Accelerator Designs

There are a number of different types of LinAcs that do not use the traditional design. The standard LinAc can be referred to as a C-arm LinAc as when it is viewed from the side it has a C shape. Some newer designs resemble that of the CT unit where the linear accelerator waveguide is mounted in-line on a rotating gantry assembly (ring gantry) or alternatively are on a robotic arm. These types of units have no need for a bending system. The units also lack an optical distance viewer as the patient setup is performed using lasers.

8.12.1 Bands

Frequencies in the microwave radio region of the electromagnetic spectrum are designated bands. In reading manufacturer's literature, linear accelerators are referred to as X or S band. Most medical LinAcs use S-band frequencies, however both the Cyberknife and Mobetron are examples of X-band linear accelerators that use a magnetron to produce the RF wave, although X-band klystrons are also now available. S-band LinAcs have a frequency of 2–4 GHz and a wavelength of 7.5–15 cm. C-band LinAcs have a frequency of 4–8 GHz and a wavelength of 3.8–7.5 cm and X-band a frequency of 8–12 GHz and a wavelength of 2.5–3.8 cm. Being X-band allows the waveguide to be shorter and therefore the head to be more compact, which is needed in ring gantry LinAcs such as the Halcyon.

8.12.2 Helical Tomotherapy

Tomotherapy means 'slice therapy', both terms being derived from the Greek language, tomo meaning 'slice' and therapy from the word *therapea*, 'to cure or heal'. The technique developed by Mackie and colleagues is the rotational delivery of radiation therapy using a fan beam of radiation collimated by slits that open and close during the treatment so giving an intensity modulate beam. Tomotherapy is possible on standard linacs with the addition of an add-on binary collimator and associated software. This allows a helical fan beam that can be intensity modulated to be delivered, but the lack of a ring gantry means that the accelerator cannot spin around the patient as fast as with dedicated hardware.

8.12.2.1 Tomotherapy Equipment

Dedicated tomotherapy equipment consists of a ring gantry that contains a megavoltage accelerator, binary MLC's, and image detector. The gantry utilises the slip ring technology of diagnostic CT units which allows continuous rotation around the patient at speeds of up to 5 rpm for treatment and 6 rpm for imaging. The accelerator produces X-rays of 6 MeV for treatment and 3.5 MeV for imaging. The beam produced is a fan beam with a maximum iso-centre width of 40 cm; no flattening filter is necessary. 64 binary MLCs then collimate the beam producing beamlets of radiation. The binary MLCs move very quickly compared to those on a conventional LinAc, with an average open to close time of 20 ms [20]. The width of the beam is limited to three different lengths, 1 cm, 2.5 cm, and 5 cm, although dynamic options are available.

The treatment couch can extend a considerable distance into the aperture, ensuring that large volumes can be made available for treatment. Cylindrical volumes of 40 cm diameter and up to 135 cm length can be treated without the need to reposition the patient or match fields. The only visible moving part in the room is the couch. The equipment combines the conformality of IMRT treatment with an inherent IGRT (image guided radiotherapy) capability. The ease of imaging presents daily pre-irradiation localization as a feasible option and in turn allows for increased confidence in target coverage with associated reduction in margins, as well as the possibility of adaptive radiotherapy and potential for dose escalation.

During the treatment the couch translates (continually moves) through the ring aperture which together with the LinAc rotation creates a continuous spiral pattern of dose delivery. A full rotation of the gantry is divided into 51 projections. Each projection therefore consists of an arc segment of 7° with each projection having its own leaf opening and closing pattern. The pitch of delivery is defined as the amount of translational couch travel (in/out) during a complete gantry rotation. Typical values for the amount of pitch are 0.25–0.5. The pitch is used to minimise the thread effect which is the ripple of doses (peak-to-trough dose relative to the average dose) as a result of the helical beam junctioning [21].

During planning three factors need to be predefined: the fixed width of the field (1 cm, 2.5 cm, or 5 cm), the modulation factor, and the pitch. All three factors can impinge on the quality of the final plan. The modulation factor is an estimate of plan complexity and can be defined as the maximum leaf opening time divided by the average (non-zero) leaf opening time. A small modulation factor value results in poorer dose distribution; a high modulation factor results in a good dose distribution, but a long treatment time. Therefore, it is necessary to set a modulation factor which balances the considerations of delivery time and dose distribution. This is important as tomotherapy planning and treatment times can be significantly longer when compared to volumetric modulated arc therapy (VMAT).

Recently the ability for tomotherapy units to deliver a static form of tomotherapy has been introduced called TomoDirect. This is brought about by moving the patient through the machine bore, modulating the beam intensity using the binary collimator, whilst maintaining specified beam angles. The use

of static field tomotherapy has been shown to produce suitable treatment plans [22] with the advantage of significantly lower optimization times [23], although issues around high dose and hotspots have been raised [24].

8.12.3 MRI Linear Accelerators

An MRI LinAc combines two technologies, a ring mounted LinAc with that of MRI scanner, so offering a therapeutic unit capable of exceptional soft-tissue imaging capabilities in real time and no additional patient dose. MRI also offers very fast volume acquisition and has no moving parts.

The main issues in the development of an MRI LinAc were the interaction of the strong magnetic fields needed for MRI imaging with the electrons needed for X-ray production, and the RF fields from the LinAc interfering with the MRI circuitry. Because of these potential issues the first MRI guided radiotherapy treatment unit, developed by Viewray, was cobalt based with a 0.35 Tesla MRI magnet and three 13 kCi cobalt-60 sources, each with its own MLC system that delivered treatment between the magnetic poles of the magnet (Figure 8.20). Using cobalt as the source of radiation removed many of the issues associated with a LinAc, particularly accelerating electrons in a strong magnetic field.

Following on from the development of the cobalt MRI guided system (Renaissance) came the first commercially available MRI LinAc, the ViewRay™ MRIdian system. The system uses a similar setup to the earlier cobalt-60 unit in that it consists of a split 0.35 Tesla superconducting magnet. In between each magnet is a 6 MV in-line standing wave LinAc on a rotating gantry assembly that can rotate 180° in each direction, giving a 360° treatment around the patient with a gantry rotation speed of 5 RPM. The radiation beam is therefore perpendicular to the magnetic field and the beam enters between the two poles of the magnet. Some other systems use parallel geometries where the X-ray beam enters parallel to the magnetic field through the holes in the magnets (see Figure 8.20).

End view (*delivery between magnet poles*)

End view (*delivery through the ring*)

Plan view (*delivery between magnet poles*)

Plan view (*delivery through the ring*)

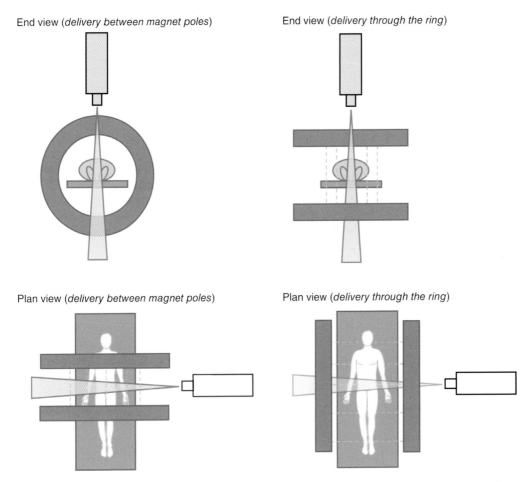

FIGURE 8.20 MRI LinAc beam transmission strategies. Beam delivery is always perpendicular to the magnetic field when the X-ray beam is being delivered between the two magnets (light grey lines) and parallel when delivering through the ring of the magnet.

Each system will affect attenuation and dosimetry of the beam and the use of the parallel system also means that the magnets (or patient) need to be rotated with the LinAc in order to treat at different angles.

The maximum field size of the Viewray system is 27.4 cm by 24.1 cm at the isocentre and the beam is collimated by a double set of curved MLCs, one set of MLCs being positioned on top of the second set giving rise to the terms 'double focused' or 'double stacked' MLCs. The upper stack of MLCs consists of 68 leaves, and the lower stack 70 leaves. Each leaf is 4 mm wide, with an offset of half a leaf width (2 mm) between the stacks to reduce interleaf leakage and the tongue and groove effect. Because of the offset nature of the leaves in the two banks this gives a resolution of approximately 4 mm at the isocentre. The gantry aperture is 70 cm with a 50 cm field of view. The Elekta system called Unity contains a 7 MV LinAc with a 160-leaf MLC system that gives a shielding width of 7.1 mm at the isocentre; the leaves move in the cranial-caudal direction giving a maximum field size of 22 cm in the longitudinal direction and 40 cm in the transverse. The gantry is able to rotate beyond 360° due to slip ring technology and rotates at 6 rpm. The Unity system has a short bore length of 145 cm which should improve patient acceptance as it will be less claustrophobic. Like the Viewray system it has a 70 cm aperture for the patient. Further groups are developing MRI LinAcs, such as the Australian consortium which has a split bore 1 Tesla magnet and uses a 6 MV Varian Linatron LinAc.

Shielding of the magnet from RF waves produced by the LinAc uses technology similar to that used in PET-MRI scanners where shielding can be achieved by encasing components with layers of carbon fibre and copper [25]. Copper reflects RF waves whilst the carbon fibre will absorb them. Magnetic shielding may also be employed where a set of magnets or coils positioned around the gantry can reduce the magnetic field strength in the cylinder during treatment which also increases the uniformity of the magnetic field.

Whilst Viewray have adopted a low field MRI 0.35 Tesla magnet, Elekta have opted for a high field 1.5 Tesla magnet. A low field magnet has the advantages of lower operational costs, and a lower fringe field (the peripheral magnetic field outside of the magnet core), and because of the lower RF excitation frequency there will be less of a heating effect in the body's tissues. A high field strength increases the signal-to-noise ratio of the MRI echo signal and allows better spatial and contrast resolution compared to low field units [26].

Although the photon beam is not affected by the magnetic field the secondary electrons created as a result of X-ray interactions will experience Lorentz forces. This is the same type of force exerted by the bending magnets on the electron stream in the head of a C-arm LinAc (see Section 8.6.2). The Lorentz forces will cause the secondary electrons to change direction and possibly be forced into a circular path. In some instances, the secondary electrons exiting a surface may be directed back towards the patient and re-enter the patient. This leads to an effect known as the 'electron return effect' (ERE) which is enhanced at tissue interfaces, typically increasing doses by approximately 30–40%. This figure was confirmed by Han et al. [27] using a 1.5 T MRI LinAc. They found that there was an increase in exit dose to the skin of approximately 34% due to this effect and that by using 1 cm bolus on the exit side of the patient the exit dose was reduced by approximately 20%. Lorentz forces can also have an effect on dose at tissue interfaces leading to dose uncertainties; the same effect can also shift the field and cause asymmetry in the crossline profiles of the beam and give a small increase in penumbra size, although the effect is reduced by the use of multiple beams. The impact of the ERE is dependent on a number of factors including field size, magnetic field strength, tissue density/interface, shape of interface shape, and geometry [28].

MRI LinAcs are able to image during treatment in real time and because of MRI's superior soft-tissue contrast, monitor both tumour and organ motion without the need for fiducials. This ability to scan during treatment and the motion tracking/management allows radiographers to account for intrafractional motion and anatomical variations and use pretreatment predicted deformations to adapt treatment. It is also possible to rapidly replan and undertake dose calculations onset, allowing online adaptive replanning during the treatment [29]. Real-time adaptive planning has the potential to further improve the dosimetry to the target and to spare the normal tissues. However, there are a number of issues still to be fully resolved. Spatial distortion during image acquisition causes distortion of the image. Although these distortions are not large, typically 1–2 mm [30], they may be a limiting factor when considering PTV margins and small adjustments on set. MRI also lacks information on the electron density, but this can be derived from the initial plan's electron density via image registration, although this must be visually reviewed prior to treatment. The use of adaptive planning will therefore increase the time the patient is on set which will impact on issues such as the patient's comfort, bladder filling, and associated patterns of work. Finally, there will be a dramatic increase in data management workload and the datasets will require efficient data storage [31].

8.12.4 Halcyon

The Halcyon linear accelerator was developed by Varian and is another ring type LinAc where the accelerator is positioned in an enclosed housing so that there no visible moving parts when the LinAc moves around the patient during treatment, similar to a CT unit.

The unit contains a 6 MV linear accelerator that operates without the need for a flattening filter (FFF beam) so the dose rate is high, approximately 800 MU min^{-1}. The ring design means that the gantry rotation speed is approximately four times faster than a C-arm LinAc allowing it to deliver 5 arcs in under three minutes [32] and as with other ring type LinAcs there is no danger of patient collision during treatment or imaging. The accelerator structure is opposite a flat panel detector and version 2 features a kV imager and associated flat panel detector positioned at 90° to the accelerating structure. This means that both MV and kV imaging including CBCT is possible, however only one imaging modality can be linked to the plan; MV imaging sizes cannot be adjusted or changed once planned and the MV imaging is limited to 28 cm^2 due to the fixed collimator. If MV imaging is used the dose is calculated within the treatment plan.

Treatment can be delivered using up to 4 rpm for IMRT fields and 2 rpm for VMAT delivery. A dual layer MLC system is utilised similar to that of the Viewray MRI LinAc with 100% over-travel (distance a leaf can travel across the midline) and 100% interdigitation (a leaf moving from one side to pass its two neighbouring leaves from the opposite side) (see Figure 8.21). The collimators give a 5 mm resolution. The treatment field volume length can be up to 28 cm with a single isocentre technique and up to 36 cm in length if a two isocentre technique is used.

The unit has a bore of 100 cm with a narrow bore depth and other than the couch there are no visible moving parts (see Figure 8.22). The pole at the end of the couch is a camera allowing the radiographers to view the patient within the bore during treatment. The unit is fully IGRT in that the unit will not let you treat unless an image has been taken and matched on set.

Because of the ease of setup and rapid imaging and delivery of treatment the unit can deliver advanced treatments much quicker than C-arm LinAcs therefore reducing the time the patient is in the room.

8.12.5 Cyberknife

Another type of linear accelerator design is offered by the CyberKnife unit. The unit comprises of a 6-MV linear accelerator mounted on an industrial robotic arm using non-isocentric beam delivery. The arm is capable of movement in any plane (6 axes of movement) allowing it to position itself around the patient and deliver radiation from virtually any angle. Collimation is done by using either fixed cones which are available in 12 different sizes ranging from 5 mm to 60 mm, or iris collimators that consist of 2 banks of 6 tungsten blocks which allow multiple-field-size treatments. Compared to the fixed cones the iris system reduces the monitor units required, increases treatment speed, and improves tumour conformation and homogeneity of treatment plans. The unit does not contain a beam flattening filter and operates with a dose rate of 800 cGy min^{-1}. The source to skin distance (SSD) can be varied from 65 to 100 cm and radiation is delivered from a discrete set of positions called nodes. The principle of field arrangement is to use non-coplanar fields, i.e. the central axis of the

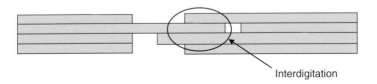

Interdigitation

FIGURE 8.21 Leaf interdigitation.

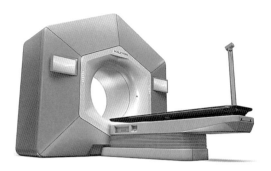

FIGURE 8.22 Halycon LinAc. (Source: image courtesy of Varian Medical Systems, Inc. All rights reserved.)

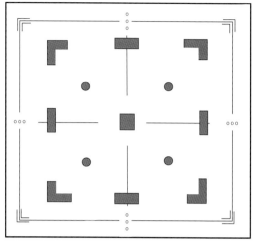

FIGURE 8.23 Position of ionisation detectors and diodes in the Daily QA ™3 instrument.

beams all lie in different planes so exit and entrance doses don't add together.

The unit has a respiratory tracking system and an orthogonal kilovoltage imaging systems mounted on the ceiling that provide the possibility of real-time IGRT. The guidance system tracks and detects motion and automatically corrects for patient and target motion with a maximum tracking error of less than 2 mm [33, 34]. This allows a very high degree of targeting accuracy meaning this type of treatment can be referred to as stereotactic. The CyberKnife system has been used successfully to treat a range of tumours and metastatic deposits throughout the whole body, using stereotactic radiosurgery (SRS) and stereotactic body radiation therapy.

8.13 Quality Assurance of a Linear Accelerator

A number of daily tests are usually performed before the LinAc can be used clinically. Some are performed by the physics department whilst others are done by the radiographers. Although the QA checks carried out by the radiographers are department specific, the following section provides an overview of the typical radiographer-based daily QA checks after the unit has been warmed up.

Output, flatness, symmetry, field size, and beam energy can all be checked using a diode and ionisation chamber-based array detector system such as Sun Nuclear Daily QA ™3. The device consists of 13 ion chambers and 12 diode detectors. For the Daily QA ™3 a field size of 20 cm by 20 cm at 100 cm FSD is set and the device aligned with the light beam using marks on the anterior surface of the detector array (Figure 8.23) and 150 MU is delivered.

The diode detectors (small white circles) are positioned on the x and y axes, three on each side of the beam, and are used to check field size. The ionisation chambers are coloured grey. Beam flatness and beam symmetry are measured using the chambers positioned on the central axis and the four rectangular ionisation chambers. The four curved detectors are used for detecting photon energy and the four circular chambers have attenuators so that they can measure electron energy. The Daily QA 3 device also contains five thermistors and one temperature sensor and so can autocorrect for temperature and pressure variations in the readings. It is important when using this type of device that it is perfectly flat on the couch in order for the reading to be accurate.

Other daily QA checks that should be performed are:

- checking the proximity detectors on the electron applicators, head, and imaging arms which can be done by simply breaking the laser or pushing against the plates and then pressing the rest button;

- the warning lights function correctly and that the door or sensor interlock interrupts the beam if opened or broken;
- MLCs can be checked against a preset image drawn on graph paper to assess leaf accuracy;
- the FSD reading is accurate which can be done by fixing a manual pointer to the head of the LinAc that has a graticule on it and comparing this distance with the optical distance indicated;
- optical field size can be checked against a 10 cm by 10 cm field on graph paper or proprietary device. Stability of the isocentre can be checked by then rotating the collimators both clockwise and anticlockwise and checking the movement of the central axis on the tool;
- all couch movements are checked to make sure that they are smooth and that the brakes engage correctly;
- the intersection of the lasers with the beam can then be measured using a plastic cube such as the ISO cube which has crosses etched on the surface. Firstly, the cube is positioned so that the crosses align with the lasers and then the couch is rotated to 90° and 270° to check that the central axis of the beam aligns to the crosses as well;
- the accuracy of the couch shifts can then be measured using the cube doing a measured offset to a new position;
- fiducials within the cube also allow checking of kV and MV imager coincidence and CBCT process accuracy;
- if respiratory gating is utilised on the LinAc this should also be assessed. This is carried out using a dynamic phantom simulating organ motion to check for temporal accuracy. Beam energy and output consistency may also be measured.

In 1997 the European Commission published Radiation Protection 91 (RP91) which contained a set of criteria for acceptability of radiological equipment. This was updated in

TABLE 8.2 Megavoltage units QA tolerances.

Dose monitoring system	Action level
Weekly calibration check	> 2%
Reproducibility	> 0.5
Proportionality	> 2%
Dependence on angular position of gantry and beam limiting device	> 3%
Dependence on gantry rotation (electrons)	> 2%
X-rays	> 3%
Movements of Patient support	**Action level**
Field size ($10 \times 10\, cm^2$)	> 1 mm
Vertical movements	> 2 mm
Longitudinal and lateral movements	> 2 mm
Isocentric rotation axis	> 2 mm
Parallelism of rotational	> 0.5°
Longitudinal rigidity	> 5 mm
Lateral rigidity	> 0.5° and 5 mm

2012 when report RP162 was published that updated and expanded the scope of the earlier publication although the criteria levels for suspension of the equipment are non-binding [35]. Table 8.2 shows examples of tolerances for various tests detailed in the report.

8.14 Cyclotrons and Proton Beams

8.14.1 Introduction

As previously described in this chapter the most common way of producing a treatment beam is to accelerate electrons onto a target to produce X-rays (high-energy photons) which are then directed at the tumour. Another less commonly used radiotherapy treatment method is to use heavy particles to treat the patient. This form of radiotherapy is called hadron therapy; a hadron being any particle that is made from quarks, anti-quarks, and gluons and includes particles such as protons or neutrons, although in radiotherapy we tend to extend this definition to include other heavy particles such as carbon ions. Electrons are charged particles, but they are not included in the definition of hadron therapy as they are a light, fundamental particle that cannot be split into any smaller particles.

Using particles for cancer treatment is not new; their first clinical use was in the late 1930s when neutrons were used to treat patients. Initially patient outcomes were not favourable, and the researchers stated that neutron treatment should not be continued, although trials still continue in some countries.

8.14.2 Particle Accelerators

When producing X-rays, we accelerate electrons, giving them kinetic energy, which can be converted into X-rays in the target material. With particle beams acceleration is usually in a circular or cyclical fashion constantly turning the particles back to the same acceleration gap.

The most common device used to produce particle beams for medical use is the cyclotron which accelerates charged particles between two hollow semicircular cavities called Dees. The two Dees are positioned opposite each other and between them is the ion source (Figure 8.24).

Each Dee is connected to an alternating voltage with a flattened waveform that creates an alternating electric field between the two Dees that can accelerate the particles across the gap. The acceleration principle is based on opposite charges attracting and like charges repelling. If the opposite Dee is negatively charged, positive particles that have reached the gap will be accelerated across the gap and also be repelled by the positively charged Dee they have just exited. Charged particles are continuously produced at the centre of the gap between the Dees and are attracted towards a Dee during half the voltage phase, effectively creating a pulsed beam. Once in

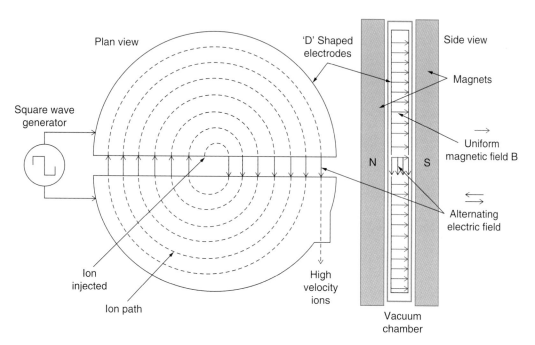

FIGURE 8.24 Schematic diagram of a cyclotron. (Source: courtesy of Electropaedia https://www. mpoweruk.com/figs/cyclotron.htm)

the Dee they undergo no further acceleration and are turned by a magnetic field using Lorentz forces back towards the gap where the particles are again accelerated across the gap because the potential difference across the gap has been reversed.

To calculate the time (T) needed for a particle's orbit we first need to know how far they are travelling, which is the circumference of a circle and is given by the formula $2\pi r$, and how fast (v) the particles are moving.

$$T = \frac{2\pi r}{v} \qquad (8.6)$$

The radius of the orbit is dependent on the mass of the particle (m) and its speed; centripetal force dictating that heavier and faster particle will take a larger orbit than within a Dee than slower, lighter particles. The radius of the orbit is also dependent on the charge on the particle (q) and the strength of the magnetic field (B). Stronger magnetic fields will force particles into a tighter orbit and if a particle has more charge it will be more strongly affected by a magnetic field than a particle with less charge.

$$r = \frac{mv}{qB} \qquad (8.7)$$

Combining these two equations a new equation is formed.

$$T = \frac{2\pi m}{qB} \qquad (8.8)$$

The new equation shows that the time T needed for a particle to complete an orbit is dependent on three factors; mass, charge, and the strength of the magnetic field, but is independent of the radius or energy of the protons. This means that if these three factors stay the same, the time for an orbit always stays the same, the inner particles moving slowly, the outer ones faster, but regardless of where they are in the cyclotron they will always reach the accelerating gap together

(isochronous), so the frequency of change of the electrical field across the Dees can always stay the same.

The premise that all three factors stay the same however is flawed; the closer particles get to the speed of light the more their mass changes and the effects of these relativistic mass changes cause the particles to get progressively more out of step with the field changes across the gap and this limits the beam energy. Because of this issue modern cyclotrons don't have a constant magnetic field and a number of different methods to overcome this issue are possible. The NHS cyclotrons are isochronous superconducting cyclotrons. An isochronous cyclotron has wedge-shaped inserts at periodic azimuthal positions of the magnet poles which produces alternating strong and weak azimuthal regions called 'hills' and 'valleys' and cause the magnetic field to change in strength (flutter) with the radius, which balances the relativistic mass increase so ensuring that the faster particles still reach the gap at the right time for acceleration. This change to the magnetic field means that the proton trajectory within the cyclotron is not a circle but more closely resembles a rounded square or diamond. Because of the use of the inserts and their position this type of cyclotron can also be called an azimuthal varying field (AVF) cyclotron. Superconducting coils are used to produce the required magnetic field, as these are more powerful than other magnets and the cyclotron can be made more compact in size because of this.

Unlike linear accelerators where one accelerator is placed in each treatment room a cyclotron is not positioned in the treatment room. The particles are transferred to the room via a 'beam line' and although it may provide protons to a single room a cyclotron can be used to supply multiple treatment rooms. The beam line contains a vacuum so that the particles are not slowed down, and the direction of the particle beam is controlled by magnets that deflect and focus the beam along the line until it reaches the desired treatment room. Because each treatment room is using protons created from one cyclotron only one room can be used for treatment at any one time, although other procedures can take place in the other rooms such as patient preparation and verification.

8.14.3 Shielding

A charged particle moving in a magnetic field radiates energy and during routine operation beam losses may occur due to the accelerating particle beam unintentionally colliding with the internal wall of the structures such as the beam line. These collisions can produce high levels of prompt neutrons and gamma rays which require shielding to be placed around the structure in order to provide a safe working environment, although neutron radiation is difficult to shield [36]. Prompt neutrons are only created when the treatment unit is on, but further radiation is also created when the beam is off from areas where the beam losses have occurred in the cyclotron itself, the beam line, and in the room: the collimators, couch, beam stopper, and patient. When protons interact with matter they interact with individual nucleons in the nucleus and produce a number of particles (protons, neutrons, and pions), a process called spallation. The released particles may go on and interact further with other nuclei producing a cascade.

8.14.4 Treatment Room

In each treatment room connected to the beam line is a treatment gantry system. The room also contains a couch and a method of verification.

8.14.5 Treatment Gantry

The treatment gantry is mounted isocentrically and can rotate around the patient, delivering the beam at any desired angle. The Varian Probeam system can rotate 190° in either direction so giving a full 360° treatment rotation. Gantries tend to be large structures

when compared with LinAcs because to direct protons with the required therapeutic energies, relatively large radii are needed. In some units this has been dealt with by the introduction of eccentric gantry systems, where both the patient and the beam line magnets move around the rotation axis. As well as the large radii needed to bend the protons the treatment gantry must also contain beam shaping and monitoring devices.

To treat a tumour effectively the proton beam must be spread out over the desired field size and the depth of the beam modified to cover the whole of the treatment volume. Two methods can be employed to do this: either passive scattering, which tends to be used in the older treatment units, and pencil-beam scanning.

8.14.5.1 Passive Scattering

Passive scattering typically uses two layers of scattering material: the first layer scatters the beam out over the required size whilst the second layer has varying thickness which modifies the uniformity of the beam so ensuring a uniform intensity across the treatment field. The field can then be modified by a field specific collimator/aperture (Figure 8.25) to the required field size. In order to spread out the dose over the required depth and shape the beam in this direction, a range modulator and compensator are used. The range modulator is a fan-shaped device of varying thickness that spins in the beam and degrades the beam energy to varying degrees; the modulator used will be dependent on the size of the tumour and depth desired and will create a spread-out Bragg peak, spreading the dose over the desired depth. Because the depth needed might not be constant due to the tumour shape, a field and patient specific compensator is also needed to shape the beam.

A disadvantage of this system is that when the proton beam interacts with the scattering material neutrons are produced from proton interactions with the various components which increases integral dose. Unique patient-specific devices are needed which have to be individually made, and because they interact

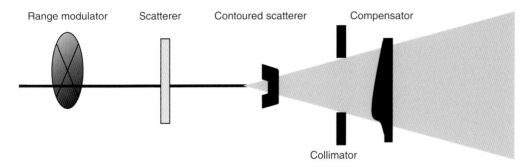

FIGURE 8.25   Beam with components (modulator, compensator).

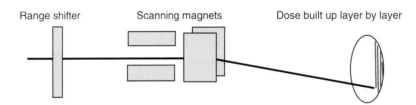

FIGURE 8.26   Beam with components (magnets).

with the beam they will become radioactive and so need special storage until their levels become safe for disposal.

8.14.5.2 Pencil-beam Scanning (Spot Scanning Proton Therapy)

The proton beam is left as a pencil-sized beam (a few millimetres in diameter), and a pair of fast scanning magnets deflect the beam moving it across the desired treatment field until all the treatment volume at that depth has been covered. The beam energy is then changed to treat the next layer and the process is repeated until the entire treatment volume has been covered (Figure 8.26). Pencil-beam scanning capability is a prerequisite for intensity-modulated proton therapy (IMPT) as passive scattering the ability to vary the dose distribution within the treatment volume is limited.

8.14.6 IMPT

IMPT using pencil-beam scanning allows for dose variation on a voxel-by-voxel basis by varying the proton beam intensity and/or the speed of the scanning beam. IMPT improves on X-ray intensity-modulated beams as the dose range can also be modulated more tightly than with photons due to the characteristics of the Bragg peak. This allows the potential for greater conformity of the dose to the target volume, better enabling treatment closer to OARs (organs at risk) and reducing the low-dose bath of IMRT plans.

8.14.7 Accuracy

As with X-rays, proton therapy poses the same requirements for accurate, repeatable patient positioning, perhaps more so; because of its accuracy and finite range the margin for error is very small in clinical use. Variation in the tumour position due to patient motion, bowel filling, or tumour shrinkage will alter the range of the Bragg peak and treatment through areas of density change lead to and increase unsureness about the exact dose distribution [37]. It is therefore essential that this risk is lessened by image guidance techniques, adaptive planning, and replanning the patient if there is significant change.

8.14.8 Rationale for Proton Beam Therapy

Particle beams interact with tissue very differently to photon beams and because of this they deposit their energy very differently in the tissues. In radiobiology, the relative biological effectiveness (RBE) is the ratio of biological effectiveness of one type of ionising radiation relative to another, given the same amount of absorbed energy. The RBE is an empirical value that varies depending on the particles, energies involved, and which biological effects are relevant. The main advantage of proton beams does not lie in radiobiological difference, which is approximately the same as X-ray interactions having an RBE of 1.1, although there is debate on this value as the RBE value changes significantly along the path rising to approximately 1.7 in the distal fall-off region of the Bragg peak [38]. The advantage of proton beams is how they spatially deposit dose in tissue; proton beams having a low entrance dose and a specific range in tissue which is characterised by the Bragg curve (Figure 8.27). Charged particles such as protons lose energy through ionisation events when passing through a material. The Bragg curve describes the rate of energy loss, or linear energy transfer (LET) as a function of the distance through the medium. Energy loss depends on the inverse square of the particle's velocity so giving the Bragg curve its familiar shape where most energy loss occurs at the end of the particles path when the velocity is low, just before the particle stops abruptly so little dose is received beyond this point. The Bragg curve tends to be sharper than that of an electron and is sometimes referred to as a Bragg peak (see Figure 8.27).

Being heavy particles also means that they are not scattered as easily as electrons and these properties allow very specific targeting of the dose within the patient, which is very important when the tumour is close to sensitive structures. It also explains why the central axis depth dose curve of a proton beam resembles a Bragg curve, whereas electrons

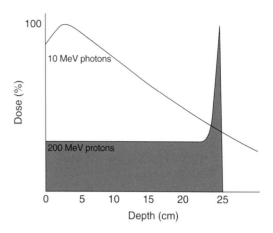

FIGURE 8.27 Bragg peak of protons compared with carbon ions and a photon central axis depth dose curve.

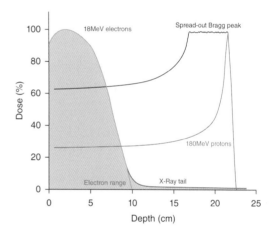

FIGURE 8.28 Central axis depth dose of electron and proton beam.

that are easily scattered do not (see Figure 8.28). Also note the extended tail on the electron beam that arises due to X-ray contamination of the beam.

Only charged particles can be accelerated in a cyclotron, but not electrons. However, it is possible to produce neutron beams from cyclotrons if wanted by accelerating charged particles such as protons or deuterons (the nucleus of a deuteron atom, an isotope of hydrogen consisting of one proton and one neutron) and firing them at a beryllium target which will knock out or strip the neutrons from the nuclei of the beryllium.

8.15 Gamma Knife

The gamma knife SRS unit is essentially a multi-headed cobalt unit. See Section 8.17.6 on stereotactic delivery for further details on radiosurgery. An array of separate cobalt sources produces multiple fine beams of gamma radiation converging in three dimensions to focus precisely onto a small treatment volume. To gain the precision needed for treatment the patient is fitted with a stereotactic head frame fixed to the outer table of the skull. This allows accurate localization of the tumour and associated structures in relation to the three-dimensional coordinates of the head frame. There are different versions of the Leksell Gamma Knife with only IPerfexion® currently available.

The isodose distribution can be modified by delivering a multiple isocentre treatment using different collimator sizes or by employing beam plugging. The gamma knife system includes a radiation unit, all components of which are static, and a movable treatment couch that provides the means for patient positioning. The beam geometry of the gamma knife unit can be hemispherical or conical in arrangement depending on the unit.

The hemispherical system such as the 4C model employs an array of 201 cobalt sources shielded in a cast iron body, each mounted in line with a beam channel. The beam channel consists of a 'source-bushing assembly', which is a pre-collimator of tungsten alloy, a primary stationary collimator, and a secondary conical collimator located in a helmet. There are four interchangeable helmets with collimator sizes of 4, 8, 14, and 18 mm. The helmet is fixed to a sliding cradle that moves into position within the unit so that the collimators are positioned under a beam channel. The radiation beams are initially focused through the primary collimator system along the conical channel and through the secondary collimator, which defines the beam diameter at the focus point. The source to focus distance is 400 mm for all sources.

Perfexion has 192 sources arranged in a cylindrical configuration of five concentric rings the geometry of which results in the SSD varying from 374 to 433 mm. The primary and secondary collimators present in the earlier units have been replaced by a single large 120 mm thick tungsten collimator which is divided into eight independent sectors each containing 72 collimators. Three collimators sizes are available in each sector, 4, 8, and 16 mm, the sources move longitudinally until the source is positioned over the required collimators. Two further docking positions are available, the sector off effectively blocking a sector or home for when the unit is not in use. No helmet is required; the couch functions as the patient positioning system moving the patient to predefined coordinates. Docking of the patient to the patient positioning system is done via an adaptor that attaches to the standard stereotactic Leksell G Frame.

8.16 Intraoperative Radiotherapy

The concept of intraoperative radiotherapy has been around for a considerable time. However, the recent technological advances have renewed interest in this field as smaller, more portable units have been developed to take advantage of the potential of intraoperative radiotherapy. Most intraoperative therapy is similar to contact therapy in that it operates at very short distances and so there is rapid fall-off of dose which allows a delivery of a high dose of radiation very precisely to the targeted area with minimal exposure of the deeper tissues, due to the rapid fall-off of dose. During the operation the access to the site is open so there is no need to go through tissue in order to reach the tumour or tumour bed and so there is no entrance dose. Fractionation, which uses the advantage of different recovery times between the tumour cells and normal cells, isn't important and doses can be delivered in a single fraction with fewer side effects. Finally, with intraoperative treatment there is no delay of treatment post-surgery so there is no opportunity for repopulation of the tumour.

Intraoperative radiotherapy is possible with brachytherapy, however this section focuses on a number of different solutions offered by different manufacturers using X-ray or electron beams. The units can deliver radiation directly to the tumour bed once the tumour has been removed during the surgical procedure, or as a secondary procedure as a day-case patient if the unit is unavailable at the hospital where the surgery was performed. Although not exclusive to breast treatments, the treatment of small, well-defined breast cancers is an area of major interest at the moment.

8.16.1 Zeiss – Intrabeam®

The unit is lightweight and small the X-ray generator body measuring $7 \times 11 \times 14$ cm, the applicator being approximately 16 cm long. The operating voltage can vary between 10 and 50 kV and has an approximate HVL of 1 mm Al. The device is mounted on mobile gantry arm which is counterbalanced to aid movement during the setup. Prior to use the unit is covered with a sterile sheath.

The unit utilises an electron gun to accelerate the electrons to the desired voltage. Once accelerated the electrons pass down an evacuated tube, eventually hitting a thin gold target. As they pass down the evacuated tube the electrons pass between a beam deflector that dithers the electrons across the target (see Figure 8.29).

The X-rays are produced isotropically and can be used with spherical, flat, surface, and needle applicators [39]. For breast treatment spherical applicators are used that maintain the tissue at a set distance from the source. Once the tumour has been removed and the margins verified, a shield is placed on the base of the incision to protect the underlying structures such as the heart and a purse string suture is applied that will hold the breast tissue close to the applicator. The intrabeam device with the appropriate spherical applicator is then put into the cavity and the suture pulled to conform the breast tissue around the top of the applicator. The applicator's solid spheres range in size from 1.5 to 5 cm, which means that the surface dose rate will vary with applicator choice. The skin's surface is then pulled back from the applicator, which can be done by the use of further sutures or a retractor clamp in order keep the skin edges away from the applicator to minimise the skin dose. A radiation shield consisting of tungsten-impregnated rubber is then placed on the patient and around the applicator to reduce the external the dose rate which means that no further shielding is required [40]. Treatment consists of a dose of 20 Gy prescribed to the applicator surface which attenuates to 5–7 Gy at 1 cm depth [41] and takes approximately 20–48 minutes. Once treatment has finished

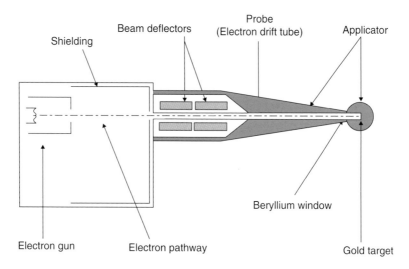

FIGURE 8.29 The Intrabeam intraoperative system.

the sutures can be relaxed, the applicator and shield removed, and the wound closed.

8.16.2 Xstrahl – Xoft Axxent

This system utilises radiolucent balloon-shaped applicators that can be filled with saline or water. The balloons which come in a range of sizes 3–4 cm, 4–5 cm, and 5–6 cm spherical shapes, and 5×7 cm and 6×7 cm ellipsoid shapes, the choice being dependent on which applicator best fits the contour of the surgical cavity. The size can be decided by balloons prior to the applicator balloon being opened.

Once selected the applicator is placed into the cavity created by the operation and inflated. Retention sutures may be used to increase the contact between the balloon and breast tissue, the position and parameters of treatment can be checked by ultrasound prior to treatment. The applicator is then attached to a controller which powers a miniaturised disposable 50 kVp X-ray source that is inserted into the catheter. The X-ray source, which is about 2.2 mm in diameter, is surrounded by a water-cooled, flexible probe assembly measuring 250 mm in length and 5.4 mm in diameter. Once treatment is started the X-ray source is moved according to preprogrammed dwell positions (see Chapter 14) within the applicator by the controller starting at the distal end of the catheter. The average time for radiation delivery is about 22 minutes and because of the low-energy nature of the X-ray source a flexible 0.4 mm lead equivalent protective drape placed over the treatment area during procedure reduces exit doses to a level that allows personnel to remain in the room during treatment.

8.16.3 Electron Beam Intraoperative Linear Accelerators

Being a linear accelerator means that these devices are considerably larger than that of the Intrabeam or Axxent systems. The Mobetron for example has a height of 198 cm, a length of 269 cm, and width of 108.5 cm, and weighs 1395 kg. All the devices however are portable and can be wheeled in and out of the operating theatre as needed. The Mobetron and Liac systems have a scattering foil to spread out the electrons whereas the Novac7 system relies on the air and the walls of the tube to provide a uniform beam. Although there is slight variation between manufacturers, applicators generally range from 3 to 10 cm in diameter. The nominal source to surface distance is 80–100 cm for Novac7, 60 cm for Liac, and 50 cm for the Mobetron unit. The Mobetron applicators are opaque whereas the Novac7 and Liac systems utilise transparent acrylic/perspex applicators, allowing a clearer view of the tumour site during setup. All the units do not require any special fixed shielding systems in the room during treatment. Applicators can come either straight edged, where the treatment distance is constant, or with an angled/bevelled end. The bevelled applicators are used when the tumour bed lies at an angle that is not within the unit's range of motion or because of anatomical constraints, however this can create gradients and offset the dose (see Figure 8.30). Plastic discs can be used as bolus to decrease the depth of the electron beam's penetration and to increase the surface dose [42]. Although electrons have a rapid fall-off of dose in tissue a protective disc made of lead and aluminium is positioned lead-side down between the deep face of the patient's residual breast tissue and the pectoral muscle in order to protect normal tissue beyond the tumour bed.

8.16.3.1 IntraOp – Mobetron

The Mobetron uses two X-band linear accelerators working in tandem. One accelerator receives one-third of the RF power producing a beam of 4 MeV. The other two-thirds of the power can either be directed into a water load or into the second accelerator guide which allows the energy to be varied [43]. The applicators can be positioned in the patient and then clamped in place. The Mobetron unit can then be positioned over the applicator and aligned using a laser-guided soft-docking

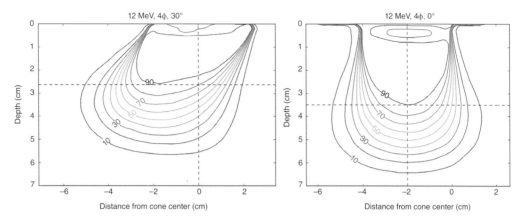

FIGURE 8.30 Comparison of in-plane profiles for a 12 MeV 4 cm applicator. (Source: Wootton et al. [43], p. 237.)

procedure that automatically positions the end of the accelerator 5 cm above the applicator, automatically adjusting the gantry's rotation angle, tilt angle, height, and two translational shifts to align with the applicator. As there is no contact between the Mobetron and applicator the position of the applicator within the patient remains true. Once in position the radiation dose can be delivered using either 6, 8, or 10 MeV electrons.

8.16.3.2 Novac7

The Novac7 is another mobile electron beam LinAc producing the following electron beam energies: 4, 6, 8 and 10 MeV. This system has a very high dose-per-pulse ranging from 2.5 to 12 cGy per pulse which is far higher than the doses per pulse produced by a conventional accelerator [44]. The unit consists of a LinAc on a robotic arm with 6 degrees of freedom and a separate treatment console. Unlike the Mobetron system the Novac7 utilises a hard-docking system between the applicators and the LinAc.

8.16.3.3 Liac

The Liac system is a third mobile electron beam LinAc which has five degrees of movement, and like the Novac7 system the device uses a hard-docking system between the LinAc and the applicators. As with the Novac7 system it has a high instantaneous dose rate. The system can come with 4

different energies, either 4, 6, 8, and 10 MeV or 6, 8, 10, and 12 MeV.

8.16.4 Intraoperative Trials

A number of trials looking at the use of intraoperative radiotherapy for early breast tumours have been undertaken. The ELIOT trial looked at 2459 patients and compared a single dose of 21 Gy using intraoperative (IO) radiotherapy with electrons (Liac and Novac7 units were used) to conventional whole breast radiotherapy. Early breast cancers with a maximum tumour diameter of up to 2.5 cm were randomly assigned to $\geq$ 48 and < 75 [45]. As expected, skin and pulmonary toxicity was reduced in the IO arm although there was greater regional failure in the IO arm (9 patients, 1.0%) compared to (2 patients, 0.3%) with EBRT (external beam radiotherapy). Overall survival at five years was nearly identical, 96.8% for the IO group compared to 96.9% for the EBRT group [46].

The TARGIT-A trial was a prospective multicentre trial looking at 3451 patients aged $\geq$ 45 years with hormone-sensitive invasive ductal carcinoma less than 3.5 cm in size using the Intrabeam® unit. Results after four years were similar in that there were six local recurrences in the IO group and five in the EBRT group. The difference in the estimate of local recurrence between the two groups was small and not significant, 0·25%, −1·04 to 1·54; p = 0·41) and as with the ELIOT trial radiotherapy toxicity (Radiation Therapy Oncology Group grade 3) was lower in the IO group (0·5%) compared to 2·1% in the EBRT group [47]. The final report Vaidya 2016 [48] supported this finding and also attributed fewer deaths from cardiovascular causes and other cancers, leading to a trend in reduced overall mortality in the IO group 3.9% compared to 5.3% in the EBRT group p = 0.099. It also suggested that use of the Intrabeam IO system was significantly less costly than EBRT, with the potential to reduce costs to the healthcare providers in the UK by approximately £8–9 million each year. NICE (National Institute for Clinical Excellence), considering the evidence for the use of the Intrabeam system, concluded that the quality of the trial and its generalizability to NHS clinical practice did not provide enough evidence for routine commissioning for adjuvant treatment in these patient groups. However, some patients if given the option by an experienced multidisciplinary team may choose this treatment and therefore treatment may continue on the existing units if patients understand and are fully informed of the options and are aware of the uncertainties about the procedure [49]. The Axxent system's results are also consistent with the finding above with a recurrence rate of 5.4% being reported [50].

8.17 Treatment Delivery Techniques

8.17.1 Alternatives to Conventional Radiotherapy

The treatment units described in this chapter offer a number of different radiotherapy techniques, some of which have already been mentioned. This section provides a brief summary of the various techniques, although fuller descriptions can be found in books aimed specifically at radiotherapy technique.

8.17.2 IMRT

The introduction of MLCs allowed us to conform the shape of the radiation beam to that of the PTV, so allowing 3D conformal radiotherapy (3D CRT) to be delivered. Although this allowed the reduction of dose to the surrounding tissue the manipulation of dose to the PTV was still limited to the use of wedges and beam angles due to the uniformity of the beam. IMRT allowed us to modulate the intensity of the beam being delivered during radiotherapy voxel by voxel across the shaped field (Figure 8.31c) so allowing better treatment of concave or complex shapes near sensitive structures.

Both conformal therapy and IMRT is possible without MLCs through the use of personalised shielding blocks and custom compensators, however MLCs and the binary collimators of the tomotherapy units offer a better option. The dose variation across the field (fluence) is achieved by a computer controlling the MLC movement during the treatment. Each pixel in Figure 8.31c is delivered by an individual beamlet of radiation. The dose delivered to each pixel being dependent on the individual weight of the beamlet. This creates a lot of variations possible for any one treatment and so planning is done using inverse treatment planning where the oncologist first defines the desired dose to the various structures and other parameters such as number of beams and the planning system computes the actual dose distribution that best meets the criteria set, see Chapter 9.

IMRT can be delivered using multisegmented static fields or dynamically. Delivery by multi-segmented static fields is also called step and shoot as the patient is treated with multiple fields. During each field the MLCs change, forming a number of subfields each with the same beam intensity; in between each sub-field the LinAc switches off as the leaves move to create the next sub-field. This is a very simple method of performing IMRT, easy to plan and deliver, but it can be time consuming. Dynamic delivery is when the radiation is on all of the time during delivery, even when the MLC leaves are

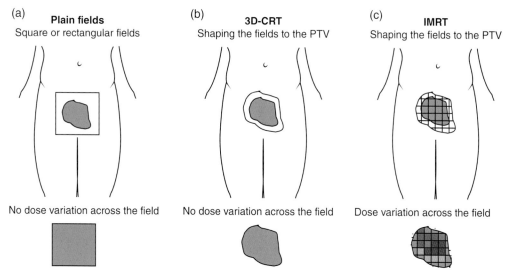

FIGURE 8.31 Development of treatment delivery from plain fields to IMRT.

moving across the target volume. As the beam remains on throughout treatment additional QA is needed, however dynamic treatment allows the production of dose distributions that are more conformal and achieve greater dose homogeneity.

8.17.3 VMAT (Volumetric Modulated Arc Therapy)

VMAT is a form of IMRT where the gantry rotation speed, dose rate, and MLC leaf speed are all continuously modulated at the same time. Instead of delivering treatment from set angles the treatment is given using one or more continuous arcs. Varian also refers to this technology/treatment as RapidArc®. Beams can be delivered in either a coplanar (co-VMAT) or non-coplanar fashion (NC VMAT) and although treatment can be done with one arc, multiple arcs offer the possibility of greater target homogeneity. When treating the breast, it is possible to treat with 2 tangential arcs of approximately 50–60° (t-VMAT) or a continuous arc of about 240° (c-VMAT).

Both IMRT and more especially VMAT can deliver beams from any angle. Data on attenuation in the patient will come at the planning stage using CT data, but consideration of the couch attenuation becomes very important due to its attenuation, especially if immobilisation devices such as an omniboard (see Chapter 7) are being used. VMAT is delivered faster than IMRT and as such there is less chance of intrafraction motion affecting the delivery. The quality of the VMAT plans are better than IMRT plans especially in reducing dose to sensitive structures [51], although the advantage over fixed field IMRT is not as clear and there is an increase in low doses of radiation to surrounding tissue (low-dose bath) [52].

8.17.4 HybridArc IMRT (HA-IMRT)

HybridArc, also referred to as FusionArc, is a combination of both step and shoot IMRT and VMAT consisting of a selection of dynamic arcs with a set of static IMRT beams at discrete intervals along the arcs. The aim of HybridArc is to combine the benefits of both forms of treatment whilst minimising the low-dose bath and direct OAR exposure within the fields. Some studies [53, 54] have shown an increased advantage in both the dose homogeneity and conformity index and also a reduction in beam-on time and monitor units of the hybrid arc plans compared to either IMRT or VMAT plans, although the difference is not always significant.

8.17.5 Adaptive Radiotherapy

Adaptive planning recognises that a single plan created before treatment commences often leads to sub-optimal treatment due to changes in anatomy over time, possibly as a result of changes in patient position, weight loss, internal motion, or tumour shrinkage. IGRT repositions the patient by applying couch shifts so that the treatment is delivered accurately, but treatment is always based on the initial treatment plan. Adaptive radiotherapy modifies the treatment plan based on observed anatomical changes found whilst imaging. These moderations can either be done 'off-line' or 'on-line'. Off-line adaptive radiotherapy is used to address progressive changes where a change such as cumulative tumour shrinkage triggers a replan which will be used for future treatments. This method suffers from the subjective assessment of the most appropriate time to intervene.

On-line adaptive radiotherapy tends to deal with random changes and occurs on-set post imaging. One current approach to on-line adaptive planning is the use of plan libraries, the so-called 'plan-of-the-day' approach. In this approach a number of different treatment plans are created that anticipate different possible anatomic variations and each treatment day the 'best' plan is selected based on the images taken. Another method used is to create a deformation field which is created from deforming the patient's 3D planning CT to that of the CBCT and so morph the treatment plan to provide an online correction of treatment [29]. This method is still a 'work in progress' and is not as yet used in routine clinical practice.

The methods above are not exhaustive and deal with time-adaptive radiotherapy, but this method of treatment also has the potential to adapt treatments based on biological considerations such as hypoxia using PET and magnetic resonance spectroscopy. Currently this form of treatment is limited by various issues such as slow accrual time and issues in the evaluation of outcome [55].

8.17.6 Stereotactic Delivery

Stereotactic delivery uses specialised equipment to localise the tumour in three dimensions so allowing a high degree of accuracy in the delivery radiation to a tumour. It is usually associated with the term radiosurgery, which is the use of high doses of ablative radiation to the PTV whilst keeping the dose to the surrounding structures low to have a minimal impact on the surrounding healthy tissue.

The rationale for stereotactic treatment is the same as for conformal radiotherapy in that it offers the opportunity for highly targeted radiation that can be shaped to match the target volume. The difference is that stereotactic localization equipment, combined with the small size of the radiation beams, allows for much more precision in the targeting of the treatment and therefore further reduction of the beam margin compared to other treatments. As with IMRT, stereotactic treatments traditionally utilise a large number of very small beams. By focusing all these beams on one volume of tissue a high dose can be delivered in a conformal manner with a low dose outside that volume.

SRS was first envisaged by Lars Leksell [56] who developed the Gamma knife for treatment of brain lesions. However, developments in areas such as CT planning, robotic control, and image-guidance technology have since allowed stereotactic-based treatments on other units and body areas. With the advent of MLCs, stereotactic radiotherapy can be given on LinAcs including cyberknife and tomotherapy units, and in some centres, proton units. If treatment is to the brain the term SRS tends to be used; in other parts of the body the following terms apply: SBRT (stereotactic body radiotherapy) or SABR (stereotactic ablative radiotherapy).

Both SRS and SBRT tend to deliver radiation in either a single fraction or a small number of fractions (1–5).

Typical conditions currently treated with stereotactic techniques are shown in Table 8.3.

Originally the high degree of accuracy was derived from the use of a stereotactic frame that was attached to the patient's skull via screws. Although this technique can still be used, frames can now be used that use reliable frames of reference such as bone or teeth, a dental mould being taken and attached to the frame.

Frameless stereotactic radiotherapy can now be given, one such system being the Fraxion immobilisation device developed by Elekta (see Chapter 7), which gives similar accuracy to the Leskell frame, but with a higher degree of comfort. Cyberknife is specifically designed to perform frameless SRS. Rather than using rigid immobilisation devices, the Cyberknife relies an orthogonal pair of X-ray cameras that can dynamically manipulate a robot-mounted LinAc, giving accuracy levels that are comparable to localization errors that have been reported using frame-based systems, Chang et al. [57] reporting a clinical accuracy of 1.1 ± 0.3 mm. Brainlab's ExacTrac shown in Figure 8.32 allows frameless stereotactic treatments on a standard LinAc with an accuracy of 1.24 mm for stereotactic radiotherapy and 1.35 mm for SRS.

TABLE 8.3	Common stereotactic treatments and doses.	
Condition	**Treatment**	**Dose**
Arteriovenous malformation (AVM)	SRS	~20 Gy single #
Brain metastases	SRS	15–24 Gy single #
Non-small cell cancer	SABR	54–60 Gy in 3–5 #

8.17.7 Total Skin Electron Beam Therapy (TSEB)

TSEB is used primarily to treat primary cutaneous T-cell lymphomas and in particular mycosis fungoides (MF). A number of different treatment options are available for MF such as corticosteroid ointments, topical

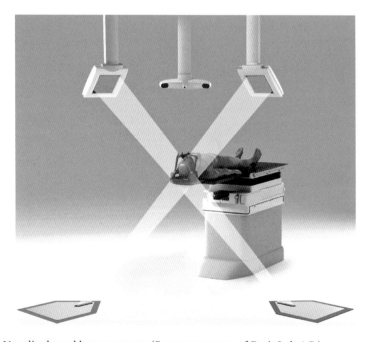

FIGURE 8.32 Novalis shaped beam surgery. (Source: courtesy of BrainLab AG.)

chemotherapy, PUVA (Psoralen + UV-A), and localised radiotherapy which may be combined with combined with immunotherapy or retinoids. TSEB, which is sometimes called Total Body Electrons (TBE) is used to try and bring the condition into complete or partial remission by treating the whole body. Typically, the total dose delivered is between 30 and 36 Gy over a period of 8–10 weeks and high remission rates are reported. However, treatment rarely induces long-term remission. Energies used are typically between 4 and 10 MeV, but because of the distance and use of a degrader this is reduced to 3–7 MeV at the patient's treatment plane [58].

The main issues with a TSEB technique are to obtain a homogenous dose across the whole of the skin's surface, and there are three main methods utilised to undertake this: large electron field techniques, rotational techniques, and techniques that involve a translational shift of the patient during irradiation.

The use of large electron fields is only possible if a large SSD is possible in the treatment room. Assuming a maximum field size of 40 cm at 100 cm, a distance of 6 m would give a field size of 2.4 m. If this is possible rotational techniques can be used where the patient stands on a motorised platform that slowly rotates during the treatment. However, most rooms are smaller than this and it is usually only possible to have a maximum SSD in the order of 4 m or less, which would give a maximum field size of about 1.6 m, which would not be large enough to cover most people in the treatment position. To overcome this limitation, most departments utilise a two-field static technique to cover the patient as shown in Figure 8.33.

The patient is positioned standing approximately 3 m from the radiation source which means that the dose rate at this distance will be 0.11 of that at 100 cm, and therefore the treatment time will be extended. This can in part be mitigated by treating at a higher dose rate compared to 'standard' treatments. In some instances, the LinAc is modified and the scattering foil in the LinAc is replaced by an external aluminium scatterer attached to the linear accelerator, but more frequently nowadays no modification is made to the LinAc and an acrylic scatterer/degrader is placed as close to the patient as possible to help with beam flatness and provide a more homogenous dose. The beams are angled 20° above and below the horizon to give the desired coverage. This angle also positions the central axis above and below the patient, which is important as most X-ray contamination of the beam is on the central axis. Reducing the patient's exposure to X-rays is important, as X-rays when present will penetrate deeper in the body than the electrons and may cause myelo-suppression. The patient is usually raised off the floor on a platform to reduce dose perturbations from the floor that would affect the dose received near the feet.

With this technique six patient positions are required, an anterior, posterior, two posterior obliques, and two anterior obliques.

Arms and legs are positioned to allow the beam to reach all parts of the body except for

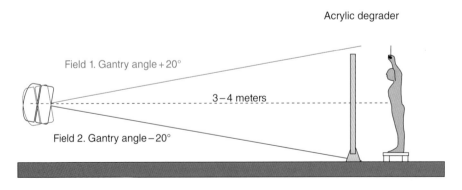

Acrylic degrader

Field 1. Gantry angle + 20°

3–4 meters

Field 2. Gantry angle − 20°

FIGURE 8.33 Machine treatment positions.

the soles of the feet, palms of the hand, vertex, and perineum, which may require additional treatment separately [59]. The arms and legs are slightly apart to allow access to the groin and the arms are raised and to the side to allow electrons to treat the axilla. To help the patient maintain their position, the patient either holds a bar suspended from above (Figure 8.33). Assisting the patient into the correct position can be time consuming as it is important to shield the lens of the eye. If the eyelids are involved internal eye shields are used, if not external eye shields can be used which can be something as simple as swimming goggles customised by the addition of lead and wax; whichever is used the patient will effectively be unable to see during the treatment and will need guidance getting into position. It is also possible to shield other areas of the body if unaffected by the disease; one area commonly shielded is the nail bed as doses are often high enough to stop nail growth or even lose the nails completely if not shielded. Hair loss will occur on all irradiated areas. Patient dignity is another aspect that must be considered as during the treatment they will only be able to wear a thin cotton smock so as not to affect the electron beam reaching the skin.

8.17.8 TBI Techniques

Total body irradiation (TBI) is a main component in the treatment of haematopoietic cancers used to suppress the patient's immune system following elimination of the cancerous cells by chemotherapy. This then stops the body from rejecting the allogeneic (from a donor), autologous (from oneself), or syngeneic (from an identical twin) transplantation of stem cells.

TBIs can be delivered either as a single fraction of approximately (4–10 Gy) or using fractionated treatments (12 Gy given in 6 fractions of 2 Gy). As with TSEB treatment one of the main issues is the size of the field needed which usually means the requirement for extended FSD treatments, although other methods such as field matching,

patient translation during treatment, and the use of a sweeping beam are possible. The most common method of treating TBIs in the UK is with static extended FSD beams. In order to cover the patient with one beam a field size of 70 cm × 200 cm is typically used which means that the treatment distance will be in the order of 5–6 m. Because of the extended FSD used the dose rate will be much reduced. With treatment distances such as this the patient can be treated supine or erect, however if the treatment distance is limited the patient may have to be treated supine or on their side with their knees bent or on a specially designed chair.

The treatment utilises a pair of opposing high-energy photon beams to the whole body, in order to give a uniform dose to the whole body (±10%), although this raises to ±30% if the skin dose is included. The patient's position is switched between each field. The photon beam energy can be selected depending on the patient's separation and dose uniformity established by the use of compensators or bolus. Separation of the body varies more in the lateral direction (approximately 50 cm) than the antero-posterio direction (20–25 cm for adults), so more consideration of dose variation is needed for lateral treatments. The organs at risk being the lungs, kidney, liver, spleen, heart, and eyes and it is possible to use shielding or compensation to reduce the dose to some of these areas, although care must be taken as circulating stem cells and bone marrow cells may also be shielded. One centre in the USA has implemented a TBI method using VMAT in order to deliver a uniform dose. One area commonly shielded is the lungs in order to reduce the median dose to this area to 8–10 Gy in order to reduce the risk of pneumonitis [60].

Patient position may also aid in protecting certain areas, for example keeping the upper arms by the patient's side helps shadow the lungs if treating supine. In order to ensure that the dose is uniform a test dose may need to be given before treatment using dosimeters such as TLDs and diodes which can be placed at different locations in order to measure the dose. If fractionating the treatment this may be done on the first treatment and later treatments adjusted.

Male patients afflicted with acute lymphoblastic leukaemia are at risk of testicular relapse, although it is not a common occurrence. If there is known or potential risk of testicular disease a boost to the scrotum might be given. Issues that may be of concern with this form of treatment is the large amount of scatter created from within the treatment room due to the large field size.

Acknowledgements

I would like to thank the following for their help and comments in the development of various sections of the chapter.

Advanced Technique: **Zankhana Jani.** Treatment Delivery Superintendent. University College Hospital London.

Cyclotrons and Proton beams: **Laura Allington.** Operational Lead for Proton Beam Therapy. University College Hospital London.

Halcyon: **Emily Borchardt.** Senior Radiographer. Queens Hospital, Romford.

MRI LinAcs: **Rebekah Lawes and Helen Creasey**. Senior MR LinAc radiographers, The Royal Marsden NHS Foundation Trust.

Tomotherapy: **Liam Mannion.** City, University of London.

TSEB: **Liz Murphy**. Clinical Specialist Therapy Radiographer. Freeman Hospital, Newcastle.

References

1. Department of Health (2004). *Manual for Cancer Services*. London: Department of Health.
2. Palmer, A.L., Pearson, M., Whittard, P. et al. (2016). Current status of kilovoltage (kV) radiotherapy in the UK: installed equipment, clinical workload, physics quality control and radiation dosimetry. *Br. J. Radiol.* 89 (1068): 20160641. https://doi.org/10.1259/bjr.20160641.
3. Klevenhagen, S.C., Aukett, R.J., Harrison, R.M. et al. (1996). The IPMEB code of practice for the determination of absorbed dose for x-rays below 300kV generating potential. *Phys. Med. Biol.* 41: 2605–2625.
4. National Institute for Health and Clinical Excellence. Grenze rays therapy for inflammatory skin conditions. *Interventional Procedure Guidance 236*. London NICE, 2007.
5. National Institute for Health and Care Excellence Interventional Procedures Programme. Interventional procedure overview of low-energy contact X-ray brachytherapy (the Papillon technique) for early stage rectal cancer. IP 1234 [IPG532] 2015.
6. Klevenhagen, S.C. and Thwaites, D.I. (1993). Chapter 3; Kilovoltage X-rays. In: *Radiotherapy in Practice* (eds. J.R. Williams and D.I. Thwaites). Oxford: Oxford Medical Publications.
7. Whelan, B., Holloway, L., Constantin, D. et al. (2016). Performance of a clinical gridded electron gun in magnetic fields: implications for MRI-LinAc therapy. *Med. Phys.* 43 (11): 5903–5914.
8. Schulz, L. (1999). Sputter-ion pumps. *Cern. Rep.* 5: 37–42.
9. Bell, K., Heitfield, M., Licht, N. et al. (2017). Influence of daily imaging on plan quality and normal tissue toxicity for prostate cancer radiotherapy. *Radiat. Oncol.* 12 (1): 7. https://doi.org/10.1186/s13014-016-0757-9.
10. Yan, Y., Yadav, P., Bassetti, M. et al. (2016). Dosimetric differences in flattened and flattening filter-free beam treatment plans. *J. Med. Phys.* 41 (2): 92–99.
11. Xiao, Y., Kry, S.F., Popple, R. et al. (2015). Flattening filter-free accelerators: a report from the AAPM Therapy Emerging Technology Assessment Work Group. *J. Appl. Cin. Med. Phys.* 16 (3): 12–29.
12. Symonds-Tayler, J.R.N. and Webb, S. (1998). Gap-stepped MLC leaves with filler blades can eliminate tongue-and-groove underdoses when delivering IMRT with maximum efficiency. *Phys. Med. Biol.* 43: 2393–2395.
13. ICRU (1976) Determination of Absorbed Dose in a Patient Irradiated by Beams of X or Gamma Rays in Radiotherapy Procedures. Report No 24. Oxford: ICRU Publications.
14. Li, H., Lee, A.K., Johnson, J.L. et al. (2011). Characterization of dose impact on IMRT and VMAT from couch attenuation for two Varian couches. *J. Appl. Clin. Med. Phys.* 12 (3): 23–31.

15. Sheykhoo, A., Abdollahi, S., Yazdi, M.H.H. et al. (2017). Effects of Siemens TT-D carbon fiber table top on beam attenuation, and build up region of 6 MV photon beam. *Rep. Pract. Oncol. Radiother.* 22 (1): 19–28.

16. Srinivasan, K., Mohammadi, M., and Shepherd, J. (2014). Applications of LinAc-mounted kilovoltage Cone-beam Computed Tomography in modern radiation therapy: a review. *Pol. J. Radiol.* 79: 181–193.

17. Parsons, D. and Robar, J. (2012). The effect of copper conversion plates on low-Z target image quality. *Med. Phys.* 39 (9): 5362–5371.

18. Broderick, M., Menezes, G., Leech, M. et al. (2007). A comparison of kilovoltage and megavoltage cone beam CT in radiotherapy. *J. Radiother. Pract.* 6: 173–178.

19. Held, M., Cremers, F., Sneed, P.K. et al. (2016). Assessment of image quality and dose calculation accuracy on kV CBCT, MV CBCT, and MV CT images for urgent palliative radiotherapy treatments. *J. Appl. Clin. Med. Phys.* 17: 279–290.

20. Binny, D., Lancaster, C.M., Harris, S., and Sylvander, S.R. (2015). Effects of changing modulation and pitch parameters on tomotherapy delivery quality assurance plans. *J. Appl. Clin. Med. Phys.* 16 (5): 87–105.

21. Kissick, M.W., Fenwick, J., James, J.A. et al. (2005). The helical tomotherapy thread effect. *Am. Assoc. Phys. Med.* 32 (5): 1414–1423.

22. Hashimoto, H., Omura, M., Matsui, K. et al. (2015). Tangent field technique of TomoDirect improves dose distribution for whole-breast irradiation. *J. Appl. Clin. Med. Phys.* 16 (3): 225–232.

23. Squires, M., Hu, Y., Archibald-Heeren, B. et al. (2017). Static beam tomotherapy as an optimisation method in whole-breast radiation therapy (WBRT). *J. Med. Radiat. Sci.* 64: 281–289.

24. Chen, Q., Mallory, M., Crandley, E. et al. (2018). Investigation of hot-spots in TomoDirect 3DCRT breast treatment. *Int. J. Med. Phys. Clin. Eng. Radiat. Oncol.* 7: 376–390.

25. Peng, B.J., Wu, Y., Cherry, S.R. et al. (2014). New shielding configurations for a simultaneous PET/MRI scanner at 7T. *J. Magn. Reson.* 239: 50–56.

26. Laader, A., Beiderwellen, K., Kraff, O. et al. (2017). 1.5 versus 3 versus 7 Tesla in abdominal MRI: a comparative study. *PLoS One* 12 (11): e0187528. https://doi.org/10.1371/journal.pone.0187528.

27. Han, E.Y., Wen, Z., Lee, H.J. et al. (2018). Measurement of electron return effect and skin dose reduction by a bolus in an anthropomorphic physical phantom under a magnetic resonance guided linear accelerator (MR-LINAC) system. *Int. J. Med. Phys. Clin. Eng. Radiat. Oncol.* 7: 339–346.

28. Lee, H.J., Choi, G.W., Alqathami, M. et al. (2017). Using 3D dosimetry to quantify the Electron Return Effect (ERE) for MR-image-guided radiation therapy (MR-IGRT) applications. *J. Phys. Conf. Ser.* 847: 012057.

29. Hunt, A., Hansen, V.N., Oelke, U. et al. (2018). Adaptive radiotherapy enabled by MRI guidance. *Clin. Oncol.* 30: 711–719.

30. Ginn, J.S., Agazaryan, N., Cao, M. et al. (2017). Characterization of spatial distortion in a 0.35 T MRI-guided radiotherapy system. *Phys. Med. Biol.* 62 (11): 4525–4540.

31. Kontaxis C. Towards real-time plan adaptation for MRI-guided radiotherapy. PhD Thesis. Utrecht University, The Netherlands. 2017.

32. Riley, C., Cox, C., Graham, S. et al. (2018). Varian Halcyon dosimetric comparison for multiarc VMAT prostate and head-and-neck cancers. *Med. Dosim.* https://doi.org/10.1016/j.meddos.2018.06.004; [Epub ahead of print].

33. Sumida, I., Shiomi, H., Higashinaka, N. et al. (2016). Evaluation of tracking accuracy of the CyberKnife system using a webcam and printed calibrated grid. *J. Appl. Clin. Med. Phys.* 17 (2): 74–84.

34. Akino, Y., Sumida, I., Shiomi, H. et al. (2018). Evaluation of the accuracy of the CyberKnife Synchrony™ Respiratory Tracking System using a plastic scintillator. *Med. Phys.* 45 (8): 3506–3515.

35. European Commission. Radiation Protection 162. Criteria for Acceptability of Medical Radiological Equipment used in Diagnostic Radiology, Nuclear Medicine and Radiotherapy. 2012. Publications Office of the European Union, Luxembourg.

36. Daugherty HM, Waaldschlager IC, Elkins DS, et al. Proton Therapy Facility Shielding. 2016 University of Tennessee Honors Thesis Projects. Available at: https://trace.tennessee.edu/utk_chanhonoproj/1936.

37. Paganetti, H. (2012). Range uncertainties in proton therapy and the role of Monte Carlo simulations. *Phys. Med. Biol.* 57 (11): R99–R117.

38. Paganetti, H. (2014). Relative biological effectiveness (RBE) values for proton beam therapy. Variations as a function of biological endpoint, dose, and linear energy transfer. *Phys. Med. Biol.* 59 (22): R419–R472.

39. Sethi, A., Emami, B., Small, W. Jr., and Thomas, T.O. (2018). Intraoperative radiotherapy with INTRABEAM: technical and dosimetric considerations. *Front. Oncol.* 8: 74.

40. Muñoz, G.H., Hany, R.P., Cosson, A. et al. (2015). Intraoperative Radiation Therapy (INTRABEAM) experience at the Mastology Unit Leopoldo Aguerrevere clinic. *J. Cancer Ther.* 6: 932–942.

41. Dutta, S.W., Showalter, S.L., Showalter, T.N. et al. (2017). Intraoperative radiation therapy for breast cancer patients: current perspectives. *Breast Cancer (Dove Med Press)* 9: 257–263.

42. Bedar, A.S. and Krishnan, S. (2005). Intraoperative radiotherapy using a mobile electron LINAC: a retroperitoneal sarcoma case. *J. Appl. Clin. Med. Phys.* 6 (3): 95–107.

43. Wootton, L.S., Meyer, J., Kim, E. et al. (2017). Commissioning, clinical implementation, and performance of the Mobetron 2000 for intraoperative radiation therapy. *J. Appl. Clin. Med. Phys.* 18: 230–242.

44. Lamanna, E., Gallo, A., Russo, F. et al. (2012). Intra-operative radiotherapy with electron beam. (Chapter 9) [online]. In: *Modern Practices in Radiation Therapy* (ed. G. Natanasabapathi), 150–152. InTech.

45. Veronesi, U., Orecchia, R., Luini, A. et al. (2008). Full-dose intra-operative radiotherapy with electrons (ELIOT) during breast-conserving surgery: experience with 1246 cases. *Ecancermedicalscience* 2: 65. Available at: https://www.ncbi.nlm.nih.gov/pmc/articles/PMC3234040.

46. Silverstein, M.J., Fastner, G., Maluta, S. et al. (2014). Intraoperative radiation therapy: a critical analysis of the ELIOT and TARGIT trials. Part 1—ELIOT. *Ann. Surg. Oncol.* 21 (12): 3787–3792.

47. Vaidya, J.S., Joseph, D.J., Tobias, J.S. et al. (2010). Targeted intraoperative radiotherapy versus whole breast radiotherapy for breast cancer (TARGIT-A trial): an international, prospective, randomised, non-inferiority phase 3 trial. *Lancet* 376: 91–102.

48. Vaidya, J.S., Wenz, F., Bulsara, M. et al. (2016). An international randomised controlled trial to compare TARGeted Intraoperative radioTherapy (TARGIT) with conventional postoperative radiotherapy after breast-conserving surgery for women with early-stage breast cancer (the TARGIT-A trial). *Health Technol. Assess.* 20: 73.

49. NICE Intrabeam radiotherapy system for adjuvant treatment of early breast cancer. Technology appraisal guidance. 2018.

50. Schwartzberg, B.S., Chin, D.T., Dorn, P.L. et al. (2018). Application of 21-gene recurrence score results and ASTRO suitability criteria in breast cancer patients treated with intraoperative radiation therapy (IORT). *Am. J. Surg.* 216: 689–693.

51. Quan, E.M., Li, X.M.S., Li, Y.M.S. et al. (2012). A comprehensive comparison of IMRT and VMAT plan quality for prostate cancer treatment. *Int. J. Radiat. Oncol. Biol. Phys.* 83 (4): 1169–1178.

52. Teoh, M., Clark, C.H., Wood, K. et al. (2011). Volumetric modulated arc therapy: a review of current literature and clinical use in practice. *Br. J. Radiol.* 84 (1007): 967–996.

53. Chen, Y.-G., Li, A.-C., Li, W.-Y. et al. (2017). The feasibility study of a hybrid coplanar arc technique versus hybrid intensity-modulated radiotherapy in treatment of early-stage left-sided breast cancer with simultaneous-integrated boost. *J. Med. Phys.* 42 (1): 1–8.

54. Li, J., To, D., Gunn, V. et al. (2018). Evaluation of hybrid arc and volumetric-modulated arc therapy treatment plans for fractionated stereotactic intracranial radiotherapy. *Technol. Cancer Res. Treat.* 17: https://doi.org/10.1177/1533033818802804, https://www.ncbi.nlm.nih.gov/pmc/articles/PMC6198396.

55. Kim, S. and Wong, J.W. (eds.) (2018). *Advanced and Emerging Technologies in Radiation Oncology Physics*. Florida, USA: CRC Press.

56. Lasak, J.M. and Gorecki, J.P. (2009). The history of stereotactic radiosurgery and radiotherapy. *Otolaryngol. Clin. North Am.* 42 (4): 593–599.

57. Chang, S.D., Main, W., Martin, D.P. et al. (2003). An analysis of the accuracy of the CyberKnife: a robotic frameless stereotactic radiosurgical system. *Neurosurgery* 52 (1): 140–147.

58. Karzmark CJ. Total kin electron Therapy: Technique and Dosimetry. Report of Task Group 30 Radiotherapy Committee AAPM Report 23. 1987.

59. Piotrowski, T., Fundowicz, M., and Pawlaczyk, M. (2018). Total skin electron beam therapy with rotary dual technique as palliative treatment for mycosis fungoides. *In Vivo* 32 (3): 517–522.

60. Wong, J.Y.C., Filippi, A.R., Dabaja, B.S. et al. (2018). Total body irradiation: guidelines from the international lymphoma radiation oncology group (ILROG). *Int. J. Radiat. Oncol. Biol. Phys.* 101 (3): 521–529.

CHAPTER 9

Principles and Practice of Treatment Planning

Pete Bridge

Aim

The aim of this chapter is to describe the fundamental physics principles underpinning radiotherapy planning. This requires an understanding of how absorbed dose is mapped in the body when a high-energy treatment beam is incident upon the surface. The basics of isodose curves, beam characteristics, and planning terminology are described along with an explanation of the steps in the planning process.

9.1 Introduction

Treatment planning has evolved from the early use of radiation for therapy, where the distribution of radioactive sources was determined from a set of rules, to modern planning techniques that rely on complex computer modelling of the dose distribution from patient data and external radiation beam parameters. The overall aim of the planning process remains the translation of the therapeutic requirements of the oncologist into a set of treatment instructions that will enable the patient to be treated accurately. The treatment plan not only provides a set of instructions for the radiographer but also provides information about the distribution of dose that enables the oncologist to assess the adequacy of the beam arrangements. This chapter describes the basic principles behind the process of radiotherapy treatment planning. No attempt is made to describe the process of producing plans for a particular tumour site, and the reader is referred elsewhere for this [1, 2]. Also, the principles of radiation dosimetry are explained in Chapter 4 and a detailed description of various systems of dosimetry calculation can be found elsewhere [3]. This chapter comprises four sections:

9.1.1 Treatment Planning Principles

The first section describes the basic principles behind treatment planning, including essential terminology, international recommendations, and aims and objectives of planning.

Practical Radiotherapy: Physics and Equipment, Third Edition. Edited by Pam Cherry and Angela M. Duxbury.
© 2020 John Wiley & Sons Ltd. Published 2020 by John Wiley & Sons Ltd.

9.1.2 Treatment Planning Process

The second section explains the key steps in the treatment planning process. A description of beam and patient data formats as well as the contouring, beam setup, optimisation, and evaluation stages of planning is provided. This section also outlines the features and tools found in modern radiotherapy planning systems to facilitate each of these stages.

9.1.3 Advanced Planning

Treatment planning systems (TPSs) are not just used for megavoltage photon calculations but across a wide range of modalities and techniques. This section outlines the additional requirements and tools necessary for proton, electron, brachytherapy, stereotactic radiosurgery treatments, and adaptive planning.

9.1.4 Quality Assurance

There is great potential for introduction of major systematic errors during treatment planning and this section outlines the quality assurance (QA) requirements that aim to reduce or eliminate these risks.

9.2 Treatment Planning Principles

9.2.1 Depth Dose

The first step to establishing the absorbed dose distribution in the patient is to determine the variation of dose along the central axis of the beam. The dose at depth depends on a range of factors including field size, beam energy, depth in the patient, distance from the beam source, and external attenuators (e.g. wedges). The dose along the centre of the field can be defined by various energy-dependent parameters, the most common of these being *percentage depth dose* (PDD) and *tissue maximum ratio* (TMR).

PDD is defined as the dose at depth in a phantom expressed as a percentage of the dose at a reference depth d_o (usually the position of the peak absorbed dose, $d_o = d_{max}$) on the central axis of the beam:

$$\mathrm{PDD}\left(d, d_o, A_d, s\right) = D_d / D_{do} \times 100.$$

The parameters shown in parentheses, as defined in Figure 9.1a, indicate the dependency of PDD on depth d, position of dose maximum d_o, area of the field A_d at depth d, and SSD (source-to-surface distance) ($s =$ SSD).

TMR is defined as the dose at depth in a phantom expressed as a ratio of the dose at the same point in relation to the radiation source but at the position of peak dose ($d_o = d_{max}$) on the central axis of the beam:

$$\mathrm{TMR}\left(d, A_d\right) = D_d / D_{do}.$$

PDD values along the central axis of the beam may be measured using a radiation detector moved to increasing depth in a phantom with the SSD kept constant (usually 100 cm). These values can then be expressed as percentages of the peak dose on the central axis.

TMR values are measured by ensuring that the source-to-detector distance remains constant with the detector always at the isocentre (usually at 100 cm), as seen in Figure 9.1b. TMR is expressed as the ratio of dose at depth to the peak dose value.

In practice, PDD requires the phantom position to remain at a constant distance from the source whilst the detector moves to the point of measurement, whereas for TMR the detector remains at a constant distance from the source and the phantom (or surface) moves to provide measurement at depth. It can be seen, therefore, that TMRs are more useful for isocentric treatments because the quantity is virtually independent of SSD,

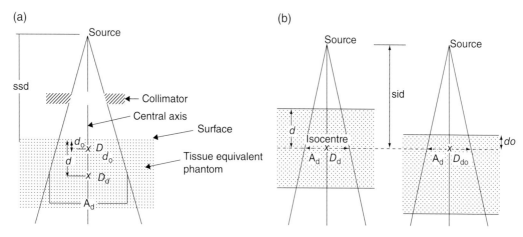

FIGURE 9.1 (a) Percentage depth dose (PDD $= D_d/D_{do} \times 100$); (b) tissue maximum ratio (TMR $= D_d/D_{do}$).

whereas PDD dose values require an inverse square correction for any change in SSD.

TPSs use PDD and TMR values for dose calculations and can be interconverted by inverse square and phantom scatter corrections. Another quantity used by TPSs is the scatter maximum ratio (SMR), which is particularly useful for calculating scatter dose from irregular field shapes in a medium. This is defined as the ratio of the scattered dose at a given point (d) in a phantom to the effective primary dose at the same point at the position of peak dose (d_o). In practice, SMR values may be obtained by subtracting the zero area field TMR, TMR (d,0), from the finite area TMR, TMR(d,A_d), and correcting for phantom scatter.

9.2.2 Isodose Curves and Dose Mapping

Isodose curves are lines joining points of equal PDD and therefore provide a means of mapping the variation in dose as a function of depth and transverse distance from the central axis of the beam. As with PDDs, the isodose distribution is affected by the beam quality (or energy), field size, SSD, attenuators, and source/collimation geometry. A detailed discussion of these parameters may be found elsewhere [3, 4].

A single beam isodose chart can be constructed for a beam and typically shows a set of isodose curves that provides incremental PDD, usually ranging from the maximum value to the 100% value in steps of 10%. An example is shown in Figure 9.2 for a 6 MV open field and a 10 MV wedge field. The isodose curves represent a field in a single plane with the beam at normal incidence to the surface of a water-equivalent homogeneous phantom. Isodose curves are an essential tool for planning and allow easy visualisation of dose distribution within the patient model. As with isodose charts, it is convenient to specify lines in 10% increments of PDD.

9.2.2.1 Normalisation
Normalisation is the process of identifying a location at which the PDD is determined to be 100%. For a single beam, this is the point of maximum dose on the central beam axis for a fixed SSD (100 cm), whilst for multiple beams this is normally the isocentre. The normalisation point, however, can be located at any point within the target volume. It should be positioned in a region where dose calculation is accurate, ideally away from areas of steep dose gradient such as a penumbra or inhomogeneity boundary. It is important that the dose is prescribed to the normalisation point in order to ensure accuracy.

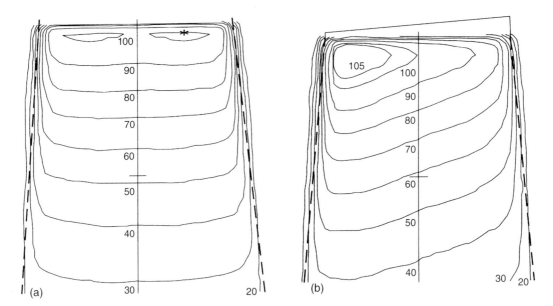

FIGURE 9.2 (a) 6 MV open field; (b) 10 MV wedged field, 45°.

9.3 ICRU Guidelines

The International Commission on Radiation Units and Measurements (ICRU) is responsible for devising and distributing recommendations for radiation dosimetry. Amongst the numerous ICRU reports are several that are of particular importance to treatment planning in describing the parameters of volume and dose when prescribing radiotherapy treatments. The publications ICRU50 [5] and its supplement ICRU62 [6] provided clear recommendations about reporting of absorbed dose distributions and set out the level of complexity of dose evaluation from basic planning techniques to complex 3D dose computation.

ICRU50 provided clear and concise definitions of *gross tumour volume* (GTV), *clinical target volume* (CTV), and *planning target volume* (PTV), which are marked on the CT images of the patient before beam placement and calculation of the plan. The later publication of ICRU62 [6] developed the concept of treatment margins by defining two categories of margin; those accounting for geometrical changes in the CTV due to anatomical uncertainties (*internal margin*) and those added to account for uncertainties on patient position (*setup margin*).

The early ICRU publications gave a general criterion for reporting dose as a point within the PTV referred to as the *ICRU reference point*; this is a point that represents the spatial variation of dose within the PTV and is generally the dose prescription point. This reference point is often, but not always (as with the case of half-beam blocked matched fields) at the treatment isocentre, which is generally the intersection of all beams. For intensity-modulated radiotherapy (IMRT), however, this point may not necessarily provide an accurate representation of dose delivered to the volume. The associated use of small-beam geometries has necessitated a different approach to evaluation of dose distributions. The 2010 publication of ICRU83 [7] specifically described a shift from point-based reporting of dose to volume-based. The concepts of D2% and D98% are helpful in this regard. D2% is the dose received by 2% of the structure volume which is the high-dose region whilst the D98% is the dose received by 98% which replaces the minimum dose recommendations.

Additional recommendations in the early ICRU Reports related to the acceptable limits of homogeneity with the PTV recommended to receive no less than 95% and no more than 107.5% of the prescribed dose. These formed the basis for plan evaluation for many years but more recently with the advent of IMRT, the concept of the minimum dose within the volume has lessened in importance, with dose–volume constraints adopted instead. Additionally, volumetric recommendations for both homogeneity and conformity have been adopted. These are outlined later.

Organs at risk (OAR) were categorised by ICRU62 into 'parallel' or 'serial' according to how dose impacts on function. Parallel structures such as the lungs are comprised of multiple subunits where organ function is reduced according to the number of subunits irradiated. For serial structures such as the spinal cord, the subunits are dependent on each other and thus if a single subunit is damaged the whole organ fails. This classification impacts on treatment planning tactics; serial structures are avoided whereas a strategy of reduction of high dose volumes is adopted for parallel structures. A planning organ-at-risk volume (PRV) is constructed for serial structures with an added margin included, along similar lines to that for a PTV.

9.4 Treatment Planning Objectives

Although individual plans will have their own patient-specific objectives, there are several key common principles guiding plan optimization and evaluation. A good plan should aim to:

- Achieve a uniformity of dose in the target volume;
- Reduce doses to critical structures as far below specified limits as possible;
- Minimise the volume of normal tissue that is irradiated;

- Ensure that the volume of the target that is underdosed is within the tolerances specified.

9.5 Treatment Planning Process

Following dose prescription and localization imaging, the principal steps involved in treatment planning are outlined in Figure 9.3.

These principles are described more fully in the following sections.

9.5.1 Contouring

The accurate delineation of target volumes and OAR is an essential element of radiotherapy planning. Inaccurate outlining can introduce systematic errors that are extremely hard to detect during treatment and have the potential to impact severely on patient outcome. The purpose of contouring is to inform the planning process as well as provide volumes for dose evaluation.

9.5.1.1 Patient CT Model

Before planning can commence it is vital to create an accurate 3D model of the patient; this not only enables visualisation of the target and critical structures but also provides the necessary tissue attenuation data to enable accurate dose calculation. The model also provides a geometric framework to enable delivery of the plan to the correct site. The most common modality for patient modelling is CT; an explanation of CT principles can be found in Chapter 6. CT provides the required heterogeneity and electron density values as well as accurate external contours of the patient. The limitations of CT mainly relate to the poor soft-tissue definition. This arises due to the similar attenuation properties of different soft tissues, giving them similar Hounsfield Units.

In recent years, these limitations have been overcome by incorporating data from

1. Contouring

Outlining of the tumour and associated target structures is performed, along with generation of appropriate ICRU margins for PTV generation. Relevant critical structures (organs at risk) that will constrain the plan are also identified and outlined.

2. Beam setup

Placing of treatment beams at appropriate angles onto the patient model and determination of optimal geometrical arrangement relative to target and critical structures.

3. Dose calculation

Calculation and display of predicted dose distribution enables the planner to identify strategies for improvement of target coverage and organ at risk dose reduction.

4. Optimisation

Varying the radiation field parameters is performed to obtain a conformal and uniform dose distribution while meeting dose constraints of organs at risk.

5. Evaluation

The resultant dose distribution is displayed in single or multiple planar views to allow assessment of the plan. Comparison of various plans enables selection of the most appropriate plan for the desired patient outcomes.

6. Plan Export

Conversion of the final plan into a format compatible with treatment deliversy systems.

FIGURE 9.3 Treatment planning steps.

magnetic resonance imaging (MRI) images. The wider range of appearance of different soft-tissue structures provided by MRI enables better tumour visualisation and enhanced information for delineation of anatomical structures. Combining the target volume information obtained from MRI and transferring this to the CT images is a complex process and involves a process of fusing (or registering) the images by matching reference points common to the two types of images. Although MRI currently lacks the geometric stability and attenuation data of CT, work is ongoing to convert MRI data for dose calculation purposes [8] to enable MRI-based planning. Additional data informing structure delineation can be provided by functional imaging modalities such as *positron emission tomography* (PET). The principles of PET are also described in Chapter 6; these images can provide additional information about the spread of the malignant disease and can enable more accurate definition of the GTV and CTV by the clinician.

Generation of an accurate patient model is challenging when additional modalities are introduced, due to variations in patient position. Accurate planning can only proceed on the assumption that the images used for planning are a true and reproducible depiction of the patient's daily position. It is important that, where possible, the patient is scanned in an identical position to the treatment position. This entails use of:

- flat-top couch inserts;
- immobilisation devices and patient alignment as used for treatment;
- marking of reference points on the patient's skin using radio-opaque markers;
- minimal distortion of the image.

The images produced for treatment planning may be transferred directly by computer network or via the *digital imaging and communications in medicine format for radiotherapy* (DICOM-RT). This format enables a common framework for data generation and exchange between radiotherapy systems although transfer between different TPSs can sometimes be problematic.

9.5.1.2 Contouring Tools and Features

TPSs commonly offer a range of tools to assist in the contouring process ranging from simple manual drawing tools to automatic and semiautomatic 'intelligent' algorithms. The simplest tools enable the freehand contouring of structures on each CT slice; this has the advantage of retaining clinical control. The ability to interpolate between contours delineated on non-consecutive slices or to copy contours between slices can shorten the process for relatively regular structures. Sequential outlining on axial slices can lead to disjointed and jagged 3D volumes. Planning system displays are accordingly commonly divided into 'windows', enabling the display of three orthogonal views. The inclusion of a 3D reconstruction of the delineated contours, with the option to hide or display individual structures, provides a helpful means of checking the continuity of structures.

Boundary detection tools can be used to contour structures that feature high contrast with surrounding structures. The lungs are a good example of this and automatic contouring tools are capable of identifying lung borders rapidly and with a high degree of success. Additional editing of these contours may be required to distinguish between lung tissue and hollow airways. These tools require priming with cutoff values for boundaries and sensible starting positions. They then grow a volume until a boundary is reached.

Other automatic segmentation tools are now available which aim to reduce the time taken to contour OAR. Many of these rely on predefined 'atlas' models of structures that can be fused with the patient model and adapted to fit [9]. Others use predefined settings for the typical CT numbers of organs such as the brain, spinal cord, and bladder, together with knowledge of the organs' typical size and shape to delineate the structures with minimal user input. Although these tools do generate volumes rapidly, most auto-generated volumes require additional manual editing. They are also unsuitable for structures that vary considerably from 'normal' appearance, such as target volumes. Evolving 'deep learning' tools [10] are showing promise for contouring and may provide a more reliable method in the near future.

Tools for the manipulation and editing of contours can improve the quality of the contouring. In addition to the simple adjustment of contours on a slice-by-slice basis, the use of

Boolean operators enables the combination or subtraction of structures (e.g. for removing contoured PTV outside the external contour). This is particularly valuable for IMRT when creating 'tuning structures'. Additional 'post-processing' algorithms for filling cavities, removing extraneous contours, and smoothing structures are particularly useful for tidying up the resulting contours. The automatic addition of user-specified margins to contoured GTV, CTV, or OAR volumes is essential for the accurate creation of the PTV or PRV, in accordance with the recommendations of the ICRU.

9.5.2 Beam Setup

In some situations, a single field is employed, usually where the tumour is superficial (e.g. spinal cord, mammary nodes). In these cases, a dose distribution is not required and the treatment is prescribed to a specified depth on the central axis of the beam. For most modern radiotherapy, the combination of two or more fields is usually necessary to meet the criteria of acceptability.

Figure 9.4a shows the simplest combination of two fields that are parallel opposed; the isodose charts are superimposed and a

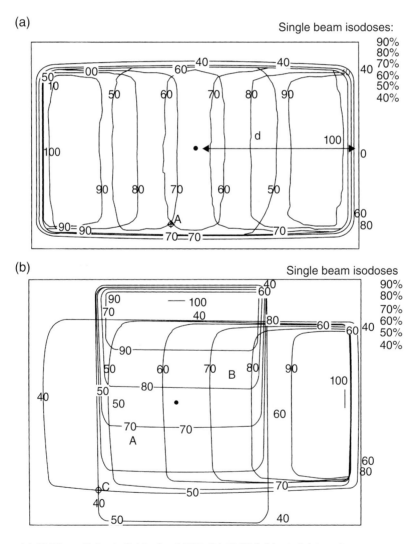

FIGURE 9.4 (a) 6 MV parallel pair fields, fixed SSD; (b) 6 MV fields at right angles.

composite chart can be produced manually by adding the dose values from each field at points where the isodoses intersect (e.g. point A in Figure 9.4a has a composite value of 130%). It can be seen that this results in a large rectangular high-dose region lying across the centre of the patient.

Figure 9.4b shows a similar exercise for two fields at right angles to each other; the resultant distribution would show a dose gradient between the bottom left corner and the top right corner when combined ($A = 120\%$ and $B = 160\%$).

These field combinations are shown for the *fixed SSD method* where the axis of rotation of the machine (isocentre) is set at the surface to which the beam is incident (generally 100 cm). Similar plans can be produced for the *isocentric method* where the isocentre is set approximately to the centre of the irradiated volume.

More complicated arrangements are common in most radiotherapy plans. Increasing the number of fields provides more options for the planner to optimise the dose. It can also lead to better matching of the shapes of the high-dose region and the PTV. Good matching of these is known as conformity; high conformity reduces the volume of normal tissue receiving a high dose. Increased beam numbers, however, increase the plan complexity and can lead to a higher volume of the patient receiving a low dose from the multiple entry and exit beams. The natural extension of increasing beam numbers is volumetric arc therapy where the gantry rotates during delivery.

Collimation of the treatment fields using multi-leaf collimators (MLCs) has already been discussed in Chapter 8. This is an essential aspect of achieving conformity during the planning process. Tools within the TPS ensure that MLCs are automatically shaped around the PTV. It is important, however, that a margin is applied to this fit due to penumbra. A penumbra occurs at the edge of the high-dose region and represents a width of tissue where the dose gradient lies. A sizeable penumbra region can be caused primarily by the size of the radiation source and increases with the distance from the source (geometrical penumbra). However, the width of the penumbra region is also dependent on scattering from both the phantom and collimator systems. For a 6 MV X-ray beam, the distance between the 20% and 80% isodoses in the penumbra is typically 4 mm at d_{max} and 6 mm at 10 cm deep. The radiation field size is defined as the lateral distance between the 50% isodoses where the field-defining light on the treatment machine coincides with these points. However, in treatment planning, the selection of field size may not be determined from the geometrical edge of the field but the position of, for example, the 90% isodose with respect to the target boundary. A great deal of uncertainty exists about the definition of field edges that are associated with dosimetric inaccuracies and beam positioning errors; particular caution should be taken when planning small fields (< 4 cm) where these uncertainties are most significant.

Care must also be taken with planning where treatment fields pass through regions of inhomogeneity. Aside from the obvious increase or decrease in attenuation caused by bone or air respectively, these regions can impact on the ability of the planner to achieve target coverage. The buildup effect in megavoltage X-ray beams is a rapid increase in dose in the first few millimetres of tissue, reaching a maximum value up to several centimetres deep depending on the incident photon energy. For a 6 MV X-ray beam, the dose increases from 20% at the surface to 85% at 5 mm deep and peaking at 15 mm depth, whereas for a 10 MV beam, the peak dose is at 25 mm depth, the dose then decreasing beyond this point. The buildup or 'skin-sparing' phenomena can be explained by the increase in secondary electrons, and subsequent energy deposition, beneath the surface, which reaches equilibrium at a finite depth whilst the photon energy fluence is continuously decreasing with depth. For superficial treatment planning it is essential to determine whether the buildup region encroaches on the target volume, in which case some external bolus may be required. For deeper target structures, particularly in the thorax, the impact of lack of equilibrium and the effective recreation of a buildup region must be considered as a potential constraint on the plan.

9.5.3 Dose Calculation

Although this is a single command within the TPS this step comprises the most complex process. The patient model, the planned beam geometry, and previously gathered beam data are combined, along with a range of correction tools, to generate as accurate a prediction of distributed dose as possible. It is essential that this is accurate as this informs all the subsequent planning decisions. Most calculation engines combine a beam model with complex correction algorithms.

It is convenient for TPSs to distinguish between the two components of absorbed dose at a point as a primary photon component and a scatter component. The primary component is easy to predict with dose depending on the effects of the inverse square law and attenuation. The scatter component is more complex and is dependent on the field size and shape.

The primary-scatter modelling process for irregular fields led to the implementation of the pencil-beam convolution algorithms. A pencil-beam kernel describes the deposition of energy around a very narrow beam, or 'pencil beam', and typically represents the scatter distribution due to the primary photon fluence and secondary electron scatter. The kernels are precalculated during the configuration of the algorithm and the dose distribution is then computed by dividing each field into pencil beams and mathematically combining (convolving) their contributions over the entire field area. It can be seen that this would naturally account for a range of field size and shapes. Making the kernels dependent upon their position within the field also enables account to be taken of any beam modifiers through which the pencil beams pass, including changes in intensity and beam hardening.

Convolution and superposition models are used to refine the shape of the kernels to increase accuracy. The traditional pencil-beam algorithm assumes a monoenergetic beam instead of the polyenergetic output from linear accelerators. The algorithm also assumes a homogeneous medium, leading to well-documented inaccuracies in depiction of dose near inhomogeneities [11]. Convolution techniques combine kernels for a range of energies to better replicate the polyenergetic treatment beam. The energy deposition kernels model the total energy imparted by the primary photons around an interaction site; this includes the energy retained by scattered photons and that transferred to charged particles (electrons). The distribution of this energy around the interaction site defines the shape of the kernels. Commonly, separate kernels are used to describe the primary energy (the primary kernel) and the scattered energy (the scatter kernel). The shape of the kernels is commonly derived for individual linear accelerators. The effect of inhomogeneities is included in dose calculations by superposition. This entails scaling the kernels, ideally anisotropically, according to the relative electron density of the tissue surrounding the interaction site. The more explicit consideration of electrons in model-based algorithms results in significant improvements in calculation accuracy over the correction-based models. The benefits of these models are evident in situations where electronic equilibrium does not exist:

- In low-density tissue such as lung, the simpler algorithms ignore the reduction in deposited dose caused by the increased range of scattered electrons and model only the reduction in attenuation of the primary photons, overestimating the dose to the low-density tissue. Model-based algorithms more accurately predict the reduction in absorbed dose; this is reflected in poorer coverage of PTVs that include lung tissue [12].
- Close to interfaces between tissues of different density (such as soft tissue and bone), correction-based algorithms fail to accurately model the changes in dose, e.g. when a beam passes from soft tissue into bone, there is an increase in the dose

in the soft tissue resulting from increased electron back scatter. Model-based algorithms model such effects more realistically, although this is perhaps the situation in which these algorithms are least accurate.

- Fields smaller than the order of 4 cm × 4 cm exhibit lateral electronic disequilibrium due to the range of the electrons relative to the size of the field. The improved consideration of the scattered electrons by model-based algorithms increases accuracy of dose prediction, which is of particular importance in IMRT treatments, which frequently comprise large numbers of very small beam segments.

Most beam models in commercial planning systems accordingly now utilise variants of convolution–superposition algorithms. Pencil-beam algorithms are still popular within IMRT planning due to their reliance on small beams.

The next generation of planning systems are likely to be based on Monte Carlo simulation, in which the individual interactions of millions of incident photons and the resultant photons and electrons are modelled with a high level of accuracy. These simulations currently represent the most accurate dose calculation model available. The latest versions of Monte Carlo algorithms in modern-day planning systems are now fast enough to be used clinically.

9.5.4 Optimisation

Optimisation is the process whereby a planner adjusts the various beam parameters to obtain the optimal plan according to the initial planning objectives. This process starts with visualisation of the planned dose distribution. As when contouring, the beam planning display of a 3D planning system generally comprises three orthogonal views, often with a 3D view (Figure 9.5). In addition, there should be a clear indication of the most important beam parameters, including field size and location, collimator, gantry and couch angles, wedge angle and orientation, SSD, and weighting. The adjustment of the field arrangement is usually done either by moving the fields on screen or by numerical entry of new values. The field size can be manually adjusted in the same way, although it is more common to automatically fit the secondary collimators to the target volume, with a user-specified margin. Non-coplanar beams, achieved through the use of collimator and couch twists, offer additional possibilities for conforming dose to the target volume.

A particularly useful display is the 'beam's eye view' (BEV) of the field. The BEV

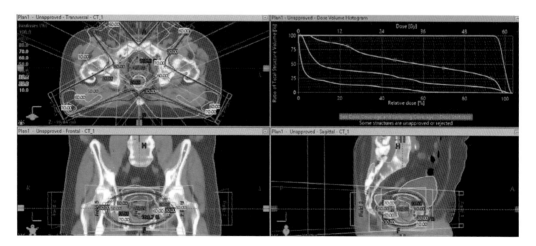

FIGURE 9.5 Typical interactive screen display of a TPS (ECLIPSE) showing orthogonal CT and dose–volume histogram (DVH) views. (Source: Copyright © 2018, Varian Medical Systems, Inc. All rights reserved.)

is a display of the internal patient contours in a plane perpendicular to the beam central axis, with the observer placed at the radiation source. The field outline is shown against a perspective view of the target and any critical structure contours. Moving the fields whilst observing the BEV is a convenient means of identifying suitable gantry angles for avoiding critical structures. Although MLCs can usually be automatically fitted to the shape of the target volume, it is often necessary to make adjustments to the positions of some leaves in order to shield critical structures. The BEV enables both this and the drawing of shielding blocks to be done easily. Some systems can generate digital radiographs from the CT data which can be displayed behind the structures in a BEV, providing an efficient method for verifying the accuracy of the plan.

The calculation options usually allow selection of the spacing between the calculation points (generally in the range 2–5 mm), the potential to choose the method of heterogeneity correction, and, in systems with more than one algorithm, which calculation model is to be used. It is essential that the user be required to recalculate the dose after any changes to plan parameters that would affect the dose distribution are made, with the exception of field weights, which simply scale the contribution of each field. Within the calculated distribution, the positions of maximum dose within the plan and reference point should be available.

A range of options for the display of the calculated dose distribution is generally available. In addition to the basic isodoses, ideally with the option to define which isodoses are displayed, it may be possible to display the dose in three dimensions, superimposed upon the 3D view of the structures. Combined with opacity control of the 3D surfaces, this enables realistic visualisation of the dose distribution within the body.

9.5.4.1 Wedges

An important optimisation tool is the wedge, which reduces the radiation intensity progressively across the beam. Historically and still in some older delivery equipment, this was performed by inserting a wedge-shaped metal block called a *wedge filter*. This causes angling of the isodose curves as shown in Figure 9.2b. Modern delivery systems replicate this effect using the movement of collimator jaws and control of dose rate to generate a wedge-shaped dose distribution. The isodose shape is the result of a summation of fields in which one independent collimation jaw is sequentially closed to create a series of decreasing field widths whilst simultaneously adjusting the monitor units per segment to achieve the required dose distribution [13].

The *wedge angle* is defined either as the angle that a tangent drawn through a specified isodose (usually the 50%) subtends to the central axis, or as the angle through which an isodose is tilted at the central axis of the beam at a specified depth (usually 10 cm). Any angle of wedge can be utilised, although to reduce QA requirements it is common to restrict this to multiples of 5°. Historically the wedge angles were set at 15°, 30°, 45°, and 60° and these are still commonly used.

In treatment planning the wedge filter is used for two purposes:

1. Deliberately to alter the dose gradient in the patient to enable a uniform distribution of dose to be produced when beams are arranged at angles to each other. This angle is known as the hinge angle. The required wedge angle can be calculated approximately by the formula:

$$\text{Wedge angle} = 90° - \left(\text{hinge angle}/2\right).$$

2. To compensate for surface obliquity off axis, by increasing the dose (thin end of the wedge) at the region of tissue excess and reducing the dose (thick end of the wedge) at the region of tissue deficiency, relative to the central axis. The wedge angle required for body curvature correction is approximately 50–75% of the obliquity angle (i.e. the angle subtended by a tangent line drawn at the beam entry point on the body contour, to a line normal to the central axis at the same point).

9.5.5 Beam Weighting

Amending the beam weighting changes the relative contribution of that beam to the total dose. This can be a very useful tool for improving homogeneity of dose. Weighting allows high-dose regions to be shrunk by reducing the contribution of the nearest beam. Changing weighting of a wedged beam impacts on the effect of that wedge on the overall dose distribution and can mimic a change in wedge angle. Weighting can be performed without the need for a recalculation as it only changes the ration of beam contributions.

9.5.6 Tissue Compensation and Intensity Modulators

Tissue compensation is often required when (i) the obliquity of the patient results in an unacceptable dose distribution, (ii) the dose to the patient's skin must be increased, i.e. sparing is not required, or (iii) the dose to a critical structure is excessive and must be reduced by shaping the dose distribution. The use of a wedge filter as a tissue compensator has already been discussed and these normally correct for obliquity in only one plane of the patient.

Tissue compensation over the full field area is simply achieved using bolus material (e.g. wax) added directly to the skin, resulting in a flat surface normal to the beam. However, such a compensator placed on the surface will result in a loss of the skin-sparing effect, which is desirable in some circumstances, although in most patients is to be avoided because of skin erythema. If the buildup effect is to be maintained, the compensating filter must be mounted on the accessory tray of the accelerator (at least 15–20 cm from the patient) and the appropriate scaling factors used.

Modern methods of dynamic collimator movement have now largely replaced the use of physical tissue compensators. *Geometrical shaping* of the radiation field is made possible by the use of the MLCs. *Dosimetric shaping* of the radiation field is made possible by intensity modulation of segments of the beam. Each field segment (or beamlet) has a specified intensity that is dependent on the required contribution at depth in the patient which itself is governed by the dose constraints to the target volumes and critical structures. The technique of IMRT is achieved by movement of the MLC leaves to specified positions whilst the intensity of the beam is controlled for each of these leaf positions. IMRT is applied using either 'dynamic MLCs' or 'step and shoot' methods. The treatment planning methods for IMRT are described in Section 9.6.1.

9.5.7 Plan Evaluation

Plan evaluation tools allow rapid appraisal of dose distributions in order to determine whether the tolerances for the target volume and critical structures have been achieved. Through their use, alternative plans for a patient's treatment can be compared and 'fine-tuning' can be performed to produce an optimal plan.

The simplest means of determining whether a plan meets the required criteria is visual assessment of the dose distribution in terms of the coverage of the target volume by the desired isodoses and the sparing of critical structures. In addition to the standard isodose display, planning systems offer a number of features to assist the visual evaluation of dose distributions. The use of a colourwash display, in which the dose levels are represented by a continuous colour gradient, may afford greater control over the display, particularly when the upper and lower displayed doses are definable. A visual indication of the location of the dose maximum within a slice or the entire calculation volume provides a convenient means of determining whether a plan's 'hottest' point is located within the target volume. Point dose tools, indicating the dose at an arbitrary point, or line profiles, indicating the variation in dose along an arbitrary line, enable more precise investigation of the planned dose distribution.

An alternative method of summarising the 3D dose distribution common to all modern TPSs is the dose–volume histogram (DVH). The most widely used form of DVH is the cumulative DVH, a plot of the percentage volume of tissue, $V(D)$, that receives a dose greater than or equal to D. The DVH for a target volume can be used to identify the percentage of that volume receiving a dose above and below the required tolerances. Higher values of $V(D)$ for doses below the prescription dose and a sharper fall-off of the DVH thereafter indicate an improved dose distribution in the target volume. Conversely, more desirable dose distributions for critical structures are represented by lower values of $V(D)$.

Implemented in a TPS, DVHs are customisable with the scales depicting either relative or absolute units. The DVH display is often accompanied by numerical summaries of the dose, such as the maximum and mean doses within a structure, which provide a clear indication of whether critical structure doses are within tolerance. A limitation of DVHs is that they provide no positional information, e.g. a target DVH may show a certain volume of tissue receiving a dose below the lower tolerance, but it does not indicate where that tissue is situated within the target.

The use of DVHs together with distributions enables an efficient evaluation of the quality of a treatment plan. The comparison of two alternative plans for a patient is facilitated by the ability to view the plans side by side on the screen or overlay their DVHs. The addition of the doses from several treatment plans enables evaluation of the total dose from, for example, a phased treatment. A useful variation on this plan-summing function is the ability to subtract one competing plan from another, the result being the volumetric dose difference between the two plans. Comparison of the plans' biological effectiveness [14] (in terms of the resultant tumour control probability and normal tissue complication probability) is a capability becoming more commonplace in commercial planning systems.

Another useful means of comparing treatment plans is the conformity index,

which quantifies how well the high-dose region coincides with the PTV. There are multiple measures of conformity but it is essentially the ratio of the treated volume to that of the PTV. ICRU83 recommended using $D_{98\%}$ as the treated volume measure. Homogeneity Index is a measure of the degree of variation of dose across the target volume and within ICRU83 it is defined as:

$$HI = \left(D_{2\%} - D_{98\%}\right)/D_{50\%}$$

The target value here is zero, which would occur when the dose is perfectly homogenous with 100% across the volume.

9.5.8 Plan Export

The accurate generation and export of the final plan and associated information are essential for successful implementation and must be an unambiguous set of accurate instructions. A dosimetry report will often accompany the plan and must contain a clear description of each field parameter, including field sizes, machine and patient angles, setting up distances, and any special instructions. The sheet should also contain a step-by-step description of the monitor unit calculation for each field from the original prescribed dose distribution. All correction factors should be clearly stated (even if the value is unity) to enable the calculation to be carefully checked before the start of treatment.

Electronic transfer of the plan data to the treatment linear accelerator reduces the possibility of transcription error that occurs when manual transfer is used. This electronic transfer of data is usually from the TPS to the *record and verify system* (RVS) but still requires checking to ensure accuracy.

TPSs tend to use a server–client architecture, i.e. the patient data and CT images are stored on a central database and pulled onto a local workstation, on which the planning is performed, before the resultant plan is pushed back to the database. The final treatment plan may be transferred electronically to other systems such as independent monitor unit checking. Accurate transfer of the plan information between systems is essential and again use of the DICOM-RT protocol helps to ensure compatibility between different manufacturers' systems.

9.6 Advanced Treatment Planning

Section 9.5 covered the most common features available in a TPS for external beam planning and many of these are available for other planning modes. The selection of beams for IMRT, electron, stereotactic radiosurgery, or brachytherapy planning will often invoke special calculation models and programme modules that provide the features required for this type of planning. In addition, the move towards adaptive planning demands a streamlined approach to planning and additional advanced tools have been developed to assist with this.

9.6.1 IMRT Planning

IMRT represents arguably the most significant advance in radiotherapy planning since the introduction of conformal radiotherapy. The various methods of IMRT delivery are capable of producing dose distributions in which the high-dose region is more closely conformed to the target volume whilst enabling greater sparing of normal tissue. A particular advantage over conventional treatments is the ability to produce concave distributions, enabling the sparing of OAR around which the target is wrapped. However, the production of IMRT plans is generally more labour intensive than conventional treatment planning. IMRT planning methods can be divided broadly into two categories: forward planning and inverse planning.

Forward planning of IMRT treatments is performed largely by the addition of smaller fields within the conventional fields in order to improve the dose distribution above that

achievable with conventional MLC fields and wedges alone. The degree of intensity modulation is limited by the number of fields used and restricts the method's ability to achieve highly conformal dose distributions. Forward planning has the benefit of requiring no more than a conventional TPS but has now largely been replaced by inverse planning techniques.

Inverse planning, as the name suggests, approaches the treatment planning process from a different angle from forward planning. Rather than positioning treatment fields as required and calculating the resultant dose distribution, the planner specifies the desired dose distribution and the TPS determines how best to deliver it. The inverse planning process is often known as 'optimisation' and the methods used vary between planning systems and according to the delivery technique but invariably requires the splitting of each beam into a large number of beamlets. A typical optimisation procedure is as follows:

- The desired dose distribution is specified in terms of a number of dose–volume constraints. For the target volume, there will generally be a minimum and a maximum constraint, defining the range of doses within which all the target tissue should lie. For OAR, a maximum dose constraint designed to limit the highest dose received by the organ and intermediate constraints to limit the dose received by a specific volume of the organ may be set;

- The TPS makes an initial guess of the required beamlet intensities (often simply uniform beams) and the resultant dose distribution within the volumes of interest is calculated. An optimisation (or cost) function quantifies the magnitude of the difference between the calculated distribution and the desired distribution – the greater the value of the function, the further the distribution is from meeting the constraints;

- The intensities of the beamlets within each field are adjusted and the dose to the volumes of interest is calculated once more. The value of the optimisation

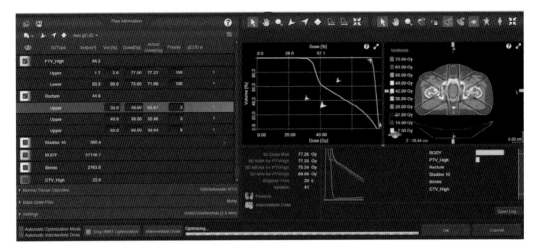

FIGURE 9.6 Typical screen from the Eclipse inverse planning module of the Varian Eclipse treatment planning system (TPS). Constraints and optimisation parameters are displayed and altered on the LHS of the screen. The RHS displays the dose–volume histograms (DVHs) of the volumes of interest (with constraints marked) at the present iteration, the current fluence for a selected field, and a plot of the optimisation function against time. (Source: Copyright © 2018, Varian Medical Systems, Inc. All rights reserved.)

function is again recalculated; if it is lower than the previous value, the new intensities are accepted; if not they are rejected;

- The iterative adjustment of intensities continues until the constraints are met, the user stops the process, or no further reductions in the value of the optimisation function (shown in Figure 9.6) occur. It may be possible for the user to interactively adjust the constraints during the inverse planning process to assist in achieving a better outcome;

- Each field's final beamlet intensities together represent the fluence required to deliver the final distribution. The inverse planning software then determines how to deliver the final fluences, in terms of the MLC patterns or dynamic MLC leaf motions;

- Finally, a forward dose calculation is performed, generally using the TPS's conventional algorithm to determine the dose distribution that will be delivered.

IMRT places additional demands on planning systems at several stages of the

planning process. The dose calculation after each iteration of the inverse planning must be performed much more rapidly than conventional algorithms are capable of, as previously described. The delivery of IMRT fields often requires more monitor units than conventional fields for the same prescription dose; the TPS must be capable of producing high-quality distributions without excessively lengthening the treatment delivery time or producing a high integral dose through high numbers of monitor units. Perhaps the greatest challenge is the frequent use of very small field segments, which requires the dose-calculation algorithm to model the penumbra and the effects of the lack of electronic equilibrium to a high level of accuracy.

The iterative optimisation methods used by most IMRT planning involve the minimisation of a cost function quantifying the difference between the desired dose distribution and that from the field fluences at each stage of the optimisation. This requires calculation of the dose distribution after each iteration. The algorithm used in this dose calculation must be accurate and calculate the dose in a sufficiently short time that the optimisations are not unacceptably slow. This latter requirement usually necessitates compromises in the accuracy of the dose calculation, such as poor consideration of scatter and inhomogeneities and widely spaced dose calculation points.

The direction of the optimisation is dependent on the dose calculations performed after each iteration; inaccuracy in the calculations will result in fields that do not produce the desired dose distribution. (For example, if the algorithm used after each iteration tends to underestimate the PTV dose by 10% and calculates a mean PTV dose of 60 Gy, the final forward dose calculation by a more accurate algorithm would reveal that the mean PTV dose was actually over 66 Gy. The optimisation would then need to be repeated with the PTV dose constraints set approximately 10% below the dose level actually desired in order to ultimately achieve the desired dose.) This variation between the desired and actual dose resulting from inaccuracies in the algorithm used during the inverse planning is known as a 'convergence error'. Until Monte Carlo can be used routinely in inverse planning, pencil-beam algorithms represent the best compromise between speed and accuracy during optimisations, ideally followed by a forward dose calculation using a more advanced algorithm.

Clearly the ability to weight different objectives within the optimization process means that there is a range of possible plans for each patient that can produce different outcomes. A high weighting of the target coverage objectives may cause higher dose to critical structures than in a plan where critical structure dose objectives are weighted higher. This has led to the development of multicriteria optimisation software [15] which produce a range of plans that are each optimal with regard to one of the objectives. The 'Pareto' optimal plan for an objective is the plan in which that objective cannot be improved without compromising another one. This range of plans can then be presented to the clinician who can select the plan that matches best to their desired outcome.

9.6.2 Electron Beam Planning

Electron planning usually involves the computation of dose distribution for a single field. The planning of electron beam treatments requires the choice of energy to achieve the required dose coverage (usually by the 90% isodose) at the maximum depth of the target volume within the dose restrictions to any critical structures. The field size selected is based on examination of the isodoses at the edge of the target volume and is particularly important for small fields where tapering of the peripheral isodoses requires the use of larger fields than normally chosen if photon fields were used. Field shaping by lead or lead alloy cutouts is a common practice in electron therapy and must be included in the dosimetric calculations. Challenges arising through use of electrons include the increased side scatter and the potential for photon contamination arising from shielding or delivery equipment. Complex modelling is required to depict these additional aspects.

The use of Monte Carlo-based dose-calculation models for electrons is gradually becoming a more common feature of commercial planning systems and offers a solution to the challenge [16]. However, most TPSs still use a pencil-beam model based on multiple-scattering theory, where the dose at a point is the sum of the contributions from all the pencil beams that make up the beam. Usually a single beam profile for each applicator at each energy is required at the depth of dose maximum to correct for the off-axis scattering that occurs within the applicator. If the applicator is not parallel to the skin surface, then correction must be made for tissue obliquity. This is achieved by an inverse square correction along the ray line from the point of calculation to the virtual source position. At angles of obliquity > 45° significant changes in lateral scatter must be allowed for in the calculation. Tissue inhomogeneity is a primary cause of electron dose non-uniformity within the body and requires careful assessment to avoid underdosing the target volume or overdosing critical structures. Correction for a slab of tissue with high (bone) or low (lung or air) electron densities can be made using an effective depth method. Small inhomogeneities produce hot and cold areas caused by scattering behind the edge of the structure and can be predicted only to an accuracy of about 10% with present electron beam models. Planning of electron fields is particularly useful for complex situations where fields are adjacent to each other, internal or external shielding is required, or bolus material must be added to achieve an acceptable dose distribution. The planning tools used for viewing and evaluation are the same as for photon beam planning.

9.6.3 Proton Planning

Proton radiotherapy treatment delivery has been discussed in Chapter 8. In terms of planning, many of the photon radiotherapy principles and processes are also relevant. The key difference lies in the different characteristics of proton dose deposition and in particular with the uncertainty over the proton range. Unlike photons, protons exhibit a finite range with most of the dose being deposited at the Bragg peak depth [17] and a very steep dose gradient immediately distal to that. This range and therefore the position of the gradient is dependent on the electron density of the tissue being traversed. Additional uncertainties can arise from inaccurate data within the planning CT [18] due to noise or artefacts; this can affect the accurate calculation of stopping power ratios. It can be appreciated that an uncertainty in the range could lead to incorrect placement of the Bragg peak and possible underdosage of the distal tumour volume. This uncertainty leads to inaccurate modelling within the TPS as well as a potential difference between planned and delivered doses.

Proton planning systems commonly utilise intensity-modulation techniques to reduce the impact of range uncertainty. For many years this was achieved by adding a 3.5% safety margin, but more recent advances have included knowledge of the errors into the process in place of a margin. There is much discussion currently regarding the value of a traditional PTV for protons and it is possible that this could be replaced with a more statistical approach [19]. Other techniques include utilising the steep lateral gradients rather than reliance on the distal gradient which can help to improve conformity. Alternative avenues of research are seeking to reduce the uncertainty arising from stopping power ratio conversion by improving CT Hounsfield Unit accuracy. Techniques such as dual-energy CT [20] or use of proton CT scanners [21] may reduce inaccuracies in Hounsfield maps and hence reduce proton range uncertainty.

9.6.4 4D Planning

Four-dimensional CT (4D-CT) introduces a time component to CT imaging which enables variations in the position of the target due to respiration to be included. The CT scan is acquired over a longer time than conventional CT, whilst simultaneously monitoring the patient's breathing either by tracking the motion of an external marker on the patient or by spirometry. The breathing is recorded as a waveform with which the individual CT slices are correlated (Figure 9.7).

On importing a 4D-CT dataset into the TPS, the images are separated into 'bins' according to the phase or amplitude of the respiratory waveform at the moment that each image was acquired. The result is a series of reconstructed CT scans, each representing the anatomy at a given stage of the respiratory cycle. Subsequent use of the scans is dependent upon the method of accounting for respiration to be used during treatment.

The movement of the target may be restricted during the times that the beam is on, either through gating the delivery according to the respiratory cycle or by a forced breath-hold method. In this situation, the planning is generally performed on a single reconstructed CT scan, corresponding to the stage of the respiratory cycle in which

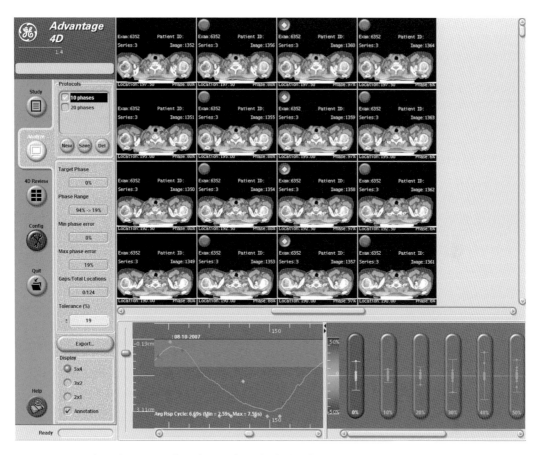

FIGURE 9.7 A four-dimensional CT (4D-CT) study display from GE AdvantageSim MD. The respiratory cycle is represented by the waveform at the bottom of the screen; each column contains images acquired during the same part of the cycle. (Source: Courtesy of GE Healthcare.)

the dose is to be delivered. Structure delineation and planning are performed only on that scan, effectively treating it as a standard 3D planning situation.

The alternative treatment technique is to adapt the treatment fields according to the position of the target throughout the respiratory cycle. To achieve this, structures must be contoured on all of the reconstructed CT scans. This process can be made significantly faster by registering the scans to each other and copying structures between them, although careful verification of the results is required to ensure that changes in location as a result of breathing are correctly accounted for, and it is wise to contour the target on each scan individually. Treatment planning becomes more involved, requiring fitting of

the fields to the target and evaluation of the resultant dose distribution on each reconstructed scan. Dynamic tracking using the MLCs throughout the respiratory cycle is generally the most straightforward means of achieving this adaptation.

The advent of MR-based delivery systems offer the potential for real-time monitoring of soft-tissue structures during treatment and it is likely that this will increase usage of gating or dynamic MLC tracking techniques. At the time of writing, the full implications of this technology have not been realised. Certainly, an important implication of 4D planning is the massive increase in data involved. Typically, at least 10 CT scans are reconstructed, resulting in a 10-fold increase in the storage required for the CT images alone.

As the technique becomes more widely implemented, it is possible that refinements to the 4D imaging process may reduce the quantities of data involved; a significant increase in required storage capacity over 3D planning will always remain.

9.6.5 Stereotactic Radiosurgery Planning

Specialist planning is required for treatment of deep-seated lesions in the brain where dedicated stereotactic apparatus, such as the Gamma Knife unit (Elekta Instruments AB) or an adapted linear accelerator, are used. More details of these delivery systems can be found in Chapter 8. Stereotactic radiosurgery or stereotactic multiple arc radiotherapy (SMART) both produce an irradiated volume that is typically the shape of a walnut with variable diameter (4–30 mm) using different collimators. Treatment of these small lesions relies on accurate localisation and positioning of the patient, which is achieved using a stereotactic frame secured to the patient's head. The frame has an orthogonal coordinate system engraved on it, which is used for localisation, dose planning, and alignment with the focal treatment point. Radiographic data is obtained from angiograms, CT, or MR images to determine the 3D coordinates of the lesion; the shape of the skull is obtained from either the surface by measuring radial coordinates and surface interpolation or the contours obtained from CT data. The planning system produces isodoses relative to the dose at the point of maximum dose, allowing for attenuation changes along geometric ray lines to each source. The dose contribution from each source is summed into a dose matrix (as for conventional treatment planning) and plotted; multiple foci with appropriate weightings may be aligned adjacent to each other to conform the dose distribution to the shape of a lesion. The dose distribution is overlaid over the image data to give anatomical perspective of the treatment.

A commercial planning system, designed to support the Leksell Gamma Knife unit, is the Elekta Gammaplan (Figure 9.8). This system can use CT and MR scans as well as projected images from angiograms. Treatment planning is performed by defining the parameters of the cranial target and the collimator helmet to be used during treatment, and of the radiation shots to be delivered by the Gamma Knife. The user interface is similar to that of a conventional TPS for radiotherapy, but includes enhanced features to set up and edit source patterns using collimator plugs.

9.6.6 Brachytherapy Planning

Brachytherapy planning systems allow calculation of individual patient treatments using various sealed sources such as iridium wire, caesium tubes or pellets, iodine seeds, and gold grains. The introduction of afterloading devices for intracavitary and interstitial radiotherapy has led to computer planning packages that are tailored to the specific needs of the treatment system. Pellet, seed, and grain sources are usually considered as point sources, where the size of the source is small compared with the distance to the point of dose calculation, requiring inverse square, tissue absorption, and scatter correction to the absorbed dose at a point. The calculation of dose distributions for line sources requires the use of integration techniques to account for the contribution of each element of the source to the dose at a point. Tables of relative dose at radial distances and angles from the centre of the source are often precalculated and known as Sievert integral tables.

Computer calculation consists of summing the dose at a point for each source, the isodose curves from a cubic grid of points being plotted as for external beam models. The isodose distribution (Figure 9.9) is usually produced from the same view as the radiographs (i.e. anterior and lateral digital images). Viewing tools are similar to external beam planning and may involve the overlay of CT data. Plans may be viewed in arbitrary planes to allow visualisation of the dose

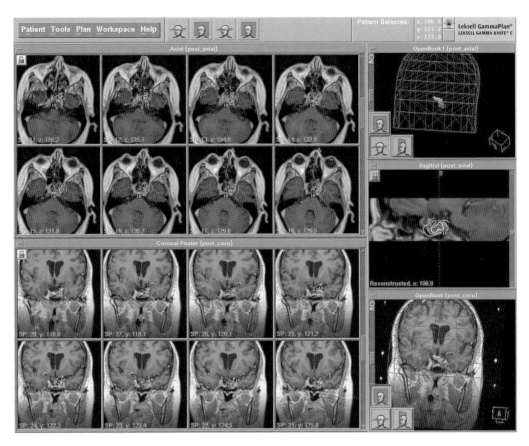

FIGURE 9.8   Stereotactic radiotherapy plan. (Source: Courtesy of Elekta Gammaplan.)

reference points defined according to the dosimetry system in use (i.e. Manchester, Paris, ICRU38 [22]). A major difference between external and brachytherapy planning is that the latter has no defined target volume and therefore the minimum dose to the target tissue is ambiguous; visual assessment of the plan and dose calculation to the reference points is vital for plan evaluation.

Optimisation tools are common in brachytherapy planning systems. These are capable of modelling stepping sources and allow definition of a required dose envelope and a calculation of the optimum source position and dwell times to accomplish this. Other planning tools that are often available are: 3D visualisation of dose surfaces; DVHs; summation of external beam dose and brachytherapy distributions; and curved plane calculations.

9.6.7 Adaptive Planning

A comprehensive discussion of adaptive radiotherapy (ART) is beyond the scope of this text and the reader is directed to specific texts for this [23, 24]. The following overview instead aims to provide an outline of the processes and additional planning requirements. Adaptive planning occurs when plans are changed after treatment has started in response to changes to the geometrical configuration of the patient. This can arise due to tumour response or growth as well as changes to tumour position as in image-guided radiotherapy (IGRT). Where ART differs from IGRT is that instead of the patient position being amended, the treatment plan is changed to reflect the new situation. There are several methods for

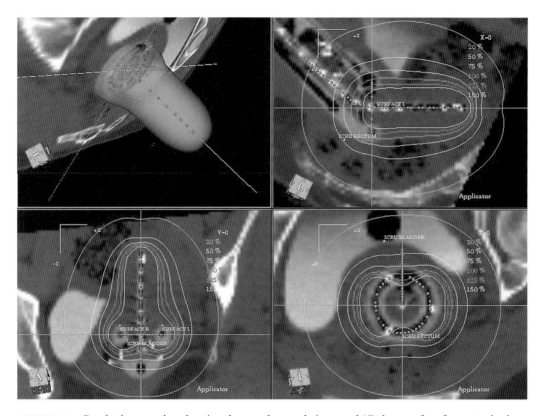

FIGURE 9.9 Brachytherapy plan showing three orthogonal views and 3D dose surface for a standard Manchester insertion. (Source: Courtesy of Nucletron.)

achieving this change in plan which can be categorised as 'proactive' or 'reactive'.

Proactive techniques include the 'plan of the day' cervix or bladder ART [25] where a range of plans are produced prior to treatment commencing. This range typically encompasses a range of possible structure sizes and the most appropriate plan for the patient on a particular day can be selected based on a daily cone beam CT (CBCT) image. This makes minimal demand in terms of planning techniques but does require multiple plans to be generated based on a range of PTV targets.

Reactive ART requires a new treatment plan to be generated, checked, and approved in a compressed timeframe. The new plan is based on updated imaging information; either from a prebooked CT scan or from daily CBCT data. Many departments schedule a single ART replanning session at a specific point within the patient treatment. This allows ART

to be conducted in a manageable timeframe and again makes minimal demands on planning techniques and technology, aside from workload and resource issues.

Emerging technology, such as the MR-LinAc or rapid kV real-time imaging, will enable reactive ART to be performed on a daily basis. Daily replanning of the patient can be performed in situations where conventional IGRT positional corrections are insufficient. Daily replanning requires a highly compressed workflow to ensure that treatment can be replanned and delivered whilst the patient is still on the couch. The process starts with daily CBCT images. Auto-contouring tools then identify the new target and OAR volumes before rapid IMRT optimization is performed and the plan is approved and delivered. Whilst still largely experimental [26], ongoing research is bringing this compressed workflow closer to being a clinical reality.

Although not restricted to ART, the increasing role of machine learning systems and artificial intelligence [27] is helping to achieve these goals of rapid contouring and planning. Most TPS manufacturers now include auto-contouring and auto-planning modules within their software. Although these tools currently require considerable clinical oversight, their capacity to 'learn' means that human input should reduce over time, creating and facilitating daily reactive ART as part of conventional clinical practice.

9.7 Quality Assurance

QA of planning data is essential to ensure and maintain the accuracy of the system. This subject is wide ranging and beyond the scope of this book; however, many radiotherapy publications provide a guide to commissioning and quality control for TPSs [28, 29]. The complexity of IMRT treatments requires additional QA measurements to ensure that the calculated dose distribution accurately reflects the delivered dose. Planning systems increasingly have facilities to assist the process and novel approaches to virtual QA for IMRT are being researched [30]. In addition to the ability to calculate the dose from the treatment fields on a user-specified phantom, enabling comparison with film, detector array, or ionisation chamber measurements, the prediction of the dose across the field as measured by an electronic portal imager allows efficient verification of the delivery.

Quality control primarily covers software performance but must also deal with the accuracy of data transfer via digital networks. Checking the consistency of data transferred between two systems involves sending a standard data set (e.g. a test plan) and determining the accuracy of the data at the receiving system by comparing against the original sent information. All aspects of the plan parameter transfer must be checked to ensure that data has not been lost or misinterpreted during the transfer. Standard data transfer protocols, such as DICOM-RT, have been adopted to ensure that all systems in radiotherapy use a common image and parameter format.

Software assurance involves testing system data integrity and the computer beam model. Beam measurements should be compared with calculations from the TPS, both at the commissioning stage and after any major upgrade of planning software. Regular quality control can be performed by comparing the output of a set of reference plans against the same distributions obtained during commissioning. These checks ensure consistency through the patient data input path and test the basic dose calculation performance.

The quality control of the system is insufficient to ensure the accuracy of treatment plans and therefore each plan must be subjected to the following (minimum) checks by a person not involved in the production of the plan:

- Check of all measurements, contouring and immobilisation device;
- Confirmation of patients' treatment prescription, as specified by the clinical oncologist;
- Check of the consistency of all field parameters throughout the planning reports;
- Independent computer calculation of the dose at the intersection of the field axes should be compared against the plan value;
- Independent calculation of the MUs performed either by a separate computer calculation programme;
- The completion of each check should be recorded and signed; any discrepancies should be investigated.

Further checks are necessary when the planning data is transferred to the RVS, before each beam exposure, and throughout the patient's treatment. Increasingly, electronic checklists are being used to organise and monitor QA and have been shown to reduce errors and improve patient safety [31].

References

1. Khan, F. and Gerbi, B. (2012). *Treatment Planning in Radiation Oncology*. Philadelphia: Wolters Kluwer.

2. Barrett, A., Dobbs, J., Morris, S., and Roques, T. (2009). *Practical Radiotherapy Planning*, 4e. Boca Raton: CRC Press.

3. Williams, J.R. and Thwaites, D.I. (2000). *Radiotherapy Physics in Practice*, 2e. Oxford: Oxford University Press.

4. Symonds, R.P., Mills, J.A., and Duxbury, A.M. (2019). *Walter and Miller's Textbook of Radiotherapy, Radiation Physics, Therapy and Oncology*, 8e. Edinburgh: Churchill Livingstone, Elsevier.

5. International Commission on Radiation Units and Measurements. *Prescribing, Recording and Reporting Photon Beam Therapy*. ICRU Report 50. Bethesda, MD: ICRU, 1993.

6. International Commission on Radiation Units and Measurements. ICRU Report 62. *Prescribing, Recording and Reporting Photon Beam Therapy* (Supplement to ICRU Report 50). Bethesda, MD: ICRU, 1999.

7. International Commission on Radiation Units and Measurements. Prescribing, Recording, and Reporting Photon-Beam Intensity-Modulated Radiation Therapy (IMRT). J ICRU 2010; 10 (Report 83).

8. Guerreiro, F., Burgos, N., Dunlop, A. et al. (2017). Evaluation of a multi-atlas CT synthesis approach for MRI-only radiotherapy treatment planning. *Phys. Med.* 35: 7–17.

9. Sharp, G., Fritscher, K.D., Pekar, V. et al. (2014). Vision 20/20: perspectives on automated image segmentation for radiotherapy. *Med. Phys.* 41 (5): 050902.

10. Lustberg, T., van Soest, J., Gooding, M. et al. (2018). Clinical evaluation of atlas and deep learning based automatic contouring for lung cancer. *Radiother. Oncol.* 126 (2): 312–317.

11. Knoos, T., Ahnesjo, A., Nilsson, P., and Weber, L. (1995). Limitations of a pencil beam approach to photon dose calculations in lung tissue. *Phys. Med. Biol.* 40: 1411–1420.

12. Bragg, C.M. and Conway, J. (2006). Dosimetric verification of the anisotropic analytical algorithm for radiotherapy treatment planning. *Radiother. Oncol.* 81: 315–323.

13. Leavitt, D.D., Martin, M., Moeller, J.H., and Lee, W.L. (1990). Dynamic wedge field techniques through computer -controlled collimator motion and dose delivery. *Med. Phys.* 17: 87–91.

14. Mavroidis, P., Komisopoulos, G., Buckey, C. et al. (2017). Radiobiological evaluation of prostate cancer IMRT and conformal-RT plans using different treatment protocols. *Phys. Med.* 40: 33–41.

15. Zieminski, S., Khandekar, M., and Wang, Y. (2018). Assessment of multi-criteria optimization for volumetric modulated arc therapy in hippocampal avoidance whole brain radiation therapy. *J. Appl. Clin. Med. Phys.* 19 (2): 184–190.

16. Chamberland, E., Beaulieu, L., and Lachance, B. (2015). Evaluation of an electron Monte Carlo dose calculation algorithm for treatment planning. *J. Appl. Clin. Med. Phys.* 16 (3): 60–79.

17. Bragg, W.H. (1904). On absorption of alpha rays and on the classification of the alpha rays from radium. *Philos. Mag.* 6: 719–725.

18. Chvetsov, A.V. and Paige, S.L. (2010). The influence of CT image noise on proton range calculation in radiotherapy planning. *Phys. Med. Biol.* 55: N141–N149.

19. Holloway, S.M., Holloway, M.D., and Thomas, S.J. (2018). A method for acquiring random range uncertainty probability distributions in proton therapy. *Phys. Med. Biol.* 63: 01NT02.

20. Wohlfahrt, P., Möhler, C., Hietschold, V. et al. (2017). Clinical implementation of dual-energy CT for proton treatment planning on pseudo-monoenergetic CT scans. *Int. J. Radiat. Oncol. Biol. Phys.* 97 (2): 427–434.

21. Giacometti, V., Bashkirov, V.A., Piersimoni, P. et al. (2017). Software platform for simulation of a prototype proton CT scanner. *Med. Phys.* 44: 1002–1016.

22. International Commission on Radiation Units and Measurements. *Dose and Volume Specification for Reporting Intracavitary Therapy in Gynecology*. ICRU 38. Bethesda, MD: ICRU, 1985.

23. Li, X.A. (2011). *Adaptive Radiation Therapy*, 1e. Boca Raton: CRC Press.

24. Timmerman, R.D. and Xing, L. (2009). *Image-Guided and Adaptive Radiation Therapy*. Philadelphia: Lippincott Williams and Wilkins.

25. Lutkenhaus, L.J., Visser, J., de Jong, R. et al. (2015). Evaluation of delivered dose for a clinical daily adaptive plan selection strategy for bladder cancer radiotherapy. *Radiother. Oncol.* 116 (1): 51–56.

26. Kontaxis, C., Bol, G.H., Kerkmeijer, L.G.W. et al. (2017). Fast online replanning for inter-fraction rotation correction in prostate radiotherapy. *Med. Phys.* 44 (10): 5034–5042.

27. Gillan, C., Milne, E., Harnett, N. et al. (2019). Professional implications of introducing artificial intelligence in healthcare: an evaluation using radiation medicine as a testing ground. *J. Radiother. Pract.* 18 (1): 5–9.

28. Smilowitz, J.B., Das, I.J., Feygelman, V. et al. (2015). AAPM medical physics practice guideline 5. a.: commissioning and QA of treatment planning dose calculations – megavoltage photon and electron beams. *J. Appl. Clin. Med. Phys.* 16 (5): 14–34.

29. Institute of Physics and Engineering in Medicine. IPEM Report 81. Treatment planning. *Physics Aspects of Quality Control in Radiotherapy.* York: IPEM Publications, 1999: Chapter 4.

30. Valdes, G., Chan, M.F., Lim, S.B. et al. (2017). IMRT QA using machine learning: a multi-institutional validation. *J. Appl. Clin. Med. Phys.* 18 (5): 279–284.

31. Berry, S.L., Tierney, K.P., Elguindi, S., and Mechalakos, J.G. (2018). Five years' experience with a customized electronic checklist for radiation therapy planning quality assurance in a multicampus institution. *Pract. Radiat. Oncol.* 8 (4): 279–286.

CHAPTER 10

Image-guided Radiotherapy and Treatment Verification

Cath Holborn and Ros Perry

Aim

The aim of this chapter is to outline the fundamental principles involved and the imaging modalities that are used to ensure accurate treatment delivery. The principles and practice of pretreatment imaging are discussed in Chapter 6.

10.1 Introduction

Treatment verification is an integral part of the treatment process. Alongside effective methods of immobilisation, it helps to ensure that the radiotherapy plan is delivered as intended and plays a crucial role in enabling us to maximise the therapeutic ratio.

Nowadays, many techniques involve the delivery of highly conformal and often intensity-modulated radiation beams. These beams, and the associated dose distribution, are precisely shaped to the target volume. Steep dose gradients (areas of high and low dose in close proximity) are often created. These may exist between the target volume and nearby organs at risk (OAR) and/or between different target volumes that have been defined and prescribed different doses. Any positional errors that occur at the time of treatment delivery could move an area of high dose into an area where only a low dose was planned, and vice versa. This could compromise the therapeutic ratio, limiting disease control and causing unwanted side effects/toxicity. Robust methods of treatment verification are needed to ensure that these techniques are delivered safely.

As treatment verification aims to detect and correct for any positional errors, it can also be used to keep the planned safety margin, around the clinical target volume (CTV), as small as possible. This helps to minimise the amount of normal tissue that is irradiated, and can enable dose escalation. Many cancers require a high dose to be delivered in order to achieve effective disease control or eradication (including hypofractionated regimes where larger doses are delivered per fraction). However, nearby OAR in close proximity to the planned target volume (PTV) can limit the amount of dose we are able to prescribe. Highly conformal planning techniques, combined with robust methods of

Practical Radiotherapy: Physics and Equipment, Third Edition. Edited by Pam Cherry and Angela M. Duxbury.
© 2020 John Wiley & Sons Ltd. Published 2020 by John Wiley & Sons Ltd.

treatment verification, can enable us to deliver the high doses required, without risking any significant side effects/adverse events.

It is also important to understand the vital role that treatment verification plays in the delivery of treatment with a palliative intent. Even if a simpler, less conformal technique is planned (for the purposes of symptom control only), palliative regimes involve the use of high doses delivered in only a single or a few fractions. Also, whilst some treatments may have a palliative intent, they may still be delivered using the above highly conformal techniques, with higher prescribed doses, in an effort to achieve a good level of disease control and improve prognosis.

This chapter aims to provide you with the fundamental principles underpinning treatment verification practice. It will then apply these principles to site-specific examples and provide an insight into future directions.

10.2 Fundamental Principles of Treatment Verification

10.2.1 Geometric Uncertainty

In order for a treatment verification protocol to be effective, a sound knowledge of the sources and types of error that may occur for a given patient population/technique is essential. The 2008 'On Target' report, published by the Royal College of Radiologists (RCR), Institute of Physics and Engineering in Medicine (IPEM), and the College of Radiographers (CoR), provides an excellent reference guide for those who wish to learn more about geometric accuracy in radiotherapy, after reading this first section on fundamental principles [1].

The safety margin around the CTV (the PTV margin) is split into two components: an internal margin (IM) and a setup margin (SM). Together these account for changes in internal organ motion and external setup/positioning of the patient. Errors (internal or external) are also either random or systematic. They can also occur in any and multiple directions. Translational errors cause a shift in position along one or more of the three axes (anterior–posterior; superior–inferior; left–right) and rotational errors can occur around each of these axes (yaw; roll; pitch) respectively.

A systematic error occurs as a result of discrepancies between the planning process and the actual treatment. It results in a fixed deviation of the target volume, from the intended planned position, over all fractions for a particular patient. Historically, this led to the use of the same fixed/stable couch tops in the pretreatment and treatment settings, in order to avoid variations in couch sag and the vertical isocentre setting. It also resulted in digital images, taken direct from the planning system, being used as a reference image against which the treatment images could be compared; as opposed to 'check films/images' taken on a simulator. It is also why we need to make sure that any immobilisation device settings are recorded accurately and replicated at the treatment stage, and why for pelvic patients, we aim to ensure the bladder and rectum status is the same (as much as possible) at pretreatment and treatment.

As the name suggests, a random error is unpredictable and can vary between fractions (interfraction) or even within a fraction (intrafraction). Factors such as poor immobilisation, poor setup, movable skin marks, and changes in internal organ position, shape, and/or size, could all contribute to the occurrence of a random error.

As systematic errors represent a consistent change/difference in position for every fraction, the dosimetric consequences of a deviation from the intended planned position are arguably more significant. However, with intensity-modulated techniques, there are often dose gradients 'across' a given treatment area, where different volumes may be defined and assigned different dose prescriptions. This means that more areas will be affected by any error that occurs. Also, for those sites where a hypofractionated regime is used, there is the larger dose per fraction and shorter overall treatment time to consider. These factors will make the dose coverage more susceptible to random error as well.

Errors may also occur or develop over a course of treatment and are sometimes referred to as a time trend error. These are more likely to occur in those sites where changes in a patient's anatomy, e.g. as a result of weight loss, are common. Gradual changes can also occur internally and introduce an error, e.g. tumour shrinkage.

The treatment site provides an indication as to what factors may contribute to geometric uncertainty. On-treatment imaging/treatment verification data can also be analysed and used to determine the systematic and random error components for a given patient population/technique. This data can then be used to ensure an appropriate PTV safety margin is allocated. Treatment verification protocols, along with robust immobilisation methods, are then applied for each individual patient, in order to ensure that the treatment is delivered within this safety margin.

It is important to note that not all imaging methods will detect all sources and directions of error. This should be taken into consideration when defining the PTV margin. It should also be taken into account when developing a specific verification/ imaging protocol for a given treatment site. Section 10.2.2 expands on this.

10.2.2 Verification Protocols

When developing a verification protocol, a number of key aspects should be determined. These include:

- The type of imaging modality;
- The method of error correction;
- The action level;
- The frequency of imaging.

Sections 10.2.3–10.2.6 expand on these and focus on the detection and correction of systematic and interfraction random errors. Section 10.2.7 will then focus on the

monitoring of intrafraction error and how this might be managed/corrected for. Finally, Section 10.2.8 will look at the concept of adaptive radiotherapy, before moving onto an overview of dosimetric uncertainty and dosimetric verification.

10.2.3 Imaging Modality

Conventional approaches to treatment verification rely on the use of two-dimensional (2D) images acquired using an electronic portal imaging device (EPID). Traditionally, these images are acquired using the megavolt (MV) treatment beam, but more recently, additional imaging devices using a kilovolt (kV) beam are now available. These kV images provide superior contrast resolution and improved image quality, as the photoelectric effect is the predominant interaction process. On modern linear accelerator treatment machines the kV source and opposing detector are integral to the treatment machine. It is also possible to purchase kV imaging equipment that is mounted separate to this, within the treatment room.

Using these 2D images, the treatment is verified based on the position of the bony anatomy, which is used as a surrogate for the PTV position. However, studies have found that for many sites, internal organ motion is evident and the target will move independently of the bony anatomy [2]. Other internal anatomy changes may also occur for some sites, for example tumour shrinkage. Verification based on bony anatomy alone will only detect and correct for external setup errors.

For those cancer sites where the target volume and/or the surrounding OAR are known to move independently of the bony anatomy, and even change their shape or size, a verification method is arguably needed that allows us to visualise this internal anatomy. As a minimum, we need a method that enables us to visualise the position of the target, but ideally one that also allows us to visualise the surrounding OAR as well. This is important in ensuring that we can fully reproduce and deliver the doses that were originally planned.

If this is not possible, then approaches to immobilisation that aim to achieve consistent internal anatomy positions are of paramount importance, for example: asking pelvic patients to attend for their planning appointment, and then daily treatment, with a full bladder and an empty rectum. Arguably, such methods are important regardless of the verification imaging modality used, as they help to avoid any large daily variations and subsequent corrections, but in the absence of an imaging modality that enables us to visualise the internal anatomy, they play a vital role in minimising this source of error.

As the imaging modalities available and approaches to verification have advanced, the term 'image-guided radiotherapy' (IGRT) is more routinely used to describe the process of treatment verification. Some use it to specifically describe those approaches that enable direct visualisation of the target and can identify and correct for positional variations in the internal anatomy, as well as the external setup/patient position.

For some sites, implanted fiducial markers in or around the target may be used to aid direct visualisation and will act as a more reliable surrogate for target position than bony anatomy. These will be identifiable on 2D portal images and therefore provide a relatively simple and cost-effective IGRT solution for many departments. Research has focused mainly on the use of fiducial markers in the prostate or breast (tumour bed). In order for fiducial markers to be a reliable method for treatment verification, it is important to ensure that any marker migration within the tissue is minimal. Any corrections made, based on movement of the markers, should be as a result of actual movement of the prostate/target. Clinicians will leave time for the markers to settle within the tissue before acquiring the planning CT (computed tomography) (approx. one to two weeks).

The 'centre of mass' (COM) of the markers may be used as a reference point, although intermarker distances and individual seed measurements can also be used. Three or more markers are more often used to act as a coordinate system for image registration. Markers cannot highlight the target contour, although assessment of marker distances over time may 'indicate' a possible change in the target's shape or size, which could be investigated further with CT if needed. Some departments may use markers as the main verification tool, but then combine this with a less-frequent CT-based method, e.g. weekly, in order to monitor for changes in the position, size, and/or shape of the target/organ that cannot be visualised using 2D portal images and markers alone.

Another benefit of using CT images for verification is that the images are matched 'like for like' with the planned CT volumes; the most common approach uses cone beam CT (CBCT). The majority of treatment machines use kV CBCT. Megavolt CBCT options are also available.

In contrast to the thin collimated beam used to take multiple slices throughout the volume in conventional CT, the X-ray source used in CBCT covers the complete volume all at once, throughout either a 180° or 360° gantry rotation (Figure 10.1). Multiple 2D images are acquired and reconstructed into a 3D volume, although they are not of diagnostic quality. Intrafraction motion can also cause reconstruction artefacts and the larger field of view (FOV) used with CBCT can cause image artefacts and streaking due to the increased amount of scattered radiation. It also means that the CT numbers (used for dose planning and calculation) are less reliable than diagnostic CT.

Kilovolt CBCT uses an additional kV X-ray source attached to the gantry, perpendicular to the MV treatment beam (Figure 10.2). As indicated above, the kV tube can be also run in plain 2D radiographic mode, and may be preferable to the MV EPID given the superior image quality. The kV tube can also run in fluoroscopic mode, and it is this that is used during the CBCT gantry rotation.

Megavolt CBCT uses the MV treatment beam and opposing detector. The increased penetration with MV energies means that more of the incident dose reaches the detector, which may be of benefit, particularly for larger patients. However, detector efficiency is low and as a result a proportion of the X-rays is not stopped and passes straight through. The high dose rate must also be lowered,

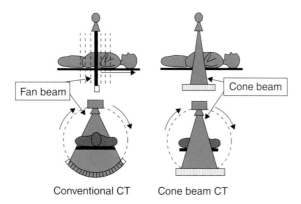

Conventional CT   Cone beam CT

FIGURE 10.1   Diagram to illustrate the differences between conventional CT and cone beam CT (CBCT). (Source: courtesy of Dr Jonathon Sykes, St James' Hospital, Leeds.)

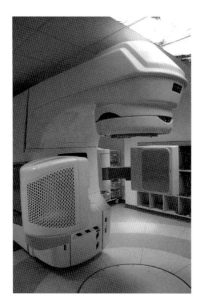

FIGURE 10.2   Varian Onboard Imager (OBI) incorporating an additional kV-X-ray source and detector. (Source: courtesy of Weston Park Hospital, Sheffield.)

otherwise the dose delivered during acquisition time would be much higher than a conventional MV 2D portal. This also means that much less radiation will reach the detector. In addition to this, the image quality with MV CBCT has a lower-contrast resolution compared with kV. This can be a benefit, however, for those patients with a hip replacement because they can be imaged without causing major streak artefacts.

Some departments may have a tomotherapy unit where the treatment is delivered in intensity-modulated slices that arc around the patient, in much the same way as a diagnostic helical CT scan is obtained. The MV treatment beam is used to acquire a CT image for the purposes of verification, however given its design, this is a MV fan beam CT. It is important to understand this difference between an MVCT and an MV CBCT.

The use of abdominal ultrasound has also been investigated, and used, as an imaging verification tool, mainly for prostate cancer radiotherapy. However, a number of notable limitations with this method were determined and it is much less frequently used nowadays. For example, the prostate could move as a result of probe pressure on the abdomen, during image acquisition, and image quality was poor. The obvious advantage of using ultrasound is the lack of radiation dose. Interest in ultrasound for managing interfraction variations still exists, but mainly as an initial bladder status assessment tool prior to daily setup for pelvic targets affected by daily changes in the bladder's position, shape, and size. The ultrasound image enables an easy, non-invasive means of checking the bladder status prior to treatment and ensuring it is comparable with what was planned. If this is not the case, the patient can be instructed to drink further fluids or empty their bladder as needed, before any verification images are taken after initial setup. This helps to reduce corrections that may be needed, and in turn can help to make the treatment more efficient [3].

Recent advances in treatment machine design have seen the emergence of image guidance using magnetic resonance images (MRI). This system has a number of potential benefits including improved soft-tissue definition and the lack of any additional radiation dose. Standard image guidance to correct for systematic and random error can be performed on these new machines, along with other more advanced forms of image guidance, i.e. intrafraction monitoring and adaptive radiotherapy [4].

Other equipment options also exist that use surface markings as a means of verifying the patient position. The term 'surface-guided radiotherapy' is used and recent systems use cameras to track the position of the skin surface (not just specific points marked on the skin), which can then be compared to the planned skin surface position, with sub-millimetre accuracy. There is a notable interest in such systems as some departments are investigating whether they can be used to guide the external setup of the patient, instead of permanent tattoos [5]. For some sites, the skin surface may also act as a reliable surrogate for the position of the target. Given its external position, this may be particularly useful for breast radiotherapy, but also for those sites where day-to-day internal organ motion is minimal, e.g. head and neck radiotherapy. Such sites may still require volumetric 3D imaging, e.g. with CBCT to detect changes over time due to tumour shrinkage, but surface-guided radiotherapy may help to reduce the amount of images required and in turn, the amount of additional dose delivered. Hoisak and Pawlicki provide a useful review of surface imaging systems in radiotherapy [6].

10.2.4 Method of Error Correction

Put simply, any shifts in the external position of the patient or internal anatomy (if the imaging method allows assessment of this), will be detected and quantified through registration of the planned reference image(s) with the treatment image taken, after initial setup. In other words, it will calculate the difference between the planned couch position and the setup couch position on treatment. Specific parts of the anatomy will be defined in both images and used as match structures for the purposes of registration. Registration can be done manually or involve the use of semi- or fully automated matching software. The automated processes help to minimise subjectivity and variability amongst those practitioners involved in image review and analysis. Practitioners may choose to register the images using the target itself as the match structure, as opposed to a surrogate for target position. However, this relies on a good image quality with sufficient contrast resolution such that the target can be accurately identified (either by the practitioner using the manual or semiautomated methods) or by the software itself (using tissue density data). Any inaccuracies may introduce an error that does not actually exist. It may be more appropriate to match to a surrogate for target position but it is important to ensure that whatever structures are used, they are subject to minimal movement. Any error calculated needs to reflect movement of the target and not movement of the surrogate. Bone is commonly used as the match structure (a necessity with 2D portal images), but if internal organ motion is an issue, this is arguably not a reliable surrogate and even when using CT-based methods, if this is the match structure used, only external setup error will be detected. However, an advantage of using CT-based methods is that the position of the target and OAR can still be assessed after an initial bone match, and if needed, the practitioners can make further adjustments to the match such that the target position is aligned with that in the reference image. A common example from practice is to perform an initial automated bone match, followed by manual adjustment of the target position. Nowadays, imaging software will calculate the error and change in couch position required to achieve the desired match.

Errors that are measured during treatment can be corrected either online or offline.

Online correction is where an image is acquired and any error is corrected before the treatment is delivered for that fraction. It is often used to identify gross errors before treatment, and is particularly useful on the first few fractions, e.g. before the systematic error is calculated and corrected. As random error varies between fractions, it can be corrected for using only online imaging.

Offline correction involves acquiring an image that is then reviewed after the treatment has been delivered. Any error is corrected for in subsequent fractions. It is used to correct the systematic error component of a patient's treatment. It cannot correct for random error.

In terms of error direction, it is possible to detect any of the three possible rotational errors, as well as the three translational error directions, if 3D imaging is used. It may then be possible to apply a 6D couch correction (as required). A specialised patient/couch repositioning system is required in order to enable this.

10.2.5 Imaging Frequency

It is also important to consider the frequency of imaging. Applying a correction based on only one image at the start of treatment provides merely a 'snapshot' of the error that day and may not be representative of the error occurring in subsequent fractions. The systematic error component can be more accurately determined by increasing the frequency of imaging in the first week. A common approach used in practice is the 'no action level' (NAL) protocol or a modified version of this. This protocol rules that a set number of initial images should be acquired and then analysed offline to determine an average setup error, i.e. the difference between the planned position and the average treatment position. As the name implies, one setup correction is then applied for all subsequent fractions, irrespective of its magnitude. A modified version would apply an action level at which the average setup error would be corrected. In terms of the number of initial images, this tends to be the first

three to five fractions. Once a correction is made for this systematic error, a final verification image on the next treatment fraction would then be used to verify the new position/setup parameters. Departments may also choose to repeat images on a weekly basis thereafter to ensure that the accuracy is maintained throughout treatment.

An alternative to systematic error correction is daily online imaging, which would correct for both systematic error as well as any day-to-day random error. The standard deviation around the average/mean (systematic) error represents the random error component. If the random error is large, then arguably a daily online imaging protocol would be preferable which corrects for both types of error. Otherwise, it is likely that the setup would still be out of tolerance on the final verification check, after initial correction of systematic error.

When designing a verification protocol for a given patient population, one must consider the source of the random error. For example, if it is mainly attributable to internal organ motion, one would have to question the benefit of daily online imaging, if a verification method was used that only based error calculation on the position of bony anatomy. This approach will only detect external setup errors.

10.2.6 Action Levels

It is important that an appropriate action level is decided upon. This is the point at which action is needed, and a measured error needs to be corrected. Action levels set minimum conditions beyond which any treatment would be deemed unacceptable [1].

The size of the planned safety margin (PTV margin) used, as well as any OAR in close proximity, would be considered. The imaging protocol being used would also need to be taken into account, in terms of what errors are actually being detected and therefore being assessed against this given action level. It would also be important to consider the inherent accuracy of the method used to measure the error, i.e. how likely it is that the error measured represents an actual error, and not one introduced through inaccuracies and uncertainty with the image registration process that takes place. This can be affected by the software itself, the image acquisition process, the resulting quality of the image, and/or the matching technique used, as well as the associated level of user involvement and potential for user variability.

More than one action level may be set in terms of the intervention required. For example, departments may have an action level for gross errors that require immediate action before delivering the treatment, and an action level for those errors that can be monitored over several fractions before taking action, i.e. when performing a systematic error correction. For many techniques, a gross error is usually around 0.5–1 cm.

10.2.7 Managing Intrafraction Motion

An increased level of accuracy is often demanded within modern radiotherapy practice where a range of advanced techniques are now being used that deliver high, precisely conformed doses to the target, with small PTV safety margins and often steep dose gradients between different targets and between the target(s) and nearby OAR in close proximity. For example stereotactic ablative radiotherapy (SABR) and LinAc-based stereotactic radio-surgery (SRS) techniques, delivering very high doses per fraction to small defined volumes. It is therefore important to consider if intrafraction error is possible, and of a magnitude beyond defined tolerances.

In the pretreatment setting (initial planning appointment) a 4DCT localisation scan is often acquired for those sites subject to motion, for example, lung cancer. This 4DCT scan is used to define an internal target volume (ITV) that encompasses the extent of movement for a given patient. Then, at the on-treatment verification stage, a 4D CBCT scan can also be acquired which allows for this planned target position over time, e.g. over the course of the breathing cycle, to be verified. Chapter 6 provides further detail on how a 4D scan is acquired.

Intrafraction motion can also be tracked 'during' treatment delivery. Such monitoring may simply be used to assess the extent of motion, or it may be combined with gated technique whereby the machine switches off if the target moves out of position (within a defined tolerance) and is switched back on (manually or automatically) once any corrections have been made, or until the target has returned to an acceptable position. Other systems provide the option of 'real-time' tracking and adjustment, and are fully automated and configured to change the treatment field position as needed in response to the changing position of the target. However, even real-time approaches need to incorporate some form of predictive tumour motion tracking due to the finite imaging frequency and system latencies between target localisation and the dose delivery [7].

There are a number of possible imaging and equipment options now available for tracking intrafraction motion. In the first instance, implanted markers within or near to the target can be monitored using the kV or MV source in fluoroscopy mode. The recently developed MR linear accelerators can also monitor intrafraction motion. Tumour motion prediction could also be facilitated by the use of cine-MRI [7]. Another equipment option available uses ultrasound to monitor intrafraction motion. Instead of using an abdominal technique, the probe is placed against the perineum and real-time images are acquired throughout treatment [8]. Surface-guided radiotherapy may also be used to monitor intrafraction motion. After its initial use for setup verification, continued monitoring throughout treatment delivery helps to ensure the patient position is maintained. These systems can also automatically signal for the treatment to be stopped if the patient moves out of the desired position.

Alternatively, for those treatment sites where intrafraction motion can occur between the treatment starting and treatment ending, but not likely to occur second-to-second (in the case of breathing motion), images may be taken less frequently throughout treatment or at the start and end of treatment. Again, these images may be used to simply assess the extent of motion, but in the case of those taken periodically throughout the treatment delivery, they may still be used to initiate a correction in couch position during treatment delivery. This imaging solution, typically using 2D kV images with or without markers, is commonly used with the type of treatment machine called Cyberknife.

10.2.8 Adaptive Radiotherapy

Adaptive radiotherapy takes into account positional changes, as well as any changes that occur in the shape or size of the target, for example changes due to tumour shrinkage or growth, or physiological changes such as bladder filling. It may include a positional correction but will also include other changes to the original plan. Adaptive radiotherapy may be 'preplanned' or undertaken 'as seen' during the course of imaging on treatment. Depending on the source of error, it may be performed daily or less frequently, i.e. once weekly. Any changes detected may be analysed offline (with any adaption to the plan applied on subsequent fractions) or online (which could also include online adaption to the plan, before treatment delivery that day).

One relatively common example nowadays is to select a 'plan of the day', at each treatment fraction (online). This is particularly useful for treating the bladder, as despite patient efforts to achieve a consistent status for each treatment, it is known to still vary. Based on the initial pretreatment planning CT, a series of plans will be created with varying PTV margins around the bladder, to account for the possible daily variations in size and shape, very often in the superior direction. For each daily treatment, any positional corrections will first be made, then a plan will be selected from the database that best matches the size of the bladder that day [9].

The above example is based on changes in size and/or shape that are predictable and can be 'preplanned'. This is not always the case, e.g. tumour shrinkage or growth, and the extent of this. However, images taken as part of the routine imaging protocol may detect such changes during the course of treatment. In these 'as seen' circumstances, online or offline review may be undertaken in order to assess the dosimetric impact of such changes (assuming the positional corrections made are still ensuring the target is covered). An example intervention would be that the PTV is then changed, and a replan is undertaken, to better match the new shape and size.

Real-time adaptive radiotherapy, using daily online imaging that incorporates positional corrections and an assessment of any changes in size or shape to the target, plus online changes to the original plan as required, is currently not commonplace. Aside from having the necessary equipment and software available, staff training and workload issues are significant considerations.

10.2.9 An Issue of Additional Dose

For all types of imaging, kV energies will deliver a lower concomitant dose than MV, and compared to 2D portal imaging, 3D volumetric images will also deliver a higher dose. When using MV 2D portal imaging it is possible to subtract the monitor units used to acquire the images from those intended for that treatment field. However, orthogonal reference images are most often acquired, so this may not be possible if the treatment fields are at oblique angles. Additional dose outside the planned treatment volume will also be incurred if a double exposure is used as a means of identifying relevant anatomy needed for the match.

As previously described, an increased frequency of imaging in the first week is needed to effectively reduce the systematic error and daily online imaging that would be needed to fully eliminate the random error. The benefits of the latter must be weighed against the potential risks of any additional dose delivered. The additional dose delivered must be justified under the regulations set out by IR(ME)R [10]. For example, if the treatment site is not significantly affected by random error, then daily online imaging is arguably not needed; especially if the random error is predominantly due to internal organ motion and only 2D portal imaging based solely on bony anatomy is being used.

10.2.10 Dosimetric Uncertainties and Verification

In addition to verifying field placement (geometric verification), dosimetric verification is of great importance, particularly considering the increased need for accuracy with conformal treatments and IMRT (intensity-modulated radiotherapy), and often high doses being delivered close to nearby OAR. Verifying the dose delivered is arguably the most obvious way of assessing the ultimate accuracy of a patient's treatment.

For conventional 3D conformal radiotherapy, or even simple non-planned techniques, 'point dose' verification is appropriate, using in vivo dosimetry. In 2008, the publication Towards Safer Radiotherapy stated that all radiotherapy centres should have protocols in place for in vivo dosimetry, as it can detect some significant errors. It was recommended that this should be in routine use at the start of treatment for most patients [11].

There are two well-known methods available for verifying point doses delivered to the patient – the use of thermoluminescent dosimeters (TLDs) and semiconductor systems – and these are most commonly used for measuring the dose to OAR such as the lens of the eye. The major advantage of semiconductor systems is that they allow real-time assessment of dose. In practice this means that, where the ratio of measured dose to expected dose exceeds a specified tolerance (typically $\pm5\%$), setup can be investigated

whilst the patient remains on the couch. Principles of these methods are given in Chapter 4. More recently developed systems, such as MOSFETs (metal oxide silicon field effect transistors), are available.

Thorough commissioning combined with the careful application of locally determined correction factors and regular calibration can result in the implementation of accurate and precise dose verification using diodes. Appleyard et al. provide comprehensive reports on the implementation of diodes for entrance dosimetry and the determination of appropriate tolerance levels [12, 13].

Another means of measuring the dose delivered to the patient (in vivo dosimetry) is with the use of the MV EPID and 'transit dosimetry'. The transmitted dose at any point within a portal image can be determined through evaluation of the pixel signals or greyscale values. These represent the portion of radiation transmitted through the phantom/patient and hence also the dose absorbed. This could be used for IMRT or non-IMRT plans, although geometric changes and uncertainties within the patient do complicate this approach.

For IMRT, point dose verification is insufficient given the varying dose gradients across a given treatment area. Pretreatment QA (without the patient) is essential in order to verify the dose fluence delivered across each of the given treatment fields or whole 3D volume.

As described above, dose fluence for each treatment field may be measured through transit dosimetry using the MV EPID and with a phantom in place. Alternatively, diode arrays (containing multiple diodes across a given plane) may be used to detect the various doses delivered across a given treatment area. Modern pretreatment QA (quality assurance) devices comprise two diode arrays at 90° angles to one another. This allows the dose delivered to be detected from all angles, and as such enables the total dose delivered to the target volume to be assessed. This is particularly useful for volumetric modulated arc therapy (VMAT) where the intensity-modulated beam continuously arcs around the patient and there are no fixed beam angles.

With the above methods, the 'measured' dose will be quantitatively compared with the 'predicted' dose, generated using algorithms and the planned CT data. A method known as Gamma analysis is used to assess the level of agreement between the two sets of doses. The Towards Safer Radiotherapy document states that each radiotherapy centre should specify action levels and the procedures to be followed for results outside of the tolerance range [11].

As IMRT delivery is achieved by the multi-leaf collimator (MLC) leaves moving during the treatment delivery, analysis of the log files from the first or subsequent treatment fractions can provide another means of confirming the treatment delivery.

CBCT images may be also used to retrospectively confirm the dosimetric plan. The CT density data is not as reliable as that from a diagnostic CT, but it may still be feasible to use CBCT images to calculate the dose delivered on treatment. This may be particularly useful if internal organs have changed in size or shape, or weight loss has occurred, potentially affecting the way the beam is attenuated through the patient, compared to what was originally planned. Emmens et al. describe the use of CBCTs for checking the plan following identified weight loss in a head and neck case [14].

10.3 Site-specific Uncertainties and Protocols

It is highly recommended that each department has a specific image guidance pathway for each tumour site [15]. A sound knowledge of the geometric uncertainties and population-based error associated with each site/technique will be used to develop these treatment verification protocols. Common issues encountered with some of the major tumour sites, as well as the implications for treatment verification practice, are outlined.

A key reference document for this section is the guidance provided by the National Radiotherapy Implementation Group (NRIG) on IGRT [15]. The reader is advised to review this document, and also the preceding 'On Target' report [1], in order to gain a full understanding of the practices recommended and the evidence base underpinning these.

10.3.1 Head and Neck

IMRT is commonly used for this treatment site. It has the potential to sculpt the high dose around complex shapes, and avoid equally complex OAR in close proximity, within this region. Lower rates of side effects for patients are now possible, for example a reduction in the long-term side effect xerostomia, due to improved parotid gland sparing. It has been stated that no locally advanced head and neck cancer patients should be irradiated in the UK without being offered IMRT [16]. However, any variation in the patient position or the internal anatomy has the potential to have a significant effect on the dosimetry of the plan when IMRT is used due to the steep dose gradients that often exist. Several studies have shown that even with a high degree of immobilisation, rotations and complex changes in patient position can be seen [17, 18].

In the head and neck region there are a number of geometric uncertainties:

- Positional Changes

An example of this can be seen where neck flexion differs from the planned position, due to patient discomfort or variation in immobilisation. The spinal cord can move closer to high-dose regions if the vertebral bodies are not in the same position as they were at the planning CT, resulting in a higher than intended dose to the cord [19].

- Weight loss

Many patients with head and neck cancer present with a less than optimal nutritional status, which may be due to the disease itself, lifestyle choices, or a combination of both of these factors. Radical high-dose radiotherapy often causes significant ulceration of the mucosa, and weight loss is often seen, even with early preventative interventions including radiologically inserted or percutaneous endoscopic gastrostomies, high levels of dietetic input, and multidisciplinary team management. If the patient loses a significant amount of weight, changes in the body contour will be seen, which can have an effect on the dose delivered compared to what was originally planned, as the beams are attenuated through less tissue. Where less tissue is present, the high-dose region may move from the planned position or dose hot spots may occur. Higher doses could then be delivered to OAR, such as the oesophagus or spinal cord. This is often a risk when there has been significant weight loss in the neck and shoulder region.

- PTV changes

With primary radiotherapy, tumour shrinkage, or indeed growth, is possible. If the PTV changes in shape or volume then the doses delivered are likely to differ from those planned for the PTV and nearby OAR that may move closer to the high-dose region. Changes are even sometimes seen at the beginning of the treatment, where changes may have occurred between the planning stage and the commencement of treatment. Changes such as a seroma shrinking, or forming, are not particularly uncommon and can have a significant impact on the dosimetry of the plan.

Despite the above uncertainties, PTV safety margins are often still small, as OAR such as the spinal cord are very often close to the target. Internal organ motion is not a significant issue for head and neck patients as structures are typically housed around and within the skull bones. Van Asselen et al., found that although the larynx moves with swallowing, no extra PTV margin was needed [20].

Image guidance is critical in this region to ensure that the precise IMRT plan is delivered

accurately on a daily basis, and given the above uncertainties and small PTV margins, it is recommended that daily online image guidance is used to ensure the treatment delivery is as accurate as possible [15]. Given the minimal daily variations in internal organ position, 2D portal imaging based on bony anatomy only is arguably sufficient, but it will not detect changes in body contour due to weight loss, or other internal changes to the PTV over time. Also, non-coplanar translations and rotations are very difficult to detect and match with 2D imaging, and are better assessed using 3D CBCT [21]. If possible, these rotations are also best corrected with a six degrees of freedom treatment couch [18]. If bolus is being used, this again can be visualised and checked with 3D CBCT imaging, ensuring no air gaps are present.

10.3.2 Breast

Current NICE guidelines indicate that there is a role for radical radiotherapy post-surgery to the breast area in the majority of breast cancers [22]. Effective patient immobilisation can generally be achieved with the use of a breast board that includes a head rest, arm supports, a bottom stop, and knee supports, and raising both arms is said to further aid reproducibility [15]. However, this region is still susceptible to a number of geometrical uncertainties. Some of these may be managed with further attempts to immobilise the target, for example a specialised bra that can help to achieve a more reproducible position (as well as provide more dignity for the patient and lift larger breasts away from the lung and heart), or the use of deep inspiration breath-hold techniques which reduce the impact of any breathing motion and also play a crucial role in lifting the breast away from the heart and lung, minimising the dose to these structures [23, 24]. Chapter 7 covers these techniques in more detail. Other uncertainties can be managed using image guidance.

- Patient position

Whilst the method of immobilisation is an effective way of stabilising patient position, it is not perfect and differences in patient position can still occur, often between planning and treatment, or planning and the first treatment, and then subsequent treatments. Very often these are due to changes in how the patient has either tensed up or relaxed down at each of these time points, altering the position of their skin markings used for setup. This can affect breast coverage as well as the amount of lung or heart in the treatment field.

• Seromas

It is not uncommon for seromas to develop following surgery, which may then reduce over time, changing the breast shape and contour and affecting the planned dosimetry [22]. A seroma may be visible with 2D planar imaging, but is more likely to be shown with 3D imaging, including the use of ultrasound. Where surgical clips are being used as a surrogate for the tumour bed, the clips may move considerably as any seroma changes [25].

• Breast oedema

Radiotherapy can cause the breast tissue to swell and will alter the external contour of the breast and position of the skin marks used to position the patient, introducing an error and affecting coverage of breast tissue. Such visible changes may be simply detected during the setup itself, but imaging will also enable assessment of any internal impact, e.g. on the lung and heart volume irradiated.

In addition to the above uncertainties, a number of different techniques may be used nowadays to treat breast cancer, depending on the stage of the disease and previous surgery. With whole breast radiotherapy, additional mini tangential fields may be used to boost the dose to certain areas of the breast and create a more even dose distribution across the tissue, avoiding any hot spots. Boost fields to the tumour bed, in addition to the whole breast prescription, may also be used for some

women. This may be done using electron fields but can also be delivered using a conformal photon plan, either sequentially as a separate treatment after the whole breast radiotherapy course has been completed, or as a simultaneous integrated boost using IMRT. There have also been a number of studies looking at the benefit of whole breast radiotherapy versus partial breast only treatment [26, 27]. Treatments using IMRT and smaller fields to boost specific areas within the breast will demand a higher level of accuracy.

For whole breast irradiation it is suggested that 2D portal imaging is sufficient, which allows assessment of breast coverage and lung depth included in the treatment field. This would be with an offline protocol used to correct for systematic setup error, with further weekly checks or as needed, to assess any further changes, e.g. in breast contour or a seroma [15].

Where partial breast radiotherapy is being delivered, either as a 'boost' to the tumour bed (sequentially or simultaneously), or as partial breast treatment only, then surgical clips are used as surrogate markers to define the tumour bed position. The raised arms and the incline used with most breast techniques may limit any CBCT imaging of the breast due to the height of the treatment couch, hence the use of planar imaging, using the kV source or a combination of kV and MV, or even a partial arc CBCT [15].

With breath-hold techniques it is important that the planned breath hold can be reproduced at the treatment stage. With this technique the image guidance needs to be performed with the patient in breath hold, and continuously acquired (cine) imaging throughout treatment delivery may be useful to confirm the treatment volume and lung position throughout the treatment. Surface-guided radiotherapy methods can also be used to monitor the breath-hold position [28].

A final consideration with breast radiotherapy and the image guidance protocol used is the dose and prescription applied.

Hypofractionated regimes continue to be researched for this cancer type and current guidance recommends the use of daily online imaging for regimes that deliver more than 2.67 Gy per fraction.

10.3.3 Chest

Radical chest radiotherapy is arguably one of the most challenging regions to immobilise and treat, due to both inter- and intrafractional motion of the tumour within the chest cavity.

- Breathing motion

Intrafraction motion is predominantly attributable to breathing motion, provided the patient is positioned sufficiently well to minimise any external body motion. Studies have shown that peripheral and lower lobe lung tumours show the most breathing motion [29–31]. Tumours closer to the mediastinum tend to move less with breathing motion, being more fixed in nature. There are a number of different approaches that can be used to manage this source of uncertainty. As previously described, this starts at the planning stage with the acquisition of a 4D planning scan, whilst the patient breathes normally, allowing assessment of tumour motion across the breathing cycle. From this 4DCT scan the maximum intensity projection of the tumour may be used to plan the ITV [29, 32, 33]. Immobilisation methods can also be used to minimise breathing motion and these are outlined in Chapter 7.

- Other inter- and intrafractional changes

Some patients who are quite frail may find it difficult to lie on the rigid treatment couch. This may introduce variations in their day-to-day position and can also make it difficult for them to remain still during the delivery of treatment. Additionally, interfractional changes may occur suddenly in this group of patients as a result of lung collapse or reinflation. In these scenarios, there is a significant risk of geographical miss in addition to the dosimetric changes seen with such notable anatomical changes. The tumour can both move significantly within the chest cavity and dosimetry can be significantly affected by changes in lung inflation [34]. As with other sites, tumour shrinkage is also possible with primary radical radiotherapy.

As much of the geometrical uncertainty is caused by internal changes in anatomy that will occur independently of any changes in the bony anatomy, it is highly recommended that volumetric imaging of the target, or implanted markers within or near to the target, is used. For some palliative treatments with larger margins and a smaller number of fractions, 2D portal imaging based on bony anatomy only may be sufficient. This is also the case for treatments close to the bony anatomy such as those for paravertebral or Pancoast tumours [15]. In terms of imaging frequency, an offline protocol is used to correct for systematic error, with regular repeat imaging thereafter to assess for those soft-tissue changes that are more likely to occur over time. However, as indicated above, some changes can occur quite suddenly and as with many other sites, IMRT is more frequently used for this treatment site, with the associated steep dose gradients that increase susceptibility to random error. SABR, which delivers very high doses per fraction over a much smaller number of fractions, is also commonly applied nowadays for certain lung cancer histologies. With all these factors in mind, a daily online correction protocol would be more appropriate in these circumstances [15].

For those treatments that were planned using 4DCT, volumetric imaging on treatment is likely to include 4D CBCT if available, even if this is just on the first few fractions as a means of verifying the planned ITV, then 3D CBCT is used thereafter. Where hypofractionated regimes are being used, such as with SABR, it may be justified to confirm the PTV coverage mid-fraction, and also post-treatment, to inform decisions for future fractions [29].

For some patients, or for techniques that demand a very high level of accuracy, gating or real-time tracking may be used (if available) to manage any intrafraction motion during the treatment delivery.

10.3.4 Prostate

Radical radiotherapy plays a major role in the management of prostate cancer. High doses are needed to achieve a good level of biochemical control. The current recommended dose prescription to the prostate is 74 Gy in 37#. More recently the CHIIP trial demonstrated the effectiveness of the hypofractionated regime 60 Gy in 20# [35]. Research is now exploring the use of SABR for prostate cancers localised to the gland, using a typical dose of 36.25–36.35 Gy in 5#, as seen in the PACE trial [36].

The major dose-limiting structure with radical prostate radiotherapy is the rectum, which is in close proximity. IMRT tends to be used along with small PTV margins, especially in the posterior region, in order to avoid excessive dose to the rectum. These factors, along with the high doses delivered, means that accuracy is of paramount importance.

- Internal organ motion

This is a major source of potential error for this group of patients. The prostate position is known to move in response to varied states of bladder and rectum filling. For this reason, departments will try to maintain a constant rectal and bladder status throughout planning and treatment, e.g. empty rectum, full bladder, but this can prove difficult, especially maintaining the same degree of bladder fullness and minimising the presence of gas within the rectum. Gas moving through the rectum also has the potential to move the prostate outside of the PTV [37]. Intrafraction error during treatment delivery is also possible if treatment times are long, e.g. with the high doses delivered during SABR.

Given the risk of organ motion, treatment verification protocols that allow direct visualisation of the target, and ideally the surrounding OAR, are required. Fiducial

markers can be implanted into the prostate gland to be used as a surrogate for the target, which can then be seen with 2D kV or MV planar imaging. Alexander et al. present a national survey of UK practice regarding the use of fiducial markers. Practice varies and standardisation is required [38]. Alternatively 3D CBCT can be used to show the soft tissue position. CBCTs have a higher associated dose compared to 2D kV images, but they will also show other soft tissue structures and can be useful for monitoring the bladder and rectal status. Even if we can ensure the target is covered with image guidance, it is still important to maintain reproducible bladder and rectal volumes, in order to ensure the planned doses are delivered as intended. If the bladder was consistently much smaller than originally planned, this could affect and increase the dose it receives throughout the treatment course. As previously described, ultrasound bladder scanners may be used to assess the bladder size prior to setup.

Volumetric soft-tissue imaging is also important when the pelvic nodes are being treated in addition to the local area of the prostate. There is some debate regarding the prostate moving independently of the nodes, and such imaging methods will ensure both the nodes and the primary target volume are adequately covered.

In terms of image frequency, a minimum standard would be to correct for the systematic error using offline correction based on images taken in the first week of treatment. As with other sites, daily online imaging in these first few days will ensure any gross error is detected and corrected for during this time before the average correction is applied. However, as the internal organ motion is arguably random in nature, a daily online correction protocol is desirable [15], especially if IMRT using small PTV margins and hypofractionated doses are applied. Indeed, if treatment times are quite long, then intrafraction monitoring may be considered. Images taken at the start and end of treatment will provide an indication of the extent of this error. Physiological changes in the bladder and rectum are not occurring second-to-second, and any error is likely to creep in over the course of treatment delivery. Alternatively, images could be taken more frequently throughout treatment delivery or real-time tracking could be used. Where implanted markers are being used, it is possible to use automatic marker detection software to track marker position and ensure they remain within a predefined tolerance of their planned position. Should any of the markers move more than this predefined tolerance, the treatment can either be automatically or manually interrupted, before starting the treatment again once marker position has been reassessed by the radiographers.

In addition to ultrasound, MR-guided radiotherapy is now in clinical use for managing both inter- and intrafraction errors.

10.3.5 Other Pelvic Examples (Bladder, Gynaecological, and Gastrointestinal [GI])

As a general rule, all pelvic treatment sites will be affected by internal organ motion as described in Section 10.3.4, as all the various structures within the pelvis are subject to variations in shape and size; either as they fill or empty, but also in response to the radiotherapy treatment, e.g. prostate gland shrinkage or a reduction in bladder capacity, or tumour shrinkage in the case of primary radical therapy for gynaecological and GI cancers.

The bladder is an organ which can dramatically change in size and shape as it fills with urine and is subsequently emptied of urine. For radical radiotherapy to the bladder, it is crucial that the patient is treated with a consistent level of bladder filling, and 3D CBCT can be used to ensure the bladder is encompassed within the PTV, although, as this is associated with an additional dose, the aforementioned pretreatment bladder scanning, using ultrasound, may also prove useful.

As outlined earlier, adaptive radiotherapy is often used for treating the bladder using a 'plan of the day' approach. Adequate staff training and audit is crucial to ensure there is a consistent approach between different members of staff, and that the chance of selecting the incorrect plan for treatment delivery is minimised. There are other methods of adaptive radiotherapy for bladder radiotherapy, and Kibrom and Knight provide a review of these [39].

For gynaecological radiotherapy, the position of the uterus and cervix can dramatically change if the patient's bladder and/or rectum change in shape or volume between fractions. Tumour shrinkage can also occur, altering the position, size, and shape of the intended target. Where highly conformal IMRT planning is being used this can again have significant effects on the dose to the target region. Again, in order to manage organ motion, many departments will adopt a bladder filling and empty rectum policy, and 3D volumetric imaging allows assessment of the target position, in addition to the bladder and rectum status. Daily online correction would be ideal for IMRT planned treatments. Offline, systematic error correction may be sufficient for non-IMRT planned treatments, but if a large random error was detected in the first week of imaging, a switch may be made to a daily online protocol [15].

For GI radiotherapy, movement of the rectum is less well understood, when this is the target structure and the tumour is present within the rectal cavity [15]. However, similar principles will tend to apply as for other pelvic sites. Where IMRT is used and/or larger doses per fraction are used with a short overall treatment time (e.g. short course pre-op RT [radiotherapy]) 3D volumetric imaging is recommended, along with daily online imaging. However, if a simpler forward planned technique is used, with standard margins, 2D portal imaging matching to bony anatomy, using an offline systematic error correction strategy, is sufficient [15]. Indeed, matching to bony anatomy is quite useful in this group of patients, where external setup reproducibility is arguably more of an issue where they are treated in the prone position that is less stable.

10.4 Record and Verify Systems and Computer-Controlled Delivery

Modern-day record and verify systems are crucial in ensuring that the correct parameters are selected for treatment. A limitation of older systems was they relied on the accurate entry of treatment parameters to start with and this was done manually. Any error introduced at this planning stage would remain throughout the treatment unless detected, resulting in a 'systematic' transcription error. Nowadays, the treatment parameters can be directly downloaded from the computer planning system to the record and verify system via the DICOM (Digital Imaging and Communication in Medicine) network, removing any transcription errors.

Record and verify systems should be fully integrated across the whole radiotherapy pathway. All geometric and physical data required for the irradiation of a specific patient is generated within the system from the beginning planning stage.

The systems allow the verification of a range of planned parameters, including:

- Patient identification details (ID);
- Mode of treatment (photons or electrons);
- Technique (static or dynamic);
- Treatment field data;
- Field size (including offset jaw positions);
- Fraction number;
- Beam energy;
- Monitor units (open and wedged fields);
- Daily tumour dose;
- Cumulative doses;
- Wedge angle and orientation;
- Gantry angles (plus start and stop angles for arc therapy);

- MLC leaf motion/log file;
- Collimator angle;
- Couch position (reliant on positioning devices being fixed at set points on the table);
- Electron applicators and field sizes.

This planned 'prescription' can then be retrieved for each treatment session. Any deviations in the daily setup from the planned parameters will be highlighted by the system and prevent the operator from initiating an exposure, unless an override is requested. Some departments choose to limit this responsibility to senior staff, as this is where an error may be introduced if an incorrect decision is made. Small, accepted, patient variations can occur on a day-to-day basis. A record and verify system must be able to accept minor deviations from values specified on the database. This is achieved by specifying maximum possible deviations or tolerances, based on a detailed appraisal of the treatment techniques employed. Tolerances determine those parameters that remain fixed, those that may vary, and others where monitoring is impractical. Tolerances that are too tight will result in the excessive need to override, and those that are too large will risk an inaccurate setup. A balance between the two is needed.

Once integrated into the planning and delivery system, the record and verify system arguably 'controls' the parameters, rather than simply verifying them. It is part of a much larger computer-controlled delivery system. Computer-controlled delivery drives our treatments. It would be very difficult to deliver IMRT and its associated multiple MLC positions, in particular those that are delivered dynamically, without this. The imaging options used for treatment verification are also guided by computer-assisted hardware and software packages and contemporary systems will use remote couch control to make the necessary positional changes.

Although record and verify systems and computer-assisted delivery are important in improving the accuracy of treatment delivery, they must not replace the diligence of the radiographer. Correct patient ID is the first critical step in this verification pathway. It is particularly important to be aware that the system cannot verify everything, for example the incorrect positioning of beam modification devices such as bolus. The human element of checking and confirming treatment delivery includes not only confirming the correct patient, but sense checks such as laterality, field entry, and exit points. The Society of Radiographers published PAUSE checklists in 2016 to help with these human factor checks [40].

10.5 Conclusion

In summary, treatment verification plays a vital role in ensuring our treatments (both radical and palliative) are delivered accurately within planned safety margins. This chapter has provided an overview of the geometrical uncertainties that we need to be aware of when developing our verification protocols for a range of sites, and has explained the key principles underpinning these practices. As a general rule, it is considered a minimum standard to ensure that the systematic error is corrected for all sites, based on a series of images taken in the first week and a subsequent offline correction. On each of these initial treatments, daily online images should be used to detect any gross errors that would require immediate action before delivering treatment that day. The type of imaging modality used should be determined based on the significance of internal organ motion for that given treatment site. Matching based on implanted markers (using 2D or 3D methods) or volumetric 3D or 4D CBCT, or even MRI (if available) is preferable if this is an issue. For some sites, ultrasound can also play a role in assessing internal organ shape and size, and like MRI, has the benefit of no additional dose. This is an important consideration that must be taken into account when developing a verification protocol and the type of imaging

modality as well as the frequency of imaging will influence this. Each protocol used, and the associated additional dose, should be justifiable under IR(ME)R. There is a vast amount of technology available nowadays for the purposes of treatment verification and departments must think carefully about what technology will be of benefit, and in what way this should be applied, for each treatment site. Aside from the aforementioned ionising radiation regulations, it would be inappropriate and costly to use everything at our disposal for all treatment sites.

As image guidance has advanced, it has also played a pivotal role in enabling us to improve the therapeutic ratio for many cancers. Combined with IMRT, which has facilitated the creation of precise dose distributions around the target, advances in treatment verification IGRT have enabled dose escalation, e.g. for prostate cancer, and subsequent improvements in disease control. It has also influenced our ability to reduce side effects as we are now able to more confidently keep our PTV safety margins small, as more errors can be corrected for.

Many of the advances mentioned in this chapter are still to become commonplace in all radiotherapy departments. The future role of verification within radiotherapy remains exciting, as the equipment available makes intrafraction monitoring and real-time tumour tracking, as well as online adaptive replanning in real time, realistic possibilities for the future for a number of cancer sites.

References

1. The Royal College of Radiologists, the Society and College of Radiographers, Institute of Physics and Engineering in Medicine (2008). *On Target: Ensuring Geometric Accuracy in Radiotherapy*. London: The Royal College of Radiologists.
2. Langen, K.M. and Jones, D.T.L. (2001). Organ motion and its management. *Int. J. Radiat. Oncol. Biol. Phys.* 50: 265–278.

3. Cramp, L., Connors, V., Wood, M. et al. (2016). Use of a prospective cohort study in the development of a bladder scanning protocol to assist in bladder filling consistency for prostate cancer patients receiving radiation therapy. *J. Med. Radiat. Sci.* 63 (3): 179–185.

4. Pathmanathan, A.U., van As, M.J., Kerkmeijer, L.G.W. et al. (2018). Magnetic resonance imaging-guided adaptive radiation therapy: a "game changer" for prostate treatment? *Int. J. Radiat. Oncol. Biol. Phys.* 100 (2): 361–373.

5. Rigely, J. and Robertson, P. (2017). EP-2338 poster: to evaluate the accuracy of delivering breast radiotherapy without tattoos. *Radiother. Oncol.* 127: S1290.

6. Hoisak, J.D.P. and Pawlicki, T. (2018). The role of optical surface imaging systems in radiation therapy. *Semin. Radiat. Oncol.* 28 (3): 185–193.

7. Seregni, M., Paganelli, C., Lee, D. et al. (2016). Motion prediction in MRI-guided radiotherapy based on interleaved orthogonal cine-MRI. *Phys. Med. Biol.* 61 (2): 872–887.

8. Richardson, A.K. and Jacobs, P. (2017). Intrafraction monitoring of prostate motion during radiotherapy using the Clarity® Autoscan Transperineal Ultrasound (TPUS) system. *Radiography* 23 (4): 310–313.

9. McDonald, F., Lalondrelle, S., Taylor, H. et al. (2013). Clinical implementation of adaptive hypo-fractionated bladder radiotherapy for improvement in normal tissue irradiation. *Clin. Oncol.* 25 (9): 549–556.

10. European Union Directive of Euratom. Ionising Radiation (Medical Exposure) Regulations. Available at www.legislation.gov.uk 2017. Accessed 4 February 2018.

11. The Royal College of Radiologists, British Institute of Radiology, Society and College of Radiographers, Institute of Physics and Engineering in Medicine, National Patient Safety Agency. Towards Safer Radiotherapy. London. The Royal College of Radiologists. 2008.

12. Appleyard, R., Ball, K., Hughes, F.E. et al. (2003). Systematic in vivo dosimetry for quality assurance using diodes. Part 1: experiences and results of the implementation of entrance dose measurements. *J. Radiother. Pract.* 3 (4): 185–196.

13. Appleyard, R., Ball, K., Hughes, F.E. et al. (2005). Systematic in vivo dosimetry for quality assurance using diodes. Part 2: assessing radiotherapy techniques and developing an appropriate action protocol. *J. Radiother. Pract.* 4 (4): 143–154.

14. Emmens, D. (2011). 1548 poster: CBCT dose calculation accuracy in head and neck. *Radiother. Oncol.* 99: S576.

15. National Radiotherapy Implementation Group report (2012). *Image Guided Radiotherapy (IGRT): Guidance for Implementation and Use.* National Cancer Action Team.

16. The Royal College of Radiologists, Society and College of Radiographers, Institute of Physics and Engineering in Medicine. Radiotherapy Board - Intensity Modulated Radiotherapy (IMRT) in the UK: Current access and predictions of future access rates 2013. Available from: https://www.sor.org/sites/default/files/document-versions/imrt_target_revisions_recommendations_for_colleges_final2.pdf

17. Perry, R., Parker, R.A., Emmens, D. et al. (2012). PD-0274: comparison of 2D kV images and 3D cone beam CT (CBCT) for positioning head and neck cancer radiotherapy patients. *Radiother. Oncol.* 103: S107–S108.

18. Kung, J., Poon, I., Chin, L., and Karam, I. (2018). An evaluation of the efficacy of corrections in 6 degrees of freedom for standard-fractionation head and neck IGRT. *J. Med. Imaging Radiat. Sci.* 49 (1): S3.

19. Hayes, J., McGarry, M., Perkins, G. et al. (2015). PD-0576: quantification of dosimetric impact of rotational displacements in head and neck VMAT radiotherapy. *Radiother. Oncol.* 115: S281–S282.

20. van Asselen, B., Raaijmakers, C.P., Lagendijk, J.J., and Terhaard, C.H. (2003). Intrafraction motions of the larynx during radiotherapy. *Int. J. Radiat. Oncol. Biol. Phys.* 56 (2): 384–390.

21. Ciardo, D., Alterio, D., Jereczek-Fossa, B.A. et al. (2015). Set-up errors in head and neck cancer patients treated with intensity modulated radiation therapy: quantitative comparison between three-dimensional cone-beam CT and two-dimensional kilovoltage images. *Phys. Med.* 31 (8): 1015–1021.

22. Clinical Commissioning Policy: Radiotherapy after primary cancer for breast cancer. 2016. Available from: https://www.england.nhs.uk/wp-content/uploads/2018/07/Radiotherapy-after-primary-surgery-for-breast-cancer.pdf

23. Comsa, D., Barnett, E., Le, K. et al. (2014). Introduction of moderate deep inspiration breath hold for radiation therapy of left breast: initial experience of a regional cancer center. *Pract. Radiat. Oncol.* 4 (5): 298–305.

24. Swanson, T., Grills, I.S., Ye, H. et al. (2013). Six-year experience routinely using moderate

deep inspiration breath-hold for the reduction of cardiac dose in left-sided breast irradiation for patients with early-stage or locally advanced breast cancer. *Am. J. Clin. Oncol.* 36 (1): 24–30.

25. Harris, E.J., Donovan, E.M., Yarnold, J.R. et al. (2009). Characterization of target volume changes during breast radiotherapy using implanted fiducial markers and portal imaging. *Int. J. Radiat. Oncol. Biol. Phys.* 73 (3): 958–966.

26. Marta, G.N., Macedo, C.R., Carvalho H de, A. et al. (2015). Accelerated partial irradiation for breast cancer: systematic review and meta-analysis of 8653 women in eight randomized trials. *Radiother. Oncol.* 114 (1): 42–49.

27. Livi, L., Meattini, I., Marrazzo, L. et al. (2015). Accelerated partial breast irradiation using intensity-modulated radiotherapy versus whole breast irradiation: 5-year survival analysis of a phase 3 randomised controlled trial. *Eur. J. Cancer* 51 (4): 451–463.

28. Alderliesten, T., Sanke, J.J., Betgen, A. et al. (2013). Accuracy evaluation of a 3-dimensional surface imaging system for guidance in deep-inspiration breath-hold radiation therapy. *Int. J. Radiat. Oncol. Biol. Phys.* 85 (2): 536–542.

29. De Ruysscher, D., Faivre-Finn, C., Moeller, D. et al. (2017). European Organization for Research and Treatment of Cancer (EORTC) recommendations for planning and delivery of high-dose, high precision radiotherapy for lung cancer. *Radiother. Oncol.* 124 (1): 1–10.

30. Peulen, H., Belderbos, J., Rossi, M., and Sonke, J.-J. (2014). Mid-ventilation based PTV margins in Stereotactic Body Radiotherapy (SBRT): a clinical evaluation. *Radiother. Oncol.* 110 (3): 511–516.

31. Sonke, J.-J., Rossi, M., Wolthaus, J. et al. (2009). Frameless stereotactic body radiotherapy for lung cancer using four-dimensional cone beam CT guidance. *Int. J. Radiat. Oncol. Biol. Phys.* 74 (2): 567–574.

32. Muirhead, R., McNee, S.G., Featherstone, C. et al. (2008). Use of Maximum Intensity Projections (MIPs) for target outlining in 4DCT radiotherapy planning. *J. Thorac. Oncol.* 3 (12): 1433–1438.

33. Underberg, R.W.M., Lagerwaard, F.J., Slotman, B.J. et al. (2005). Use of maximum intensity projections (MIP) for target volume generation in 4DCT scans for lung cancer. *Int. J. Radiat. Oncol. Biol. Phys.* 63 (1): 253–260.

34. Møller, D.S., Khalil, A.A., Knap, M.M., and Hoffmann, L. (2014). Adaptive radiotherapy of lung cancer patients with pleural effusion or atelectasis. *Radiother. Oncol.* 110 (3): 517–522.

35. Prof Dearnaley, D., Syndikus, I., Mossop, H. et al. (2016). Conventional versus hypofractionated high-dose intensity-modulated radiotherapy for prostate cancer: 5-year outcomes of the randomised, non-inferiority, phase 3 CHHiP trial. *Lancet Oncol.* 17: 1047–1060.

36. Morrison, K., Tree, A., Khoo, V., and Van As, N.J. (2018). The PACE trial: international randomised study of laparoscopic prostatectomy vs. stereotactic body radiotherapy (SBRT) and standard radiotherapy vs. SBRT for early stage organ-confined prostate cancer. *J. Clin. Oncol.* 36 (6_suppl): TPS153–TPS153.and On Behalf of the PACE TMG.

37. Nederveen, A.J., van der Heide, U.A., Dehnad, H. et al. (2002). Measurements and clinical consequences of prostate motion during a radiotherapy fraction. *Int. J. Radiat. Oncol. Biol. Phys.* 53 (1): 206–214.

38. Alexander, S.E., Kinsella, J., McNair, H.A., and Tree, A.C. (2018). National survey of fiducial marker insertion for prostate image guided radiotherapy. *Radiography* 24: 275–282.

39. Kibrom, A.Z. and Knight, K.A. (2015). Adaptive radiation therapy for bladder cancer: a review of adaptive techniques used in clinical practice. *J. Med. Rad. Sci.* 62: 277–285.

40. Society of Radiographers. 'Have you paused and checked?' 2016. Available from: https://www.sor.org/learning/document-library/have-you-paused-and-checked/have-you-paused-and-checked-downloads

CHAPTER 11

Quality Management in Radiotherapy

Renee Steel

Aim

The aim of this chapter is to outline the fundamental principles and processes of quality assurance, management, and control, and its associated legislation.

11.1 Introduction

Radiotherapy is a technical intervention involving the expertise of many different professionals. It is delivered in a context where there is rapid technological development coupled with pressure on resources. Evidence-based practice, guidelines, and regulation are continually evolving. A high degree of accuracy and reliability is essential at each of the multiple points along the radiotherapy pathway to ensure the standard of the resultant treatment. In addition, there are many communication interfaces to consider due to its multi-disciplinary nature. The challenge, therefore, for individuals working within this system is to manage this complexity in order to deliver high quality care for patients.

Quality management provides a framework with which to do so.

11.2 What Is Quality?

Quality may be defined as 'the degree or standard of excellence' (Collins Concise Dictionary, 5th edition, 2001). The degree or standard of excellence for any given process or procedure is relative to one's own perspective, experience, and relationship to that procedure. This holds true for radiotherapy. For instance, whilst on treatment a patient may describe the quality of radiotherapy as a function of information provision, comfort, side effects experienced, and time spent waiting. A radiographer may describe the quality of radiotherapy as a function of the reproducibility of the patient setup and proximity to the target following image verification. A dosimetrist may describe the quality of radiotherapy as a function of dose conformation to the target and dose to the organs at risk. This chapter will consider the systems and processes within a radiotherapy service which contribute to quality.

Practical Radiotherapy: Physics and Equipment, Third Edition. Edited by Pam Cherry and Angela M. Duxbury.
© 2020 John Wiley & Sons Ltd. Published 2020 by John Wiley & Sons Ltd.

11.3 Quality Assurance and Quality Control

There is a clinical requirement for quality throughout all points of the radiotherapy pathway in order to safely achieve an optimum treatment outcome with maximum tumour control and minimal dose to normal tissue [1–3]. In 1988, the World Health Organisation defined quality assurance (QA) in radiotherapy as:

> *all procedures that ensure consistency*
> *of the medical prescription, and*
> *safe fulfilment of that prescription,*
> *as regards to the dose to the target*
> *volume, together with minimal dose*
> *to normal tissue, minimal exposure*
> *of personnel and adequate patient*
> *monitoring aimed at determining the*
> *end result of treatment [4].*

In order to ensure quality in radiotherapy the steps in the pathway should be defined and the accuracy and reliability of these steps should be independently assured.

The terms QA and quality control (QC) refer to the processes undertaken to ensure that a piece of equipment, procedure, or system is functioning as intended or can be made to be so (see definitions Table 11.1). QA and QC are essential in providing confidence in and maintaining the quality of the physical and technical aspects of equipment, dosimetry, and treatment delivery. Colloquially, the terms QA and QC may be used interchangeably as both serve to ensure the quality of an output.

Under both the Ionising Radiation (Medical Exposure) Regulations 2017 (IR[ME]R) [5] and the Ionising Radiation Regulations 2017 (IRR) [6], radiotherapy services must have programmes in place that address QA. The QA programme will be specifically designed for the equipment and systems available within a particular radiotherapy service. Medical physics experts (MPEs) working in the service will be responsible for coordinating the QA programme and defining the appropriateness, frequency, and action level associated with each check [2].

The QA programme will incorporate checks performed by different users (medical physicists, technicians, and radiographers), with checks being performed at specified intervals. Equipment checks will be routinely performed to ensure that the equipment is operating within established parameters (i.e. those defined during commissioning).

TABLE 11.1 Quality terms – definitions.

Term	Definition
Quality assurance (QA)	'All those planned and systematic actions necessary to provide adequate confidence that a structure, system, component, or procedure will perform satisfactorily' [5]
Quality control (QC)	'The set of operations (programming, coordinating, implementing) intended to maintain or to improve quality and includes monitoring, evaluation, and maintenance at required levels of all characteristics of performance of equipment that can be defined, measured, and controlled' [5]
Quality management	All those activities undertaken to ensure service quality and consistency, incorporating: • quality planning; • quality assurance; • quality control; • quality improvement.

These checks will include dosimetric, mechanical, and electrical parameters. Checks of the treatment planning system (TPS) and other computer systems will also be included in the QA programme.

The frequency of required checks will be dependent on the equipment or the system being tested and as such may be performed daily, weekly, monthly, or annually (see Table 11.2 which demonstrates a sample of the frequency of linear accelerator checks). If the likelihood of an out-of-tolerance result is high or a significant impact on quality is likely with such a result, then checks will be performed more frequently. Some checks such as

a door interlock check will simply have a pass/fail result, as the check performed is to ensure that it is functioning as intended.

Performance criteria or levels will be set for each parameter based on commissioning data, and the desired or achievable level of accuracy. The values specified for tolerance and suspension limits (see Table 11.3) will also take into consideration the anticipated impact of an out-of-tolerance result [2]. The results obtained from QA processes require analysis and are assessed for consistency, discrepancy, and the requirement for remedial action. Electronic recording methods assist with this process.

TABLE 11.2 Examples of linear accelerator quality assurance (QA) checks [2, 7].

Linear accelerator test type	Test example	Frequency	Action limit
Safety check	Access interlock – door/maze	Daily	Functional
	Radiation warning lights	Daily	Functional
	Emergency off switches	Monthly	Functional
Output check	Dose constancy	Daily	±3%
	Output calibration	Annual	±1%
Mechanical check	Laser alignment	Daily	2 mm
	Couch movement	Monthly	2 mm
	Machine isocentre	Annual	2 mm diameter

TABLE 11.3 Performance tolerance definitions [2].

Term	Performance acceptability
Tolerance level	Results or performance within this range are acceptable (i.e. within the tolerance limit).
Action limit	A result above this value requires some form of action but clinical treatments may continue (coincident with tolerance limit).
Action/Notification level	Results or performance within this range are escalated for further monitoring, possibly leading to planned remedial action.
Suspension limit	A result beyond this value requires clinical treatment to be halted. It represents significant deviation from acceptable performance (the lower limit of the suspension level).
Suspension level	Results or performance within this range are unacceptable and require remedial action.

It is worth noting that increased treatment complexity and increased accuracy requirements increase QA overheads [7]. For example, specialist techniques such as stereotactic radiosurgery (SRS) or stereotactic radiotherapy (SRT) necessarily require additional time spent to ensure that radiotherapy equipment is operating within narrower tolerances.

Comprehensive guidelines for radiotherapy QA programmes are available. The Institute of Physics Engineering and Medicine have published the second edition of Report 81, Physics Aspects of QC in Radiotherapy [2] which covers processes that may be included in a QA programme in radiotherapy. The reader is directed to this document for further detail of technical QA requirements.

11.4 Quality Management

At its inception, QA and QC within radiotherapy centred on providing assurance that equipment operated within established limits. Over time and as radiotherapy became more complex, the scope expanded to include other elements such as treatment planning software, data transfer, and patient factors such as setup reproducibility [8–10].

From the late 1980s there was a drive within radiotherapy to enhance quality and safety initiatives in response to significant radiation incidents. In the UK, following an incident at the Royal Devon & Exeter Hospital in 1988 in which over 200 patients were overdosed by 25% (as a result of an error in the calibration of a Cobalt-60 treatment unit), a Department of Health working party was convened to advise on QA. The initial *Quality Assurance in Radiotherapy (QART)* report devised 18 quality standards (criteria to demonstrate in order to maintain quality) and was intended to provide a framework for radiotherapy services to implement a quality system [11]. The use of the proposed standard was piloted in Manchester at the Christie Hospital and at the Bristol Oncology Centre. The results from the implementation of the quality standards in these services were published as a QART manual in May 1994 [12], and radiotherapy services throughout the UK were encouraged to implement this.

The ethos of a comprehensive approach to quality within radiotherapy builds on the existing strengths and scope of a QA programme. All elements of the radiotherapy pathway, from new patient referral through to follow-up and operational requirements such as staffing levels and staff training and competency are considered [8–13]. Attention is given to all streams of work within a service – clinical, technical, and administrative [7], as all impact on quality. Underpinning this is a focus on quality planning and improvement. An overarching term for this approach is quality management.

Just as radiotherapy takes a multidisciplinary team to deliver, so too does quality management. Engagement from all members of the team will help to ensure the benefits of quality management are realised such as:

- Adherence to best practice;
- Process standardisation and improved efficiency;
- Ensuring technical accuracy and reliability of equipment and systems;
- Reducing the likelihood of errors;
- Increasing the probability that errors will be found and corrected;
- Improvement identified through feedback (patient, staff, and system), learning from errors, and auditing.

Why is it important?

- Patient expectations;
- Staff expectations;
- Organisational (wider-hospital) expectations;
- Regulatory requirements.

Quality management helps to negotiate radiotherapy's complexity and a quality management system (QMS) provides a framework to support this approach.

11.5 QMS

A QMS may be thought of as a framework or database of policies, procedures, and records which describe the purpose of, responsibilities for, and processes undertaken within an organisation or service. A QMS should focus on delivering outputs of a consistently high standard, quality improvement, and service user satisfaction [14]. There will be a defined set of documentation levels in the system (see Table 11.4).

11.6 ISO 9000

The International Organization for Standardization (ISO) develops and publishes International Standards. A standard is a set of characteristics or specifications for a product, service, or system that aims to ensure quality, safety and efficiency. ISO 9000 is the name given to the group of standards pertaining to quality management [14].

ISO 9001:2015 [15] is the current standard for QMSs. Central to the standard is a focus on continual improvement. To facilitate this, use of a quality improvement tool is embedded in the standard. The Plan-Do-Study-Act (PDSA) cycle (or Plan-Do-Check-Act [PDCA] cycle, Table 11.5) presents an iterative approach to quality improvement [16] and fits naturally with the feedback processes established within the quality system such as QA/QC, audit, and clinical incident reporting. The study of risk is also central to the standard and aims to improve the resilience of the QMS [15] (see Section 11.11). A QMS that meets the ISO 9001:2015 standard will have demonstrated it assists in ensuring the quality, safety, and consistency of services provided.

A radiotherapy service may be certified to the ISO 9001:2015 standard. Certification is a way to provide assurance (a sense of confidence) to service users, the wider organisation, and to regulators that the requirements of the standard have been appropriately demonstrated and that the service is focused on quality improvement. To achieve this, a radiotherapy service will have been audited against the requirements of the standard by an independent certification body.

TABLE 11.5 Plan-Do-Study-Act (PDSA) cycle [15].

Cycle stage	Action required
Plan	Define the service objectives, processes, and resource requirements
Do	Carry out the plan
Study/Check	Monitor and measure
Act	Make changes for improvement, as necessary

TABLE 11.4 Documentation levels.

Level	Documentation type
1	Quality Policy/Manual/Operational Policy: these documents provide a general statement or set of statements that define what the service does and should clearly show intent to nurture quality improvement.
2	Policies: documents in this level give the overall detail of 'when' a process should occur, 'what' will need to occur, and by 'whom'. Unless outlining a small process the 'how' is left to separate level 3 documents (which will reference each other).
3	Procedures/Work Instructions/Standard Operating Procedures (SOPs): these documents provide the detail of how to complete a process or task.
4	Forms, records etc.

11.7 The Radiotherapy QMS

The importance of a QMS in radiotherapy is long established. Development of a radiotherapy QMS based on the ISO standard was initially recommended in the QART report in 1991 [11, 12] and was recognised as fundamental to satisfactory service delivery in the Manual of Cancer Services in 2004 [17]. In 2008 a key recommendation made in Towards Safer Radiotherapy (TSRT) was for radiotherapy services to have an externally accredited QMS which included all documentation related to radiotherapy processes [13]. A comprehensive radiotherapy QMS will assist an organisation in demonstrating compliance with the radiation regulations IRR and IR(ME)R.

A QMS will define the scope of the service, including for whom radiotherapy will be provided and what types of radiotherapy are available. It will clarify such questions as: Does the service only treat adult patients, or does it also provide radiotherapy for paediatric patients? Does the service provide all treatment modalities, or are patients who require brachytherapy referred elsewhere? A QMS will define who is responsible for the service delivered (for example the joint Heads of Service: clinical oncology, radiotherapy, and medical physics) and it will detail the service's approach to quality improvement, risk management, clinical governance, and health and safety. A QMS will provide detailed information about what, when, and how things are done within the service and by whom (in policies and procedural documents). It will also provide the supporting documentation required for the processes to be undertaken within the service (records such as tabulated machine data or forms for tasks such as referral or consent).

The QMS is a resource and its overall aim is to improve practice. It focuses on processes and will address all aspects of radiotherapy, including:

- Service structure;
- Patient pathways;
- Timely delivery of care;
- Competencies of personnel involved in radiotherapy;
- Performance of the planning and treatment equipment (QA/QC);
- Policies and procedures (document control);
- Incident monitoring and reporting;
- Quality improvement (feedback loops, audit).

To be robust and effective the QMS needs to be supported and accessible. This means that there needs to be a level of participation and ownership from those working within a radiotherapy service. It also means that the QMS needs to be understood and the information it contains needs to be easily available. Staff need to work together, to make it a user-friendly and relevant system, and providing feedback will help to improve it. During radiotherapy clinical site visits undertaken by the Medical Exposure Group (MEG) (part of Public Health England [PHE]), good practice was noted in departments which had comprehensive documentation in the QMS and provided training in the use of the system to staff during induction [18].

11.8 Document Control

Documents within a QMS are controlled. This means that there are processes in place to ensure that only valid documentation is available to the user. Prior to being issued (released for use) within the QMS, documentation will be checked to ensure that it is acceptable and will be authorised. Documentation will be produced following a standard format and will be assigned a unique document code together with an issue date and version number.

Once in the QMS, documentation will have a set review date (nominally two years, however this may vary), at which point it will be assessed to ensure it still reflects current practice. If it does then this will be recorded and the document will continue to be used. If not, the document will be updated and reissued (following the checking and authorisation process). There will also be a process for staff to follow in order to provide feedback on documents that may require update prior to the set review (i.e. following a change to practice or identification of an error).

The current version of a document must be identifiable in order to prevent the use of any obsolete versions and only the current version should be available at the point of use. Electronic systems therefore facilitate version control as hard copies of obsolete versions do not need to be removed from use. This is especially pertinent across multi-site services.

11.9 Concessions and Non-conformances

The term concession is used to describe a planned and authorised change or deviation from documented procedures contained within the QMS [13]. For example, during the planning of radiotherapy a clinical oncology consultant may decide to alter the established dose and fractionation regime to limit the dose to organs at risk that lie adjacent to the treatment volume. They will record this change and the rationale for it in the patient's clinical record. In comparison a non-conformance is an unintended change or deviation from documented procedures [13] (see Section 11.14).

The QMS will document what steps need to be taken in response to both concessions and non-conformances. For concessions the process for recording, justifying, and authorising will be outlined. For non-conformances the process for recording, investigating, and determining corrective actions as necessary in order to prevent recurrence will be outlined.

11.10 Clinical Governance

The concept of clinical governance was first introduced to the National Health Service (NHS) in 1998 and was defined in *A First Class Service: Quality in the New NHS* [19] as:

> *A framework through which NHS organisations are accountable for continuously improving the quality of their services and safeguarding high standards of care by creating an environment in which excellence in clinical care will flourish*

Clinical governance frameworks focusing on quality improvement, high standards of care, and patient safety are now embedded in NHS organisations. Clinical governance should be designed to bring policies and approaches together across an organisation so that quality improvement activities have visibility and are of recognised importance. It should promote the dissemination of good clinical practice and promote sharing of lessons learned from instances where there has been a failure to meet expectations (i.e. clinical incidents or complaints) [20].

The clinical governance responsibilities may vary between organisations, however the following activities should be considered:

- Risk management (patient safety, clinical incidents – reporting and learning);
- Patient/carer involvement (experience, complaints, and feedback);
- Quality improvement;
- Clinical audit;
- Clinical effectiveness;
- Training and personal/professional development;
- Use of information (information governance and clinical informatics).

Clinical governance provides an assurance mechanism within an organisation that quality management processes are being undertaken by individual services. Radiotherapy services are likely to have all of the activities listed above defined within the QMS. In turn, the outputs of the QMS will link in to the clinical governance framework of the wider organisation.

11.11 Risk Management

The management of risk is essential for every healthcare organisation. Risk may be defined as the chance of an adverse event occurring, such a threat, injury, or loss. The source of risk may be internal or external to an organisation and may affect differing domains including patient safety, operational performance, financial performance, staffing, etc. Risk management is the system of clinical and managerial activities that assess such events and acts to minimise the risk [1]. It is important to note that risk management activities feed into the governance framework within a healthcare organisation. Within this section risk and risk management will be considered with respect to the radiotherapy pathway and not the wider concept of risk that impacts on all processes within an organisation.

Risk management is one of the key functions of a QMS and assists in ensuring patient safety and quality of care within a radiotherapy service. There are three main components: proactive risk assessment; reporting of adverse events; and reactive risk assessment [21]. Risk management aims to minimise harm to patients by:

- identifying what can and does go wrong during care;
- understanding the factors that influence this;
- learning lessons from any error or near miss;
- ensuring action is taken to prevent recurrence;
- putting controls in place to reduce risks.

Risk identification is undertaken to establish what the risks are and this process may be proactive (i.e. the risk is identified before it occurs) or reactive (i.e. the risk was identified because it occurred). Risks are then reviewed to determine the associated likelihood (frequency/probability) and severity (seriousness of the consequences). Typically, the likelihood and severity of the risk are each assigned a numerical value which are either multiplied together to establish a risk score or plotted on a risk matrix to assign a risk level (see Table 11.6). Strategies and priorities for managing the risks are then evaluated with the assigned risk score or risk level being used to inform this assessment. Decisions will then be made regarding the actions that will be

TABLE 11.6 Example of risk matrix indicating likelihood and severity scores.

Likelihood	Severity				
	No harm (1)	Minor (2)	Major (3)	Severe (4)	Catastrophic (5)
Almost certain (5)	5	10	15	20	25
Likely (4)	4	8	12	16	20
Possible (3)	3	6	9	12	15
Unlikely (2)	2	4	6	8	10
Rare (1)	1	2	3	4	5

taken to prevent or minimise (i.e. to control or 'treat') the risk.

For risk management to be effective, risks and the associated controls must be monitored. This provides assurance that these are being handled appropriately and effectively. It is essential to communicate to staff so that they are aware of the risks that have been identified. Risk will also be communicated through the clinical governance framework. This is especially important for risks that may not be able to be managed solely at the service level.

11.11.1 Risk Management in Radiotherapy

Risk is inherent in radiotherapy due to the nature of the treatment and the complexity of the context within which it is delivered. In the World Health Organisation's Radiotherapy Risk Profile, 81 risks were identified which were considered to have the potential to result in high- or medium-impact adverse events if realised. The risks were categorised as relating to patients, staff, systems, information technology, or a combination of these [3].

Assessment of risk within radiotherapy is required under the radiation regulations IRR and IR(ME)R [1, 5, 6]. IRR stipulates that an employer must undertake a risk assessment prior to the introduction of any new activity involving ionising radiation [6]. Regulation 8 of IR(ME)R stipulates the risk of accidental or unintended exposure must be assessed within the QA programme and that 'a system for recording analyses of events involving or potentially involving accidental or unintended exposures' must be implemented [5].

11.12 Risk Assessment

Risk assessment and the maintenance of a risk register (a document that details the assessed risks) are important tools that assist in patient safety and quality improvement.

There are two broad approaches for assessing risk: proactive and reactive.

11.12.1 Proactive Risk Assessment

A proactive risk assessment occurs prior to a risk being realised (i.e. before it happens). A risk assessment of this type is required when risks are identified during routine review of the service or when changes are proposed within a service – for instance, the introduction of new pathways, processes, techniques, or equipment [1, 13]. These changes must be evaluated to determine the impact (both positive and negative) and to ensure that measures (risk treatments/controls) to minimise any foreseeable risk are incorporated into the implementation plan. The outputs will be recorded in a risk assessment – a document which defines the risk, its analysis and evaluation, and the decisions made regarding risk treatments or controls.

11.12.2 Reactive Risk Assessment

A reactive assessment of risk is undertaken after an adverse event has occurred (such as an error or near miss). The purpose of a reactive assessment is to analyse the event to determine causes and to prevent recurrence [1]. The resource assigned to the response will be dependent on the severity or potential severity of the consequences and the likelihood of recurrence. Those events more likely to cause harm or be repeated will require extensive analysis in order to distil the learning and identify appropriate actions to prevent recurrence.

A common form of reactive risk assessment is a root cause analysis (RCA). An RCA looks to establish what happened and why. Information will be gathered from many sources to assist with this process including accounts from staff, patient records, documentation from the QMS, clinical guidelines, and correspondence. A report will be produced and will outline:

- Contributory factors (factors which influenced the event);
- Root cause (the factor which caused the event);
- Learning derived from the event;
- Actions to prevent recurrence.

It is essential following any reactive assessment that the findings are communicated widely. Dissemination of information helps to ensure that more staff are able to learn from the event.

11.13 Reducing Risk

There are many approaches to reducing risk within a radiotherapy service. Safety barriers are used to limit the probability or severity of an event (see Table 11.7). These can also be thought of as a risk treatment option or control. These may be inherent in the design of the equipment or system or may require the operator to act in order for the safety barrier to work [1].

Independent checking is a safety barrier that is frequently utilised within the radiotherapy pathway and is one of the top interventions for risk reduction identified by WHO [3]. Utilisation of checklists, staff training, equipment QA, and audit are other common examples.

11.14 Clinical Incidents: Reporting and Learning

As discussed previously, the context in which radiotherapy is delivered is complex and delivering treatment requires several multidisciplinary interactions with multiple communication interfaces (between both individuals and systems). Due to this complexity radiotherapy pathways and processes need to be risk assessed and safety barriers implemented in order to minimise the chance of error occurring. However, despite our best intentions, clinical incidents will still occur and may be attributable to multiple factors, whether equipment, system/organisational, or human [22]. Although each adverse event is unique, similarities in the source of risk may be established over time [23]. It is therefore important that these adverse events are reported and analysed so that learning is derived to prevent repetition and improve patient safety.

11.14.1 Regulatory Requirement to Report

Reporting of incidents is mandated under the radiation regulations. Adverse events affecting staff or the public are reported under IRR and events affecting patients under IR(ME)R. Under Regulation 8 of IR(ME)R, employers

TABLE 11.7 Types of safety barriers [1].

Barrier type	
Interlock	Inherent in design; does not require operator action to work; for example access interlocks, performance interlocks
Warning	Prompts the operator to take action; for example warning messages displayed in the record and verify system
Instruction	The operator follows a documented process; for example a verbal cross-check to ensure bolus has been placed on the patient prior to treatment

must have processes in place to record and analyse 'events involving or potentially involving accidental or unintended exposures' and are required to report any accidental or unintended exposure 'significantly greater' or 'significantly less' than intended [5] to the Care Quality Commission.

11.14.2 Radiotherapy Error Terminology

There is variation in the literature with regards to the terminology used to describe clinical incidents. Adverse event, error, adverse-error event, and patient safety incident are used interchangeably. In the UK in 2008, a taxonomy for error reporting within radiotherapy was provided in TSRT. TSRT proposed terminology to describe errors, defining a radiotherapy error (RTE) as:

A non-conformance where there is an unintended divergence between a radiotherapy treatment delivered or a radiotherapy process followed and that defined as correct by local protocol [13]

It provided an error classification grid (see Figure 11.1 and Table 11.8) and coding system (an index of points along the radiotherapy pathway) to assist in the standardisation of error reporting. The aim of this standardisation was to facilitate comparison of errors and trend analysis both within a service and nationally [13, 23, 24]. In 2016, the pathway coding was updated, safety barriers (points along the pathway that aim to detect error) were identified, and an additional taxonomy for causative factors (root causes) was introduced [24]. These changes were made to enhance the learning able to be derived from analysis of RTEs.

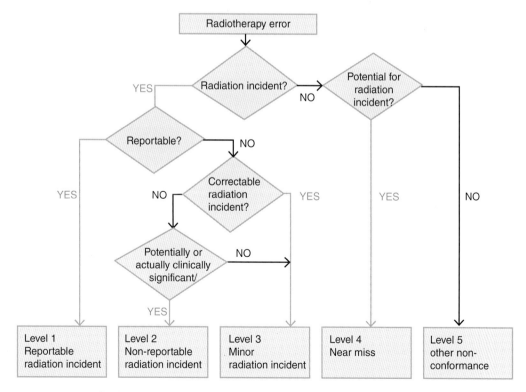

FIGURE 11.1 Radiotherapy error (RTE) classification grid – reproduced from Towards Safer Radiotherapy (TSRT) Royal College of Radiologists [13].

TABLE 11.8	Radiotherapy error (RTE) definitions reproduced from Towards Safer Radiotherapy (TSRT) [13].
Term	**Definition**
Reportable radiation incident (RI) Level 1	An RI that falls into the category of reportable under any of the statutory instruments, i.e. IR(ME)R, IRR
Non-reportable RI Level 2	An RI not reportable as above, but of potential or actual clinical significance
Minor RI Level 3	An RI in the technical sense but one of no potential or actual clinical significance
Near miss Level 4	A potential RI that was detected and prevented before treatment delivery
Other non-conformance Level 5	None of the above; that is, non-compliance with some other aspect of a documented procedure but not directly affecting radiotherapy delivery

11.15 Why Is it Important to Report?

The purpose of reporting is to promote learning and improve patient safety. All staff have a professional responsibility to report. Reporting and learning systems (RLS) aim to increase risk awareness, and to decrease the likelihood of repetition and severity of the associated consequences of adverse events. RLS are a tool that can be used to analyse the radiotherapy pathway to identify areas of greatest risk and to inform quality improvements including the strengthening of safety barriers. RLS have been shown to be an effective way to prevent major incidents [3, 25].

11.15.1 Voluntary Reporting

TSRT also recommended that a national voluntary reporting system be established for radiotherapy services to contribute to [13]. In England and Wales, radiotherapy services voluntarily submit RTE reports to the National Reporting and Learning System (NRLS). These reports are then forwarded to PHE under a data sharing agreement. There is a system for radiotherapy services in Northern Ireland and Scotland to submit data to PHE directly. Publications based on the analysis of these submissions are generated by the MEG at PHE and include both biennial reports and quarterly newsletters. The purpose of the provision of this analysis and dissemination of information is to assist the wider radiotherapy community to establish and maintain safe practice and may also be used as a learning tool when establishing the risk profile of new technologies and techniques [23].

11.16 Clinical Audit

Clinical audit is an important quality improvement tool used within healthcare to enable services to measure how well practice adheres to an evidence-based standard [26] and to establish what action needs to be taken to improve practice. Clinical audit is cyclical; following the implementation of any recommendations identified in an audit, remeasurement is required [27] to establish the effectiveness of the change.

Clinical audit is about improving patient care and involves:

- Agreeing best practice criteria;
- Measuring current performance against those criteria;
- Making changes to improve performance;
- Remeasuring to make sure there has been improvement.

Clinical audit of medical radiological procedures is required under Regulation 7 of IR(ME)R [5], therefore radiotherapy services must participate in audit. A radiotherapy service will typically develop an audit programme which will consist of:

- Quality system audits (to ensure documented procedures are fit for purpose);
- Dosimetric audits;
- Clinical audits;
- National audits (such as those undertaken under the auspices of the Royal College of Radiologists).

Participation in dosimetric audit networks is a key recommendation from TSRT aiming to facilitate interdepartmental comparison of dosimetry against a standard and dosimetric assessment of specific techniques [13].

Audit should be undertaken regularly and forms part of the quality improvement feedback loop in the QMS. The PDSA cycle and its iterative approach to improvement fits well with the requirements of clinical audit and can be used to help to plan and undertake audit.

References

1. EC (2015). *Radiation Protection N° 181 in General Guidelines on Risk Management in External Beam Radiotherapy*. Luxembourg: European Commission (European Union).
2. IPEM, ed. Physics Aspects of Quality Control in Radiotherapy – IPEM Report 81, 2nd edition. Patel, I. (ed.). 2018, Institute of Physics and Engineering in Medicine.
3. WHO (2008). *Radiotherapy Risk Profile*. Geneva: World Health Organisation.
4. WHO (1988). *Quality Assurance in Radiotherapy*. Geneva: World Health Organization.
5. European Union Directive of Euratom. *The Ionising Radiation (Medical Exposure) Regulations*. 2017: UK. Accessed 4 February 2018.
6. European Union Directive of Euratom. *The Ionising Radiations Regulations*. 2017: UK.
7. Hartmann, G.H. (2006). Quality management in radiotherapy. In: *New Technologies in Radiation Oncology. Medical Radiology (Radiation Oncology)* (eds. W. Schlegel, T. Bortfeld and A.L. Grosu), 425–477. Berlin, Heidelberg: Springer.
8. Papakostidi, A., Tolia, M., and Tsoukalas, N. (2014). Quality assurance in health services: the paradigm of radiotherapy. *J. BUON* 19 (1): 47–52.
9. Kehoe, T. and Rugg, L.J. (1999). From technical quality assurance of radiotherapy to a comprehensive quality of service management system. *Radiother. Oncol.* 51 (3): 281–290.
10. Scorsetti, M., Signori, C., Lattuada, P. et al. (2010). Applying failure mode effects and criticality analysis in radiotherapy: lessons learned and perspectives of enhancement. *Radiother. Oncol.* 94 (3): 367–374.
11. Bleehan, N.M. (1991). *Quality Assurance in Radiotherapy Report from the Standing Subcommittee on Cancer*. Department of Health.
12. DOH (1994). *Quality Assurance in Radiotherapy. A Quality Management System for Radiotherapy*. Department of Health.
13. RCR, Towards Safer Radiotherapy. 2008, The Royal College of Radiologists, Society and College of Radiologists, Institute of Physics and Engineering in Medicine, National Patient Safety Agency, British Institute of Radiology: London.
14. ISO. ISO 9000 family-Quality Management. [cited 2018 21st October 2018]; Available from: https://www.iso.org/iso-9001-quality-management.html.
15. ISO (2015). *ISO 9001:2015, in Quality Management Systems — Requirements*. Geneva: International Organisation for Standardisation.
16. Taylor, M.J., McNicholas, C., Nicolay, C. et al. (2014). Systematic review of the application of the plan–do–study–act method to improve quality in healthcare. *BMJ Qual. Saf.* 23 (4): 290.
17. DOH (2004). *Manual of Cancer Services*. Department of Health.

18. PHE (2018). *Learning from the Past 10 Years of the Radiotherapy Clinical Site Visit*. Public Health England.

19. DOH (1998). *A First Class Service: Quality in the New NHS*. Department of Health.

20. Scally, G. and Donaldson, L.J. (1998). The NHS's 50 anniversary. Clinical governance and the drive for quality improvement in the new NHS in England. *Br. Med. J.* 317 (7150): 61–65.

21. Malicki, J., Bly, R., Bulot, M. et al. (2014). Patient safety in external beam radiotherapy – guidelines on risk assessment and analysis of adverse error-events and near misses: introducing the ACCIRAD project. *Radiother. Oncol.* 112 (2): 194–198.

22. Shafiq, J., Barton, M., Noble, D. et al. (2009). An international review of patient safety measures in radiotherapy practice. *Radiother. Oncol.* 92 (1): 15–21.

23. Findlay, Ú., Best, H., and Ottrey, M. (2016). Improving patient safety in radiotherapy through error reporting and analysis. *Radiography* 22: S3–S11.

24. PHE (2016). *Development of Learning from Radiotherapy Errors (Supplementary Guidance Series)*. Public Health England.

25. Kalapurakal, J.A., Zafirovski, A., Smith, J. et al. (2013). A comprehensive quality assurance program for personnel and procedures in radiation oncology: value of voluntary error reporting and checklists. *Int. J. Radiat. Oncol. Biol. Phys.* 86 (2): 241–248.

26. Brain, J., Schofield, J., Gerrish, K. et al. (2011). *A Guide for Clinical Audit, Research and Service Review*. Healthcare Quality Improvement Partnership.

27. NICE (2002). *Principles for Best Practice in Clinical Audit*. Oxon: Radcliffe Medical Press Ltd.

CHAPTER 12

Radiation Protection

Pete Bridge

Aim

The aim of this chapter is to provide an introduction to the principles and practice of radiation protection as well as explaining the key aspects of radiation protection legislation, with a focus on the UK regulations.

12.1 Dangers of Ionising Radiations

Ionising radiation is hazardous to humans. Radiation protection practices and equipment aim to enable safe use of ionising radiation by reducing the risk of harm to those working or otherwise coming into contact with it. It is important for clinicians working in radiotherapy to understand the dangers of ionising radiation in order to reassure patients and ensure that respect for the radiation leads to safe working practices. Sadly, much of our knowledge concerning the hazardous nature of ionising radiation has been gained at the expense of early radiation workers and victims of nuclear accidents and weaponry. Common practices in the early days of radiography seem foolhardy today, but stemmed from a lack of understanding of the hazards associated with these new unseen 'magical'

rays [1]. Early radiotherapy delivery entailed clinicians passing patients radioactive isotopes for them to hold next to their tumours until erythema was evident. Diagnostic X-ray workers commonly checked functioning of fluoroscopy screens by watching to see if an image of their watch was visible when placed on the opposite side of their head to the source of X-rays. Unsurprisingly, radiodermatitis of the hands was common in these early workers, often leading to necrosis and amputation. Overtreatment of patients in the early days, as well as use of radiation for treatment of benign conditions such as ringworm [2], led to many cases of overdosing and development of side effects drastically worse than the original symptoms. Induction of cancer is a common long-term effect of radiation exposure as history has demonstrated. In the 1930s it was common practice for painters of radium dials on watches to lick the ends of their brushes to produce neat dots on the watch face. A retrospective study linked this ingestion of the radium paint to increased bone cancer incidence [3]. More recently, long-term follow-up studies of the survivors of the Nagasaki bomb [4] showed an increased leukaemia incidence of 1.5 extra cases per million people per cGy per year. Dangers are not restricted to cancer induction, however, and a total body exposure in the order of 8–10 Gy will cause lethal radiation syndromes arising from a failure of body systems.

Practical Radiotherapy: Physics and Equipment, Third Edition. Edited by Pam Cherry and Angela M. Duxbury.
© 2020 John Wiley & Sons Ltd. Published 2020 by John Wiley & Sons Ltd.

Radiation dose received by gonads will also increase the chance of genetic abnormalities in children conceived following exposure.

12.2   Rationale for Radiation Protection

Despite the medical benefits of radiotherapy, it is clear that it is a double-edged sword capable of causing a range of acute and long-term problems to those exposed or their future families. These effects are categorised as either 'stochastic', meaning 'random in nature', or 'deterministic'. Stochastic effects can occur with even a small radiation dose, with the incidence of the effect increasing with higher doses. Deterministic effects occur only after a 'threshold' dose has been received, and then the severity of the effect increases with higher dose. In radiotherapy deterministic effects in patients who have been prescribed radical doses are common; skin erythema and diarrhoea are common examples of this. Radiotherapy practitioners however are unlikely to receive doses high enough for deterministic effects to occur. The aim of radiation protection practices and legislation from a staff perspective is to reduce dose in order to minimise the chance of a stochastic effect occurring.

12.3   Radiation Protection in Practice

12.3.1   Risks and Benefits

Clearly, the safest approach to dose reduction is to avoid use of ionising radiation at all costs. In medicine, however, there are clearly proven benefits associated with radiation. Potential benefits of ionising radiation include cure of disease or improvement in quality of life, accurate diagnosis, early disease detection, or accurate placement of catheters and stents.

It is important to consider for an individual patient the extent to which these benefits outweigh the risks for their exposure. Ionising radiation should only be used where there is clear justification, meaning that there is an overall benefit compared with the level of risk. The use of non-ionising radiation alternatives should also be considered.

12.3.2   ALARA

If radiation is justified then it is essential to use the minimum possible dose, according to the principle of ALARA (or ALARP). This stands for 'as low as reasonably achievable' (or 'practicable'). Adoption of ALARA ensures that those working with radiation will keep their exposure and that of others to a minimum and therefore reduce the chance of stochastic effects occurring. It is important to ensure that dose is not reduced to such an extent that it compromises the aims of the exposure and necessitates repetition of the exposure. This is achieved by following established protocols and procedures using modern and well-maintained equipment. Prior determination and ongoing evaluation of dose levels and procedures is an essential aspect of ALARA and this is embedded in radiation legislation within the UK Ionising Radiation (Medical Exposure) Regulations 2018 (IRMER 2018). Dose limitation to radiotherapy patients cannot be performed with regard to tumour dose, which must be maintained at a therapeutic level. Dose to non-target tissues must, however, be kept ALARA through careful and conformal planning along with effective immobilisation and image-guidance procedures. For non-radiotherapeutic procedures, reduction of dose is possible, so settings must be carefully chosen to ensure that images do not need repeating and equipment such as image intensifiers, auto-exposure controls, and image-capture software must be used. Furthermore, employers have a responsibility to ensure that each exposure is evaluated and recorded; the verification and recording software usually performs this task.

12.4 Radiation Protection by Design

There are a number of protective measures that may be employed to limit the amount of radiation personnel are exposed to. The three main principles of radiation protection are time, distance, and shielding.

Time: the dose someone receives when exposed to radiation depends on the dose rate of the source and the time spent exposed to it. As a consequence, anything that can be done to limit the time exposed to a radiation source will minimise the exposure.

Distance: the radiation arising from a point source reduces in intensity in proportion to the square of the distance from the source (inverse square law). This means doubling your distance from the source would quarter your exposure.

Shielding: by placing an appropriate protective barrier or shielding between the radiation source and the area you are trying to protect, the level of radiation reaching that area will be attenuated and reduced.

12.4.1 Equipment Design

There are three main sources of radiation associated with any radiation generator: the primary beam, scattered radiation produced by interactions of the primary beam, and leakage radiation from the radiation generator itself. Manufacturers have a responsibility to maintain radiation leakage levels as low as possible. It is down to the room design to minimise the impact of the primary and scattered radiation.

The primary factor affecting room design is the type of equipment that is to be located in it. With the exception of simulator and CT equipment, kilovoltage equipment is non-isocentrically mounted, so the main beam can be aimed in any direction. This presents a different challenge for radiation protection than isocentrically mounted megavoltage equipment which inherently restricts primary beam

directions. For proton beams, it is the neutron scatter that is the major radiation protection challenge.

Proton facilities bring additional challenges to radiation protection depending on the delivery mechanism. Passive scattering equipment generates significant additional scattered neutron dose arising from the scattering mechanism and range compensator, whereas scanned beams are much more efficient and most of the dose is absorbed by the patient. The patient is the source of most of the scattered radiation for scanned beams. For both mechanisms there is likely to be scatter contribution arising from the range modulation system. Neutrons demand high levels of protection as they are capable of penetrating shielding materials. There is an additional challenge associated with 'activation' of the equipment and room itself with residual radiation hazards persisting after the beam has switched off.

12.4.2 Barrier Design

For isocentrically mounted radiation generators, the primary beam is only capable of irradiating a rigidly defined section of the room (Figure 12.1). For gantry systems this encompasses a band of walls, floor, and ceiling which is known as the *primary barrier*. The remaining boundaries of the room that receive only secondary (leakage) radiation from the delivery system and scattered radiation from the patient and other materials are known as *secondary barriers*. It is important to distinguish between these barriers because only the primary barrier needs to be thick enough to attenuate the primary beam and choosing a thinner secondary barrier can save money.

A variety of building materials can be used for barrier construction as seen in Table 12.1 and the density of the chosen material will clearly affect how thick the barrier needs to be.

Major factors affecting barrier thickness include the daily workload and energy of the machine. This will determine the dose rate at the isocentre, and it is the aim of the barrier to

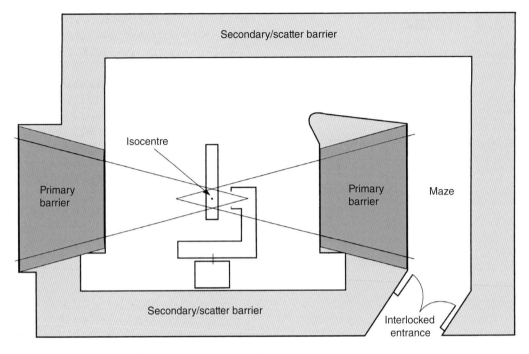

FIGURE 12.1 Primary and secondary barrier location.

TABLE 12.1	Barrier construction material characteristics.

Material	Density (kg m³)
Brick (common red)	1920
Breeze block	1200
Concrete	2370
Barytes concrete	3100
Earth fill	1520
Glass	2580
Glass (lead)	4360
Steel	7849
Lead (solid)	11 340

reduce the dose rate outside the room to no more than the safe limit (for public areas this should be around 0.3 mSv year⁻¹) [5]. Typical thickness requirements are 6 or 7 tenth value layers (TVLs) for a primary barrier and around 3 TVLs for a secondary barrier. The TVL is the average amount of material needed to absorb 90% of all radiation, i.e. to reduce it to a tenth of the original intensity.

The size of the room will influence barrier thickness, with the inverse square law reducing intensity and therefore barrier thickness for a large room. Conversely to this, a larger distance to the barrier will necessitate a wider primary barrier due to beam divergence.

The width of the primary barrier is dependent on the maximum area that can receive the primary beam. Beam divergence, collimator rotation, and multiple gantry angles need to be considered when determining how much of the room needs to be a primary barrier. Penetration of barriers for cable access, for example, needs to be planned using angled access tubes and shielding to ensure that radiation cannot escape through the ducts.

For non-isocentrically mounted apparatus such as kilovoltage radiotherapy units, the primary beam direction is not so constrained and the entire room has to act as a primary barrier. As a result of the relatively low beam quality however, the walls can be much thinner than those required for megavoltage installations.

12.4.3 Treatment Room Entrance

The room entrance design plays a large role in radiation protection. There are many factors impacting on the design and the reader is directed to more specialist texts [6] for an in-depth discussion of this. Clearly any treatment or simulation rooms where patients are left alone need to be accessible in case of emergency, yet an entrance presents an opportunity for radiation to escape. For this reason, treatment rooms using high-energy megavoltage photons or protons will usually use a maze entrance [6] to attenuate radiation via scatter processes (see Figure 12.1). This allows for ease of access but denies scattered radiation or neutrons passage out of the room. At lower kV energies, a shielded door may be sufficient, but, as the energy increases, the required door thickness presents technical difficulties such as the need for a motorised opening mechanism. When using photon energies over 20 MeV or high-energy protons, neutron generation is a significant problem. Shielded doors impregnated with boron are then necessary to absorb neutrons. The choice of entrance will largely be dictated by availability of space whilst balancing the need for protection against the need for easy access to the patient. The control area must be remote to the radiation generator, with CCTV (closed-circuit television) or lead glass screens allowing visualisation of the patient at MV and kV respectively.

12.4.4 Treatment Room Location

Another important factor affecting radiation protection is the position of the room itself in relation to its surroundings. Adjoining treatment or simulation rooms can benefit from sharing of primary barriers, thus saving on shielding materials. Any other rooms need to be shielded according to their typical occupancy. Rooms that are used sporadically, such as toilets or corridors, have a lower 'occupancy factor' than offices or wards so

shielding needs to reflect that. Apart from being adjacent to other radiation generators, bunkers can benefit from being single-storey buildings (thus avoiding the need for reinforced and shielded floors and ceilings). Backing into a hill is ideal because earth fill can be used as a cheap shielding material.

12.4.5 Additional Safety Features

Any controlled areas must have warnings in place identifying prohibited access and displaying the radiation caution trefoil, as illustrated in Figure 12.2. In addition to *warning signs*, there should be *warning lights* and an *audible alarm* to alert visually impaired visitors. For proton facilities, a neutron monitor, or more commonly a gamma monitor, is recommended. A range of *interlocks* should be present to ensure that the patient is the

(a)

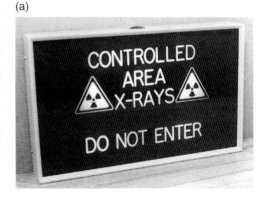

(b)

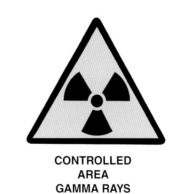

CONTROLLED
AREA
GAMMA RAYS

FIGURE 12.2 (a) and (b) Warning signs.

only person being irradiated and that he or she is receiving the correct dose. *Access interlocks* such as barriers, infrared beams, doors, or motion sensors will terminate the exposure if broken by an intruder. Various systems such as verification software, 'select-and-confirm' protocols, and accessory interlocks ensure that the correct parameters are used in the exposure. *Performance interlocks* within the radiation generator are designed to maintain correct beam quality, intensity, and dosimetric consistency.

12.5 Personal Monitoring

It is common practice for all staff members working in the radiotherapy departments to participate in *personal dose monitoring*. Principles of personal dosimeters have already been detailed in Chapter 4. It is important that these devices are portable, tough, sensitive, reliable, and relatively cheap. Monitoring is performed whenever people could receive 10% of the annual dose limit. Therapy radiographers rarely receive any more than background dose (2.6 mSv year^{-1}) [7] so the main aim of personal dosimetry in most areas within the radiotherapy department is to check for problems with radiation shielding and local rules or staff compliance/understanding with the local rules. The exception to this is, of course, brachytherapy, where the nature of the radiation is such that dose to staff is more likely. Radiation protection issues relating to this area are covered in more detail in Chapter 14.

12.6 Radiation Protection Legislation

It can be seen, therefore, that there are a great number of design features and principles that enable radiation protection to be achieved in the radiotherapy department. These can only

be effective, however, in the context of commitment to staff training and compliance with legislation, local rules, and protocols. Section 12.6.1 addresses the relevant legislative framework with an emphasis on UK regulations. The principles of the legislation, however, share similarities with those in place internationally.

12.6.1 Ionising Radiations Legislation

In 2017 and 2018, the legislation governing the use of ionising radiations in the UK was updated. These are the Ionising Radiation Regulations (IRR 2017) [8] and the Ionising Radiation (Medical Exposure) Regulations (IR(ME)R 2018) [9].

The IRR 2017 deals with the protection of workers and members of the public from ionising radiations from any source. The Approved Code of Practice: 'Work with ionising radiation' [10] supports the legislation. These documents are legally enforceable and breaches of their requirements could lead to prosecution by the regulators, normally the Health and Safety Executive (HSE) [11].

The IR(ME)R 2018 are designed to protect a patient undergoing treatment or diagnosis with ionising radiation; they also cover persons exposed to radiation as part of research and medico-legal procedures, such as preimmigration chest radiographs. These regulations are policed by the Care Quality Commission. A set of amendment regulations were published shortly after the publication of the 2017 regulations in relation to safety measures with regard to radioactive substances and the emission of ionising radiation.

12.7 Radiation Protection Organisations

The International Commission on Radiological Units and Measurements (ICRU) is an international body established in 1925 to ensure consistency in radiation measurement and reporting. The International Commission on Radiological Protection (ICRP) is an international advisory body founded in 1928 to advise on radiation protection issues and form recommendations.

This chapter focuses on the aspects of IRR 2017 that are directly relevant to radiotherapy as well as providing a comprehensive overview of the IR(ME)R 2018. The UK reader is urged to read the regulations in conjunction with this chapter.

12.8 IR(ME)R 2018

12.8.1 Overview

In the IR(ME)R 2018, there is an emphasis on justification of doses and keeping them as low as possible to minimise the chance of stochastic effects. Throughout the regulations, there is reference to 'practical aspects'. This term refers to exposing someone to radiation or any supporting task that is contributing to the delivery of that exposure. It encompasses such diverse tasks as handling of the equipment, identification of the patient, and patient positioning.

12.8.2 Role Definitions

A key aspect of legislation is an understanding of terms and definitions. Within IR(ME)R 2018 there are a number of defined roles that are important, as seen in Table 12.2. In most of the definitions, there is reference to 'the employer's procedures'. These procedures are written by the employer and include:

- Patient identification;
- Identification of referrers, practitioners, and operators;
- Check for female patients' pregnancy status;
- Quality assurance (QA) programmes;
- Assessment of patient doses;

- Provision of patient information and written instructions;
- Dose evaluation;
- Investigation and reporting of clinically significant unintended or accidental exposure;
- Reduction of chance of accidental exposure.

12.8.3 Duties and Responsibilities

A major part of the IR(ME)R 2018 is the clear delineation of duties and responsibilities for each of the roles. The employer, as has already been determined, has to write the procedures listed in Section 12.8.2 and ensure compliance with them. The employer also has to write protocols (or work instructions) and recommendations for QA checks and dose levels. Other responsibilities include staff training and investigation of incidents, with associated notification of authorities.

The practitioner, operator and referrer must all comply with the employer's procedures, highlighting their importance within the IR(ME)R 2018. The practitioner must be able to justify all exposures, whilst the operator is responsible for practical aspects and, depending on the employers' procedures, can authorise exposures under certain conditions. The referrer has the responsibility to provide all relevant medical data in order to prevent repeat exposures being undertaken.

12.8.4 Justification

The IR(ME)R 2018 outline when an exposure can be justified. It is the responsibility of the practitioner to determine if there is sufficient net benefit to the exposure and this is the main source of justification. Authorisation is also dependent on women having been asked if they are pregnant or breastfeeding and on the referrer's medical data having been used. The IR(ME)R 2018 also highlight the importance of keeping doses low. Clearly

TABLE 12.2 IR(ME)R 2018 role definitions.

Role	Definition
Employer	Any person who, in the course of a trade, business, or other undertaking, carries out (other than as an employee), or engages others to carry out, those exposures described in regulation 3 or practical aspects, at a given radiological installation.
Medical physics expert (MPE)	A state-registered clinical scientist with corporate membership of the Institute of Physics and Engineering in Medicine (MIPEM) or equivalent and at least six years of experience in the clinical specialty. An MPE is a legal requirement, they must be full-time contracted to the radiation employer and available at all times for radiotherapy practices. Their roles in radiotherapy are, amongst other things, to provide consultation on the suitability of treatment techniques, with responsibility for the dosimetry and accuracy of treatment, optimization of treatments by ensuring that equipment meets adequate standards of accuracy, and the definitive calibration of radiotherapy equipment and dosimeters.
Operator	Any person who is entitled, in accordance with the employer's procedures, to carry out practical aspects including those to whom practical aspects have been allocated, MPE and, except where they do so under the direct supervision of a person who is adequately trained, persons participating in practical aspects as part of practical training.
Practitioner	A registered healthcare professional who is entitled in accordance with the employer's procedures to take responsibility for an individual exposure.
Referrer	A registered healthcare professional who is entitled in accordance with the employer's procedures to refer individuals for exposure to a practitioner.

radiotherapy doses cannot be low in order to ensure tumour kill, but doses must be planned in order to ensure that normal tissue doses are low. Non-radiotherapy doses arising from simulation or image guidance must be minimised with equipment and methods chosen to assist with this. All doses must be recorded and evaluated, even in the pretreatment area. Another key element of dose minimisation is provision for clinical audit and the IR(ME)R 2018 state that this should be an integral part of practice.

12.8.5 Advice

IR(ME)R 2018 ensure that the medical physics expert (MPE) and other MPEs are available in all departments and are closely involved with all radiotherapy practice. They must be involved to optimise treatments, help with dosimetry and QA, and advise on radiation

protection for medical exposures. They are also charged with providing advice on compliance with regulations in a similar role to the IRR 2017 Radiation Protection Advisor (RPA) (see Section 12.9.4).

12.8.6 Training

IR(ME)R 2018 clarifies that neither practitioners nor operators can carry out medical exposures or practical aspects without adequate training and certification. Provision is made for students to train so long as an adequately trained person supervises them. Employers must keep records of staff training and, when agency staff are employed, the agencies must give their employee records to employers. Schedule 3 of the IR(ME)R 2018 outlines the key knowledge and understanding that should be included in training programmes.

12.9 IRR 2017

12.9.1 Overview

IRR 2017 comprises a more extensive set of legislation than IR(ME)R 2018 because it covers all uses of ionising radiations. They contain sections concerned with arrangements for control of radioactive items and details of how radioactive quantities of different substances are to be stored. Clearly these sections are essential reading for those departments that routinely use sealed or unsealed sources. There are also details of organisational arrangements and procedures, dose limits and personal monitoring, and duties of employers, which need to be applied to all radiotherapy departments.

12.9.2 Registration

There is a new three-tier system of authorisation for work with ionising radiation which has a sliding scale of requirements depending on the risk. This also encompasses different levels of regulatory control and consent from HSE.

12.9.3 Local Rules

A central aspect to IRR 2017 is the requirement of the employer to write local rules using the advice of the RPA (see Section 12.9.4). The purpose of these rules is to inform employees of the correct practices that must be used to minimise exposure. In radiotherapy, the dose to staff is negligible so the purpose of radiotherapy department local rules is to prevent accidental irradiation. Local rules list the relevant radiation protection personnel, detail where radiation protection hazards and protective features are, as well as outline systems of work. There are general rules to be followed everywhere and area-specific rules. General rules ensure that warnings are heeded, dosimeters are worn, and that the patient is alone in the room when radiation is present. Furthermore, the operator must not be distracted, faults must be listed, and the machine must remain supervised when switched on. Area-specific rules describe safety devices and procedures, e.g. the 'closing-up' procedure for ensuring that the patient is alone when the beam is on.

12.9.4 Personnel

Once a controlled or supervised area has been defined, then it is necessary to have written local safety rules, referred to as local rules. These should be drawn up taking into account the findings of the prior risk assessment. These rules must be drawn to the attention of any worker who needs to enter a controlled or supervised area. Amongst other things, they should contain written schemes of work for safe entry into the controlled areas and contingency plans for any foreseeable accident, e.g. radioactive source spillage. They should also contain the name of the RPA, who needs to be appointed by any employer who has set up a controlled area. Their duty is to advise the employer on compliance with the regulatory requirements, assistance in undertaking a prior risk assessment of areas where ionising radiation is to be used, the correct identification of controlled and supervised areas, the prior examination of plans for radiation installations, and the acceptance into service of new or modified sources of ionising radiation. In the Health Service, an RPA is normally an experienced radiation physicist. An RPA is required to have a certificate of competence to act as an RPA, which is issued by an HSE-approved certification body every five years to candidates who can prove they are suitably competent to act as an RPA. In addition, the name of the Radiation Protection Supervisors (RPS) for the area should be included in the local rules. Their responsibility is to supervise that the work with radiation that is being undertaken on a day-to-day basis is in compliance with the local rules. They should also be involved in the preparation of the local rules for the area that they supervise in order to ensure that they are both practical and not prohibitive. To act as an RPS, the person must have received training in a core of knowledge that has been specified by the HSE. They should also be someone in a position of authority and familiar with the work of the area they are supervising. The HSE has also indicated that there should be approximately one RPS for every 20 members of staff working in the radiation areas in order for adequate supervision to be undertaken.

12.9.5 Dose Limits

The annual dose limit has remained largely unchanged for the past 40 years and, despite the new dosimetric evidence, the absolute whole body dose limit per year remains at 50 mSv. However, such a level of dose is only allowable in special circumstances as the dose averaged over a 5-year period and must not exceed 20 mSv year^{-1} for those occupationally exposed and aged over 18 years old. For those employees under 18 years old, the whole body dose limit is 6 mSv year^{-1}. Women of reproductive capacity working with ionising radiation are subjected to a further dose constraint that the equivalent dose to the abdomen shall not exceed 13 mSv in any consecutive calendar quarter.

12.9.6 Area Designation

According to the IRR 2017, employers are responsible for designating areas of their department by radiation risk. 'Controlled areas' are those in which people working there are likely to receive an effective dose greater than 6 mSv a year, which is 3 tenths of the limit for a classified worker. In the radiotherapy department, this includes treatment rooms, mazes, and pretreatment rooms containing simulators or CT scanners. People entering these areas need to follow special procedures in order to restrict their exposure. An example of this is the 'closing-up procedure' to ensure that no one is in the room when there is radiation present. Controlled areas must be described in the local

rules, be obviously demarcated, and highlighted with suitable and sufficient warning signs (Figure 12.2). The only people who can enter a controlled area are *classified people* (those receiving >6 mSv year^{-1}), patients receiving an exposure, Health and Safety Inspectors, and employees following a written system of work (e.g. local rules). Therapy radiographers are not classified employees because they receive minimal dose and are able to enter controlled areas via the latter provision. Entry to a 'supervised area', on the other hand, is less strict, although these need to be constantly under review to check whether they should be controlled or not. People working there are likely to receive an effective dose >1 mSv a year. Examples of these in radiotherapy departments are the control desks and any waiting rooms immediately adjacent to treatment rooms.

References

1. Mould, R.F. (1993). *The Early Years of Radiotherapy with Emphasis on X-ray and Radium Apparatus*. Bristol: Institute of Physics Publishing.
2. Ron, E., Modan, B., and Boice, J.D. (1988). Mortality after radiotherapy for ringworm of the scalp. *Am. J. Epidemiol.* 127: 713–725.
3. Polednak, A.P., Stehney, A.F., and Rowland, R.E. (1978). Mortality among women first employed before 1930 in the US radium dial-painting industry. A group ascertained from employment lists. *Am. J. Epidemiol.* 107: 179–195.
4. Finch, S.C. (2007). Radiation-induced leukaemia: lessons from history. *Best Pract. Res. Clin. Haematol.* 20: 109–118.
5. Allisy-Roberts, P. (ed.) (2002). *Medical and Dental Guidance Notes. A Good Practice Guide on All Aspects of Radiation Protection in the Clinical Environment*. London: Institute of Physics and Engineering in Medicine.
6. Horton, P. (2017). *Design and Shielding of Radiotherapy Treatment Facilities*. London: Report 75, 2e. London: IPEM.
7. Hughes, J.S. (1999). *Ionising Radiations Exposure of the UK Population: 1999 Review*. London: Health Protection Agency.

8. Statutory instrument 1075 (2017). *The Ionising Radiations Regulations 2017*. London: The Stationery Office Limited.

9. Statutory instrument 1332 (2017). *The Ionising Radiations (Medical Exposure) Regulations 2018*. London: The Stationery Office Limited.

10. Work with Ionising Radiations. Approved Code of Practice and Guidance. L121 HSE. 2 March 2018.

11. Health and Safety Executive (2007). *Statistics of Fatal Injuries 2006/07*. London: Health and Safety Executive.

CHAPTER 13

The Use of Radionuclides in Molecular Imaging and Molecular Radiotherapy

Paul Shepherd OBE and Terri Gilleece

Aim

The aim of this chapter is to introduce the fundamental principles and practice of the use of radionuclides in molecular imaging and molecular radiotherapy.

13.1 Introduction

Radionuclides play a dual function in the management of cancer. Radionuclide imaging is used for the diagnosis, staging, and monitoring of cancer, and in radiotherapy or brachytherapy radionuclides have been at the forefront of cancer treatment for decades. A good example is the use of radioactive iodine in both the imaging and the treatment of thyroid cancers.

A therapeutic radiographer is required to have an understanding of the physical principles underpinning and the potential hazards associated with the use of radionuclides in imaging and radiotherapy practice. Radionuclides are localised to the desired tissue by

being chemically attached to, or incorporated into, a compound that is designed to follow a known biodistribution in the body. There are a number of different mechanisms by which this is achieved. The radionuclide and compound together is known as the radiopharmaceutical (RP). By introducing RPs into the body that follow specific physiological pathways whilst emitting radiation, it is possible to detect and map penetrating radiation from outside the body to produce images or to use non-penetrating radiation for therapy. In therapeutic applications the activities administered are much higher than for imaging. In recent years, methodologies have been developed specifically for tumour imaging (molecular imaging) and the targeting of tumours with radionuclides or molecular radiotherapy (MRT). This chapter provides an understanding of the science, technology, and safety relating to radionuclide imaging and in the therapeutic use of radionuclides. These activities bring with them safety and radiation protection challenges as patients who are administered radionuclides become radiation 'sources' (and sometimes leaky ones) for periods of time.

Practical Radiotherapy: Physics and Equipment, Third Edition. Edited by Pam Cherry and Angela M. Duxbury.
© 2020 John Wiley & Sons Ltd. Published 2020 by John Wiley & Sons Ltd.

The regulations and procedures for managing this are also summarised.

13.2 Radionuclides

13.2.1 Radionuclides for Therapy

For therapy, the energy imparted from the ionising radiation should be deposited in the target tissue that is to be destroyed. Depending on the volume of the target tissue, radionuclides with a desired energy/range of particle emissions, beta rays, or occasionally alpha particles, can be selected. The range of particle emissions has to be considered because if they are too small, there may be incomplete irradiation of part of the target volume leading to failure and tumour repopulation. If they are too large, the surrounding normal tissue will be unnecessarily irradiated with consequent damage.

If pure alpha or beta emitters are used, the radiation will not be emitted from the patient's body. This is clearly an advantage in radiation protection terms. If, however, the nuclide also emits gamma rays, it enables simultaneous imaging of the biodistribution.

13.2.2 Radionuclides for Imaging

For imaging, the emissions need to leave the body to be detected. To minimise the patient radiation absorbed dose, ideally nuclides that emit only gamma rays should be used. The radionuclide must decay slowly enough that the activity remaining will still be adequate for imaging when the RP has reached its destination. However, it must be expelled from the body or decay at a rate where it will not expose the patient to radiation for prolonged periods after the imaging study has been completed. The element has to have a chemical affinity for the compounds to which it is to be labelled and it must be nontoxic.

Synthetic isotopes with optimum characteristics for imaging and for various therapies are continually sought and produced. For most imaging purposes, technetium-99 m (^{99m}Tc) is used, which is a pure gamma emitter with 140 keV characteristic energy and a half-life ($t_{1/2}$) of six hours. The 'm' in ^{99m}Tc indicates that this radionuclide is metastable. Metastability can be defined as an excited state of an atom with a measurable half-life or a nucleus that takes time to decay.

13.2.3 Radioactive Decay

Radioactive substances decay at an exponential rate. Despite decaying by different decay schemes, with different emission(s)/particles and varying energies, the decay process always follows the exponential decay pattern. The rate of decay cannot be altered and is not affected by such things as heat, magnetic, or electrical fields. Radioactive isotopes are known as *radioisotopes*. When discussed in relation to nuclear medicine, they are commonly known as *radionuclides*. Radionuclides bound to pharmaceuticals are known as *RPs*.

Radioactive decay is an event originating in the nucleus of the atom, hence it is sometimes described as nuclear decay. The physical half-life of a radioisotope is the time taken for the amount of radioactivity of a substance to reach half its original value. This is a distinctive time for each individual type of radioisotope. Radioactive decay is a random event but the law of averages enables us to determine physical half-lives. This can vary from microseconds to thousands of years depending on the type of radioisotope involved.

Radioactive decay can be calculated using the equation:

$$A = A_0 e^{-\lambda t}$$

where A = amount of radioactivity present at a given/desired time (t), A_0 = initial amount of radioactivity present, or at time zero, t = time, and λ = the transformation (or decay) constant.

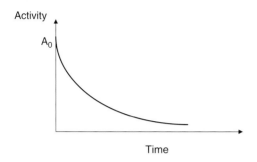

The exponential decay can more conveniently be expressed as the half-life ($t_{1/2}$) which is the time taken for radioactivity to decrease by one half.

Consider an example when t equals the half life of a radionuclide. The amount of radioactivity, A, will equal half of the initial radioactivity A_0. If $A_0 = 1$ then A equals 0.5, therefore $A/A_0 = 0.5/1 = 0.5$.

The equation $A = A_0\ e^{-\lambda t}$ can be transformed to $0.5 = e^{-\lambda t}$. Apply logarithm to the base e to both sides of the equation: $\log_e 0.5 = -\lambda t$ or $-0.693 = -\lambda t$ or $\lambda = 0.693/t$;

t equals the half-life of the radionuclide and by adding this to the modified equation the decay constant for that particular radionuclide can be determined.

The half-life for ^{99m}Tc is six hours or 21 600 seconds. Therefore, the decay constant for ^{99m}Tc = $0.693/21\,600 = 0.000\,032 = 3.2 \times 10^{-5}$ (with units of time in seconds).

Knowing the initial activity in Bq (A_0) it is possible to determine how much activity in Bq (A) will remain after a period of time t in seconds. This enables the therapeutic radiographer to prepare suitable quantities of activity in advance when they can accurately estimate the period of time from preparation of the radionuclide until the time for patient administration.

The transformation constant is the same for all radionuclides with the same physical half-life. The SI unit for measuring radioactivity is the *becquerel* (Bq): 1 becquerel equates to one radioactive disintegration per second.

Doses (activity) used in diagnostic nuclear medicine are usually stated in megabecquerels (MBq), whereas those used for radionuclide therapy, where higher doses are used, can be stated in gigabecquerels (GBq). The non-SI unit used in some countries is the *Curie* (Ci): 1 mCi is equivalent to 37 MBq.

13.2.4 Radionuclide Generator Systems

Logistically, to use radionuclides that have half-lives of less than a day, a local source is necessary. One way of doing this is to keep a supply of one radionuclide (the parent or mother) that decays to another, useful radionuclide (the daughter) in a form in which parent and daughter can be separated. This storage and separation system is called a generator.

Most commonly used nowadays is the molybdenum/technetium (^{99}Mo/^{99m}Tc) generator. The parent is ^{99}Mo, which decays to ^{99m}Tc. The ^{99m}Tc decays in turn to ^{99}Tc which has a half-life of 2.1×10^5 years and can thus be considered effectively stable (Figure 13.1). The generator system allows the technetium to be separated from the molybdenum in radiation and microbial safety (Figures 13.2 and 13.3). As the daughter radionuclide is to be administered to patients, it is essential that the entire internal generator system is a sterile environment.

The ^{99}Mo, as ammonium molybdate $(NH_4)^+(MoO_4)^-$, is adsorbed onto an alumina column on which the ^{99m}Tc is formed as ^{99m}TcO$_4$ and which can then be removed by ion exchange. When physiological saline (0.9% saline) is passed through the column, a process known as elution, the chloride ions exchange with the TcO$_4$ but not the MoO$_4$ ions as these are more tightly bound to the column and a solution of sodium pertechnetate Na$^+$TcO$_4^-$ is produced and known as the eluate. The saline can be pushed or pulled over the column in either a positive or negative pressure system. Negative pressure is

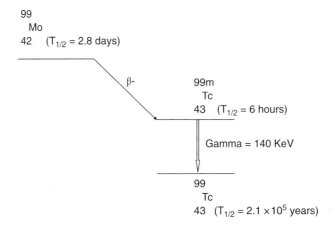

FIGURE 13.1 Simplified decay scheme for ⁹⁹Mo showing production of ⁹⁹ᵐTc and associated decays.

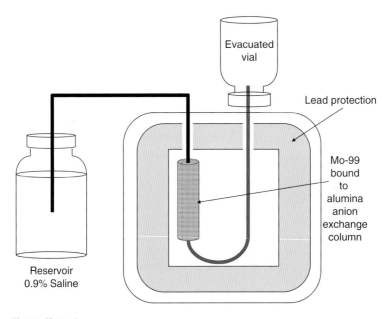

FIGURE 13.2 ⁹⁹ᵐMo/⁹⁹ᵐTc dry generator system.

safer for radiation spill but may draw in bacteria so microbial filters are included. Generators can be supplied as dry generators with the requirement to connect saline on site (Figure 13.2) or as wet generators with saline reservoirs already sealed inside (Figure 13.3).

After elution there is very little ⁹⁹ᵐTc left on the column and this needs time to build up again before the process can be repeated. The maximum individual yield from a column is obtained 23 hours after the last elution, after which time the rate of decay matches that of

buildup and the level does not increase but decreases with the decay rate of the parent radionuclide (Figure 13.4). Generators can be eluted more frequently, yielding less activity each time but providing more activity in total over the course of a day. The amount of activity obtained depends on the time since the previous elution, the size of generator delivered (the original activity of the parent), and the age of the generator (how long it has been in the department). ⁹⁹Mo/⁹⁹ᵐTc generators are replaced weekly.

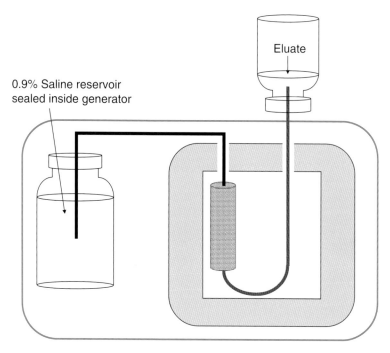

FIGURE 13.3 ^{99m}Mo/^{99m}Tc wet generator system.

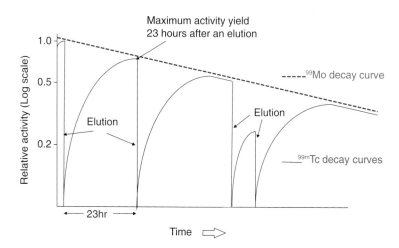

FIGURE 13.4 Decay curve for molybdenum-99 and ingrowth curves for technetium-99m.

Before patient use, the eluate undergoes several quality control checks, either on a daily or a weekly basis. These include checks for ^{99}Mo and aluminium breakthrough into the eluate, as well as radiochemical purity and sterility.

Departments buy the minimum-size generator possible for their activity needs, not just for financial reasons but also to reduce the amount of activity they are storing and to minimise the risk of radiation exposure to operators. Germanium-68/gallium-68 (^{68}Ge–^{68}Ga) and strontium-82/rubidium-82 (^{82}Sr–^{82}Rb) generators are also available to generate radionuclides for use in positron emission tomography (PET).

Furthermore, radionuclides less commonly used in nuclear medicine can be obtained from other sources. Iodine-131 (^{131}I), used mainly for therapeutic applications, can be obtained from nuclear reactors. ^{131}I is a superfluous by-product of common fission reactions and as a result is usually inexpensive to obtain. Other radionuclides, including indium-111 (^{111}In) and gallium-67 (^{67}Ga), are cyclotron produced. Cyclotron-produced radionuclides are relatively expensive to purchase compared with other radionuclides.

13.3 Imaging Equipment

13.3.1 The Gamma Camera

After the administration of a RP, the radioactivity circulates within the patient in a distribution corresponding to a physiological process. This is mapped into an image using a gamma camera. Although there are several producers of gamma cameras internationally, the components and construction of the gamma camera are essentially the same. The following is an outline description of the design of the gamma camera.

The collimator is used to select the desired rays for use in the image. Gamma rays are emitted from a patient in all directions. When they are detected in the crystal there is, therefore, no way of knowing where they came from and so the distribution cannot be mapped. It is necessary to confine the rays reaching the camera face to those perpendicular to it, thus producing a 1 : 1 map of the distribution in the body. As can be seen in Figure 13.5, this is done by cutting out as many of the other rays as possible by absorbing them in lead. To do this, a collimator or lead block is interposed between the patient and crystal; this collimator contains a honeycomb of equally sized and spaced holes, the size, spacing, and thickness of the block differing according to use. Collimators are interchangeable on a given camera and different ones are used for different characteristic energies,

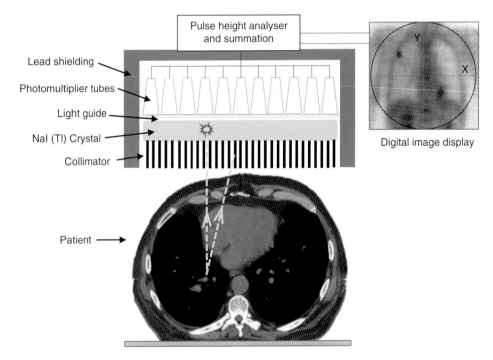

FIGURE 13.5 Schematic diagram of the gamma camera demonstrating the collimation of gamma rays emitted from the patient.

different fineness of detail or *resolution* (better resolution can be gained only at the expense of the images taking significantly longer), and sometimes to manipulate the shape of an image.

The crystal is located directly behind the collimator. It is made of sodium iodide (NaI) into which impurities of thallium (Tl) have been introduced. This material will *scintillate* or give off flashes of light when a gamma photon imparts its energy into it. Crystals are fragile and the camera has to be handled with extreme care, especially when the collimator is being changed because the crystal is particularly vulnerable to mechanical damage. The crystal is also highly sensitive to moisture (hygroscopic) and light, and for protection is encapsulated in a thin aluminium cover.

Once the *gamma photon* enters the crystal, its energy is transformed into a shower of light photons by a process in which electrons excited by the gamma ray are liberated from the valence band and move into a higher-energy level band and a 'hole' created in the forbidden gap by the atoms of the impurity, thallium. Their excess energy is emitted as flashes (or photons) of light or a scintillation. The number of light photons released is proportional to the energy deposited. All the energy of the gamma ray must be used up in this process to make the system work. This usually happens as a result of Compton scatter events in which kinetic energy is lost and is followed by a photoelectric interaction. These interactions occur within a very small distance so that they can be considered as happening at one point on the camera face. Light close to the crystal edges is reflected from the sides of the aluminium casing, allowing it to be included. Some photons pass straight through the crystal and are not detected. For any given crystal substance, the efficiency (proportion of the activity detected) depends on the thickness of that crystal and the energy of the incident ray.

Each gamma event is processed separately but as the luminescence decay is in the order of nanoseconds, the camera is ready to process the next incoming photon so rapidly

that count rates up to $10^4 s^{-1}$ can be handled. The time that it takes the camera to generate and process a reading from a single photon interaction is known as dead-time (the camera cannot detect any further gamma events during this time). This is usually only a problem with very high count rate studies and rarely occurs.

The light is directed to the next stage, the photomultiplier tubes (PMTs), by a light guide. This is made of Plexiglass and optically couples the crystal to the front face of the *PMTs* (Figure 13.5). The light flashes are detected by the PMTs adjacent to it, which ultimately turn that flash into a detectable current by converting light energy to usable electrical energy. The light guide diffuses the light around it to increase the number of PMTs involved in detecting light and improves positioning efficiency. The number of PMTs per camera head varies for different manufacturers and camera head dimensions.

Inside an evacuated glass tube the PMT contains the *photocathode*, which is made of caesium antimonide. Light energy ejects a few electrons from this material in a manner analogous to the photoelectric effect (Figure 13.6). When it receives a flash of light from the crystal, the number of electrons ejected is still proportional to the incident light and hence the energy of the photon.

Inside the tube are a number of *dynodes* or metal plates also coated with caesium antimonide and positively charged because there is an applied voltage between cathode and each successive dynode of about 200 V. This causes an electron to be accelerated towards the dynode. When it strikes the dynode, a secondary emission occurs, i.e. several electrons are ejected for each one that impinges. This happens at each succeeding dynode thus multiplying the number of electrons at each stage. If there are 10 dynodes the current will be increased by 10^6. This is a respectable current and the proportionality of this current to the characteristic energy of the photon is maintained.

These bursts of current are converted into voltage pulses and shaped in the preamplifier. They all need to be multiplied by the same

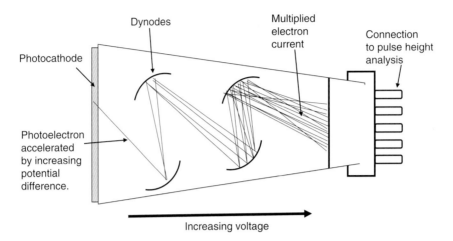

FIGURE 13.6 Photomultiplier tube (PMT).

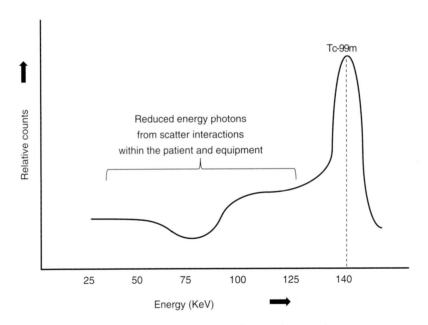

FIGURE 13.7 Spectrum for Technetium-99m emanating from within a patient.

factor before sorting and positioning. The amplifier converts millivolts to tens of volts.

Pulses from a gamma event arriving at the end of the amplifier part of the circuit are then examined in two ways. *Pulse height analysis* and summation circuitry are used to select and position the events into an image. Only those gamma rays that had the original characteristic energy need to be recorded in the image. Figure 13.7 illustrates the spectrum of energies detected from 99mTc gamma rays emanating from within a patient and

detected using a gamma camera with a collimator in place. Only photons with energies close to 140 keV need to be processed. Pulses corresponding to other energies are from either scattered rays or electronic noise and are not required. Before a pulse is accepted as part of the image, the total amount of current from all PMTs is summated and passed to the *pulse height analyser* (PHA).

The system is not perfect and there is a small variation in amplifications in the pulses, so a range of voltages corresponding to energies about 10% above and below the characteristic energy are likely to correspond to genuine events. Thus, only pulses corresponding to energies between these preset levels should be accepted for further processing. The PHA looks at the size of the incoming pulse and compares it with the *lower level discriminator* and rejects it if it falls below that level. It then compares it with the *upper level discriminator* and again rejects it if it is greater.

To detect the position of the original photon, the strengths of the signals from the various PMTs are compared in the summation circuitry, e.g. if the light flash happens on the right side of the field, the signals from the combined PMTs on the right will be larger than those on the left. The difference in signal size will give a measure of how far to the right of the midline the event occurred. This procedure is repeated for each event accepted for left and right (or X) coordinates and top and bottom (or Y) coordinates. This positions the flash of light onto a cathode ray tube or in a computer matrix, which then forms the final image. The forming image can usually also be seen on a persistence scope so that the position can be adjusted before the image acquisition is started.

The signals are digitised in an *analogue digital converter* and assigned to a certain *pixel* (short for picture cell) in a computer matrix. The memory in this pixel then increases by one unit so that a distribution of numbers in different cells is collected over the period of the acquisition; these numbers can be translated into intensities on a screen. This can be viewed directly and stored digitally for future display and manipulations. In the past, the images were recorded on film, but are now stored digitally on acquisition stations and on systems such as PACS (picture archiving and communications system). As the information now consists of a series of numbers in a matrix it can be manipulated and different areas numerically compared, e.g. left and right kidney uptakes. This is called *quantitation* and allows for numbers equating to physiological function to be obtained as well as images.

13.4 Single Photon Emission Computed Tomography (SPECT)

Just as computed tomography (CT) added an extra dimension to conventional planar radiography, single photon emission computed tomography (SPECT) uses analogous techniques and reconstruction algorithms to extend the usefulness of radionuclide imaging and produce cross-sectional images of the distribution of a RP in the body.

There are several advantages to SPECT. Similar to all tomography it removes overlying structures from the image and also gives more information on the position of a structure. It can determine size and more importantly, volume, which allows for quantification, and it can reduce the effects of attenuation. These advantages can be very important for relative uptake measurements.

The gamma camera gantry needs to be structured to be capable of rotating around the patient and acquiring data at varying angles over 360°. Increasing the number of camera heads used simultaneously increases the amount of information collected in a given time. Cameras with two camera heads (Figure 13.8) are most common, but other multiple-head configurations are possible. Heads can be set in various positions depending on what body area is being imaged and how much information is required.

13.5 Positron Emission Tomography (PET)

13.5.1 PET Imaging

PET is based on similar principles to general nuclear medicine scanning. The main differences are in the type of radionuclide used and the image acquisition equipment.

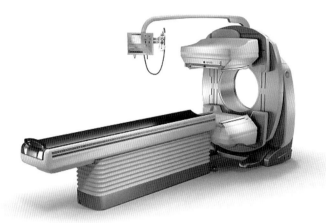

FIGURE 13.8 A multi-headed gamma camera. Source: NM 830 – Image courtesy of GE Healthcare.

Positrons are emitted from a nucleus that has too many protons. A proton will decay to a neutron with the emission of a positron and a neutrino. The positron travels only a very short distance before combining with an electron. An annihilation event occurs at this time with the creation of two 511 keV gamma photons travelling at 180° to each other (Figure 13.9). It is these photons that are detected as they interact with the crystal of the detector. The gamma ray photons in PET are always of 511 keV, much higher energy than most radioisotopes used with gamma cameras. Therefore, the scintillation crystals must have a much higher stopping power than sodium iodide. The crystals most often employed are either bismuth germanium oxide (BGO), gadolinium orthosilicate (GSO) or lutetium orthosilicate (LSO).

PET scanners are composed of a ring of detectors within which the patient is positioned (Figure 13.9). Rather than register the gamma photons as two separate events, the PET machine registers them as a paired or coincidence event. It does this through the establishment of time windows. If two gamma photons are detected within the same time window (typically 12 ns), the camera records them as coming from the same annihilation event. This is known as electronic collimation. As the gamma photons travel at 180° to each other, the computer draws a line of flight between the two events and determines that the annihilation

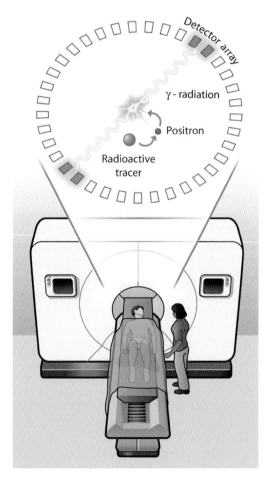

FIGURE 13.9 PET camera detector array and diagram of annihilation event after positron emission (top). Source: Image by Jiang Long, Science Creative Quarterly, is licenced under CC BY-NC-SA 2.5.

must have occurred along this line. This type of acquisition is not faultless and some errors do occur, especially at high count rates, resulting in noise and background in the image.

13.6 Hybrid Imaging Systems

Images acquired using both gamma cameras and PET scanners provide excellent functional information. However, differentiating anatomical detail on either type of scan can be challenging and coupled with issues linked to attenuation and scatter of gamma rays in surrounding organs, hybrid imaging has been introduced as a means of improving accuracy of diagnosis. Increases in sensitivity and specificity have been achieved by combining anatomically useful diagnostic imaging modalities with nuclear medicine instrumentation. Most centres now have SPECT-CT cameras and stand-alone PET scanners are no longer in manufacture.

13.6.1 SPECT-CT

The combination of a gamma camera with a CT scanner has two benefits. The CT images allow the application of non-uniform attenuation correction to the nuclear medicine image, therefore helping to compensate for patient variables such as obesity and giving a more accurate representation of radionuclide distribution. CT also assists with accurate localisation of RP within organs. This can be important for, amongst other things, differentiating localised from extracapsular tumour spread – thus providing functional (nuclear medicine) and structural (CT) information.

Initially the CT component of such machines was generally considered non-diagnostic. Now manufacturers are producing hybrid machines with truly diagnostic CT components so that patients can potentially undergo their molecular imaging study and diagnostic CT study in one appointment (Figure 13.10).

13.6.2 PET-CT

The addition of CT has provided the benefits of attenuation correction and coregistration of functional and structural elements in PET imaging. The CT component has increasingly become diagnostic which offers the possibility of combining PET, CT, and planning for radiotherapy into a single appointment and therefore has the potential to speed up the process between diagnosis and treatment.

Although the development of PET-CT heralded great improvements in molecular imaging it is not without limitations. Whilst the patient is imaged by both PET and CT on the same couch/in the same position, both sets of images are acquired sequentially rather than simultaneously and differences

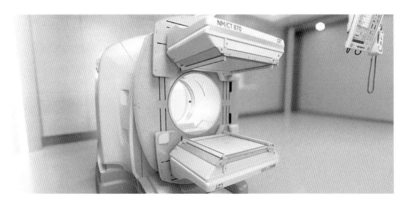

FIGURE 13.10 NM/CT 870 CZT single photon emission computed tomography/computed tomography (SPECT-CT) system. Source: Image courtesy of GE Healthcare.

associated with breathing and peristalsis in the PET scan compared to CT must be considered. The additional radiation dose imparted by addition of the CT must also be justified.

13.6.3 PET-MRI

Magnetic resonance imaging (MRI) is superior to CT for some applications; it offers better soft-tissue contrast and functional imaging capabilities with functional magnetic resonance imaging (fMRI). It also has the advantage of utilising non-ionising radiation. A PET-MRI system (Figures 13.11 and 13.12) offers the ability to acquire PET and MRI images simultaneously, unlike PET-CT, partly because of the similar independent imaging times [1, 2]. But MRI poses significant challenges when attempting to develop hybrid combinations either in molecular imaging or external-beam radiotherapy (EBRT)

(a)

(b)

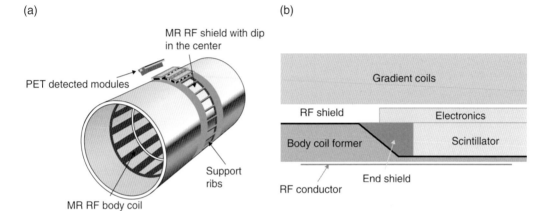

FIGURE 13.11 (a) Schematic of prototype of the GE SIGNA™ PET/MR. (b) Arrangement of RF conductor of the body coil, RF shield, and PET detector so that attenuation of PET data by the body coil is minimised. Source: Image courtesy of GE Healthcare.

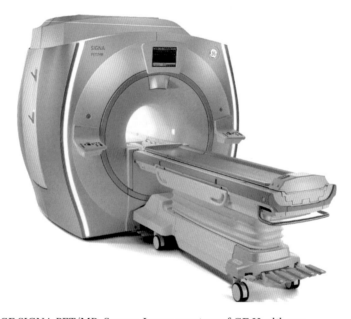

FIGURE 13.12 GE SIGNA PET/MR. Source: Image courtesy of GE Healthcare.

equipment because of the magnetic field. Manufacturers have overcome these issues in part with the development of solid-state photo detectors to replace the PMTs. Consideration must be given to attenuation in PET-MRI due to the hardware and the MRI coils within and close to the field of view which degrades the PET image. MR-based attenuation correction (MRAC) or PET-based attenuation correction can be utilised. The process of combining PET RPs with magnetic resonance (MR) (where ^{18}F-FDG is tagged with Gd-DTPA) allows visualisation of the perfusion of tissues alongside molecular information of the metabolism of those tissues. Thus the future of PET/MRI as an imaging modality looks promising.

13.6.4 SPECT-MR

Work is ongoing to develop a clinical SPECT-MRI system [3].The main work is being undertaken as part of the Integrated SPECT-MR for Enhanced stratification in Radio-chemo Therapy (INSERT) project. The biggest problem is the collimators that are used in SPECT systems (an issue which didn't present itself with PET-MRI systems). Currently a miniature preclinical system has been developed, but this utilises a pinhole collimator with magnification which is suitable for small objects only. It is envisaged that the main application for SPECT-MRI will be with brain imaging but some opponents refute the clinical need for a simultaneous SPECT-MRI.

13.7 Radiopharmaceuticals

13.7.1 For Gamma Camera/ SPECT Imaging

The most widely used radioisotope is the metastable form of technetium; ^{99m}Tc. As stated in previous sections it is a pure gamma emitter with a photon energy of 140 keV. It is widely available and economically viable. It is easily tagged to numerous compounds to allow imaging of a variety of target tissues and organs within the body. When the radioactive isotopes have been 'tagged' with pharmaceuticals they will concentrate in specific organs within the body, e.g. phosphonates such as HDP (hydroxymethlyene diphosphonate) will take ^{99m}Tc to bony tissues, DMSA (dimercaptosuccinic acid) will take the ^{99m}Tc to the kidneys. It should be noted that the pharmaceutical is only added in trace amounts and is considered sub-pharmacological – it has no action and does not change the physiological processes within the body in any way.

Other RPs can also be used with standard gamma camera/SPECT systems but if they produce higher-energy gamma rays, special collimators which contain thick lead septa will be required to prevent scatter radiation from interacting with the crystal of the camera, e.g. ^{68}gallium citrate or ^{111}indium.

13.7.2 For PET

The production of radioisotopes for PET imaging requires a cyclotron. When combined with or 'tagged' to trace amounts of substances naturally taken up by the human body they become useful for accurately showing natural biodistribution within the body. They are usually short-lived radionuclides (short physical half-lives) ranging from seconds to minutes. As a result, departments need to be close to the supplying cyclotron, or use a suitable generator that is stored in the department.

The most widely used radiotracer for PET purposes is ^{18}F-Fluorodeoxyglucose (^{18}F-FDG). It is particularly useful for oncology applications as it is an analogue of glucose that is required as an energy source for the mitotic cancer cells, which divide more rapidly than normal cells. Unlike normal glucose the radioactive FDG is trapped within the cells. ^{18}F-FDG has been used for cancer detection, staging, planning, therapy monitoring, and restaging. However, being an analogue of glucose, ^{18}F-FDG is not a specific radiotracer for malignancies and can demonstrate increased uptake in sites of inflammation/ infection and active muscle contraction. Malignancies with low glucose metabolism such as neuroendocrine tumours, mucinous tumours, differentiated teratomas, many prostate carcinomas, lobular breast cancer, some renal and hepatocellular carcinomas, and most bronchioloalveolar carcinomas have relatively poor FDG uptake. For these reasons additional PET imaging agents (Table 13.1) have been developed.

13.7.3 For PET-MRI

MRI can image specific nuclei; ^{1}H, ^{19}F, ^{23}N, ^{31}P. The signal of these nuclei is sensitive to their microenvironment, allowing detection of changes and related metabolic information from the molecules that contain them. MRI images can be further enhanced using contrast agents. By utilising MRI contrast agents along with, or combined with PET RPs, the advantages of both modalities can be synergistically combined (bimodal agents). The most

TABLE 13.1 Positron emission tomography (PET) imaging agents.

Biochemical/ biological process	Radiopharmaceutical (RP)	Acronym
Proliferation	Carbon-11-thymidine	^{11}C-Thy
	Fluorine-18-fluorodeoxythymidine	^{18}F-FLT
Amino-acid transport	Carbon-11-methionine	^{11}C-MET
	Fluorine-18-fluoroethyltyrosine,	^{18}F-FET
	Fluorine-18-fluorometilthyltyrosine	^{18}F-FMT
Hypoxia	Fluorine-18-fluoromisonidazole	^{18}F-FMISO
	Fluorine-18-fluoroetanidazole	^{18}F-FETA
	Fluorine-18-fluoronitroimidazole	^{18}F-FETNIM
	Fluorine-18-fluoroazomycin-aribinoside	^{18}F-FAZA
	Copper-60- diacetylmethylthio-semicarbazone	^{60}Cu-ATSM
	Copper-62-diacetylmethylthio-semicarbazone	^{62}Cu-ATSM
	Copper-64- diacetylmethylthio-semicarbazone	^{64}Cu-ATSM
Receptors	Fluorine-18-octreotide analogues	^{18}F-DOTATOC
		^{18}F-DOTANOC
		^{18}F-DOTATATE
	Gallium-68-octreotide analogues	^{68}Ga-DOTATOC
		^{68}Ga-DOTANOC
		^{68}Ga-DOTATATE
	Fluorine-18-fluoroestradiol	^{18}F-FES
	Fluorine-18-galacto-RGD(Arg-Gly-Asp	^{18}F-galactoRGD
Dopamine metabolism	Fluorine-18-fluorodihydroxyphenylalanine	^{18}F-FDOPA
Lipid and fatty acid metabolism	Carbon-11-choline	^{11}C-CH
	Fluorine-18-fluorocholine	^{18}F-FCH
	Carbon-11-acetate	^{11}C-acetate
	Fluorine-18-fluoroacetate	^{18}F-acetate

common approach is to add a radioactive isotope to the surface of a small superparamagnetic iron oxide (SPIO) particle. Oncology is the most promising field for these new contrast agents with the detection of sentinel lymph nodes and the targeting of tumour neoangiogenesis. Future prospects include the use of specific antibodies and hybrid multimodal PET-MRI-ultrasound-fluorescence imaging with the potential to provide overall pre-, intra-, and postoperative patient care.

13.8 Tumour (Molecular) Imaging and Molecular Radiotherapy (MRT)

A considerable application of nuclear medicine is in oncology and in radionuclide therapy. Several RPs are used for this purpose. The most recent developments have involved the use of theranostics, receptor, and antibody imaging.

13.8.1 Theranostics

One of the most recent advances in medicine has been in the field of nanotechnologies [4]. Nanoparticles are materials with at least one dimension below 100 nm. Some of these substances allow the combination of imaging and therapeutic agents in a single material. Gadolinium has been used as a contrast agent in MRI for many years but it has a future in the development of gadolinium-based nanoparticles. These nanoparticles of gadolinium focus in the areas of disease for imaging using MRI scanning (diagnostic) but are combined with other therapeutic agents to deliver drugs or radiotherapy (therapeutic) producing a 'theranostic' (combined therapeutic and diagnostic) application. They produce a radiosensitising effect. Gold nanoparticles have previously been shown to be useful in

increasing the effects of EBRT but the gadolinium nanoparticles serve the dual purpose of acting as a contrast agent for MRI and increasing the effectiveness of the EBRT. Given the development of MRI/LinAcs, this could be an important step for radiotherapy.

13.8.2 Radiolabelled Receptors

A receptor is a molecule of integral protein in the cell membrane that can identify and attach to a specific molecule, such as a hormone or neurotransmitter, which has some function of that cell. A molecule that specifically binds to a receptor in this way is called a *ligand* for that receptor. When a receptor and ligand interact they can either inhibit or stimulate cell function. Hormone-dependent tumours have receptor sites typical of the tissue from which the tumour arose and sometimes to a greater degree than the normal tissue.

The ligand, or a biological analogue that does not cause cell activity, may be included in the molecule of the RP. The radionuclide labelling the ligand has to have a half-life suitable for the accumulation and clearance rates of the individual ligand on the receptors. When injected into a patient the ligands will attach to the receptors and the distribution of radioactivity follows that of the receptor density. Increased density implies the presence of tumour tissue. The same technique can potentially be used with suitable radionuclides to target and destroy tumour cells.

One example of receptor imaging is the study of neuroendocrine tumours. Potentially three different RPs may be used for this purpose: ^{111}In-labelled octreotide, ^{123}I-labelled mIBG (*meta*-iodobenzylguanidine), and ^{99m}Tc-labelled depreotide. Neuroendocrine tumours vary in the type of receptors present in their cells and therefore the degree of uptake of each of these RPs will vary. Two patients with the same type of neuroendocrine tumour may show different biodistribution for each of these RPs. By replacing the radionuclide attached to each pharmaceutical with beta-emitting radionuclides, these RPs can then also be used for therapeutic purposes; the avidity of the tumour for each RP will help determine which radionuclide therapy treatment to administer. If different RPs demonstrate different tumour biodistribution in the same patient, the patient may receive two different radionuclide treatment types. This is more common with octreotide- and mIBG-avid tumours.

Repeat treatments can also be administered if needed. This is especially important for tumour location or spread that cannot be dealt with surgically or by other means, particularly for those patients with widespread metastases.

13.8.3 Radiolabelled Antibodies

A similar methodology uses the body's own immune system. An antibody is a protein produced by the lymphocytes in response to the presence of a foreign substance or antigen. Many antibodies may be produced in response to one antigen but each lymphocyte produces a single type of antibody. Antigens may be expressed on the walls of tumour cells and may be tumour specific or (more usually) typical of the tissue from which the tumour arose. When antibodies that attach to these antigens are radiolabelled and injected into a patient, their accumulation can be imaged. When labelled with a beta-emitting radionuclide, the use of radionuclide therapy also becomes possible [5].

Monoclonal antibodies are produced by the hybridoma technique and are usually murine (mouse) derived. A mouse is injected with the relevant antigen for the tumour being sought. Specific B lymphocytes are then taken from the animal's spleen or lymphoid tissue and manipulated, isolated, and radiolabelled. Hundreds of different antibodies have been produced in this way and are identified by letters and numbers but not all are suitable for radiolabelling. Antibody fragments and subfragments, as well as full antibodies, are used for radiolabelling. These may be labelled with ^{99m}Tc and ^{111}In (which has a longer half-life of 2.8 days and thus enables imaging over longer periods of time to allow the antibodies

to accrue onto the tumour) and for therapeutic purposes ^{131}I (iodine: half-life 8.1 days) and yttrium-90 (^{90}Y). When used as a therapy agent, this approach is known as radioimmunotherapy. Current research is also looking at the possibility of radiolabelling antibodies with alpha particle-emitting radionuclides as therapy agents.

Zevalin is one example of a monoclonal antibody that has been developed specifically to treat refractory B-cell non-Hodgkin's lymphoma. Zevalin is taken up at the CD20 receptor of normal and cancerous lymph cells. When labelled with ^{111}In, a diagnostic image can be acquired showing biodistribution of the RP. For therapeutic purposes, Zevalin may be labelled with ^{90}Y. As ^{90}Y is a pure beta emitter and excretion rates of this RP are low, these patients are often treated on an outpatient basis. It is administered together with the drug rituximab to increase its efficacy. Unfortunately, the relatively high cost of this treatment has meant that it is currently underused, despite the fact that very good partial and complete response rates show it is an effective tool in fighting this disease.

Another, lesser-used approach is to administer a radiolabelled antibody before sending the patient for surgery to remove the tumour. A small probe detector system can be used to identify affected lymph nodes during the operation. By monitoring but not imaging radiation the surgeon can check directly if all tumour tissue has been removed from the area and adjacent nodes.

13.9 Radiation Protection Related to Radioactive Substances

European Directive 2013/59/Euratom in Dec 2013 required changes to UK legislation in relation to the Ionising Radiation Regulations (IRR) and Ionising Radiation Medical

Exposure Regulations (IR[ME]R). These changes will be unaffected by the UK's departure from the European Union.

IRR 2017 [6] and IR(ME)R 2017 [7] replace a number of previous pieces of UK legislation; IRR99, IR(ME)R 2000, and Medicines (Administration of Radioactive Substances) Regulations (MARS), which have now been revoked.

Two licences are now required for the administration of radioactive substances. Each department within the UK must hold a licence listing the RPs permitted in that department alongside the purpose for which they may be administered. Each practitioner who administers the RPs must also hold a licence; the facility licence and the individual's licence must match. The Administration of Radioactive Substances Committee (ARSAC) who previously issued certificates now take on an advisory role and licences are issued by Public Health England and corresponding authorities in the other regions of the UK.

In both molecular imaging and MRT, potential hazards can arise from preparation of RPs, administration to patients, radiation emitted from the patients, disposal of medicinal waste products, and from radioactive excreta. Radiation protection must therefore be applied for the safety of patients, staff, and the environment.

13.9.1 Patient Safety

The administration of RPs results in patients becoming a radiation source. This should not cause significant problems since the doses are always administered in line with the ALARP (As Low As Reasonably Practicable) principle in accordance with IR(ME)R 2017. Local Rules within departments will dictate the protocols for each trust but generally patients undergoing imaging procedures should be advised to avoid unnecessary contact with pregnant women and young children for 24 hours (longer for imaging with ^{111}In or ^{68}Ga). In addition to checking pregnancy status before injecting RPs, patients should also be asked whether they are breastfeeding since the radioactive tracers will pass into the breast milk. Clinicians will always justify the use of RPs in any patient but this is even more important for patients who are pregnant or breastfeeding. There are times where imaging is in the patient's best interest, but the doses administered will be reduced to the minimum possible by increasing scanning time to achieve a useful number of counts. If the patient is breastfeeding she will be advised to express and dispose of the milk for at least 24 hours after injection (the time will be increased for longer half-life radioisotopes). If babies or children are being imaged the parents must be given adequate information, particularly in relation to nappies and bodily fluids to ensure the dose to them and other members of the family are minimised.

Hospital inpatients will follow procedures dictated by the Radiation Protection Adviser (RPA) as laid out in the Local Rules. The ward staff will be informed of the patient's status and this will ensure that pregnant staff will not work with such patients. The patient's urine, faeces, and incontinence products are afforded special considerations as dictated by the RP half-life and dose administered to the patient.

13.9.2 Staff and Public

The three main principles of radiation protection for staff working with unsealed radioactive sources are:

1. Distance: keep as far away from sources (including patients) as possible – remember the inverse square law!
2. Time: reduce the handling time with injections, prepare everything in advance, give patients instructions, and answer questions in advance of administering RPs.
3. Shielding: use syringe shields, lead glass screens, shielded sharps disposal containers.

There are defined dose limits for staff and public who come into contact with radioactivity which have been reviewed in IRR 2017 and IR(ME)R 2017. The limits are shown in Table 13.2.

TABLE 13.2	Annual dose limits (IRR 2017 [6]).	
	Workers (mSv)	**Public (mSv)**
Skin (1cm²)	500	50
Extremities	500	50
Whole body	20	1
Lens of eye	20	15

13.9.3 Pregnant Staff

Staff who are pregnant should declare their pregnancy to their employer as soon as they are aware of their condition. Employers MUST then adjust duties to ensure that the foetus receives a dose of not more than 1 mSv during the declared term of the pregnancy. Staff are also assumed to be breastfeeding for six months after giving birth and again the employer must alter duties to limit the possibility of contamination through breast milk. If staff wish to continue to breastfeed beyond this time the employer should be advised and the same arrangements will continue.

13.9.4 Molecular Radiotherapy (MRT)

The amount of activity administered to patients undergoing MRT is significantly higher than that administered for imaging purposes but many therapeutic procedures involve only β particles and so the patient only needs to give attention to urine contamination to ensure the safety of others. The administration of treatment doses of gamma emitters poses a risk to patients, staff, and the public.

To safeguard the public (family, carers, work colleagues), restrictions will be placed upon the patient and hospitalisation will be required until radioactivity has decayed sufficiently or been excreted [8]. This will be assessed by measuring the effective dose at a distance of 1 m from any point in the patient's body to estimate the residual activity.

Restrictions for inpatients:

- Patient rooms: these should be specially designated and preferably single.
- Patient movements: these must be confined to the room/suite and rooms should be left only with permission from the RPA and with a suitably knowledgeable expert.
- Beds: these should be marked with radiation warning signs.
- Walls and floors: these must be easily cleaned.
- Bathroom and toilet: these should be exclusive or the patient should have exclusive use of bottles or bedpans. Disposable items are preferable.
- Crockery and cutlery: these should be separated from other utensils and the patient should wash these up if disposable items are not available.
- Waste and soiled linen storage: these should be segregated in little-used areas.
- Contaminated bedding or personal clothing: these should be changed as soon as possible and the affected bedding/clothing segregated in little-used areas.
- Protective clothing: staff should use gloves and aprons at all times.
- Contact time for nursing staff and visitors: this varies with radionuclide and activity and is determined individually by radiation protection staff. It should, in any case, be the minimum consistent with proper nursing care. Non-urgent nursing procedures should be postponed until the levels drop.
- Pregnant staff: should be allocated other duties wherever possible.

When patients travel home or move between hospitals, rules still apply. If they are transferred, information on levels of activity must go with them. There are four categories of activity levels that determine the allowable means of transport and restrictions on their activities (Table 13.3). An instruction card stating restrictions and the times for which

TABLE 13.3 Restrictions on high-activity patients leaving hospital by category.

Category	Effective Dose Rate μSv/hour	Estimated Remaining Activity MBq	Restrictions
1	< 3	< 10	Safe to leave hospital; No restrictions
2	3–5	10–50	Avoid prolonged contact with children and radiosensitive work
3	5–10	50–150	Do not return to work if close contact is involved; Avoid close contact generally, e.g. places of entertainment
4	10–20	150–300	Do not return to work; Do not use public transport
5	>20	>400	Cannot leave hospital

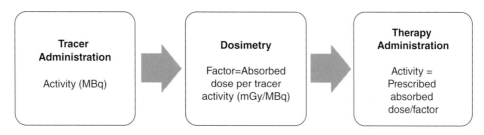

FIGURE 13.13 Flow diagram for planning absorbed dose in molecular radiotherapy (MRT) treatment.

they apply have to be issued where indicated. There are also procedures for patients dying with high levels of radioactivity in them in order to protect the public.

13.10 Dosimetry

In EBRT and brachytherapy, radiation will be prescribed in terms of absorbed dose delivered to target tissues and organs at risk. In MRT (also referred to as unsealed source or radionuclide therapy) the source is diffuse since the RP is administered systemically and circulates around the patient's body. The amount of RP that is concentrated over time in different organs will vary between patients depending on their individual metabolism; the effects of MRT are governed by the absorbed activity rather than the administered activity (see Figure 13.13).

The treatment team must therefore consider the specific properties; path through the body, how long it remains in the body; biological half-life, ($T_{1/2bio}$), and the physical half-life ($T_{1/2phys}$) of the radioisotope (how long it takes to decay), as well as the type of radiation emitted and the energy of the emissions. We must also consider that as the radioactivity moves into each organ that organ becomes another radioactive source, e.g. if the RP passes through the liver on its way to the kidneys the liver will both receive a dose of radiation and emit radiation to surrounding tissues, even though that is not the target organ. As with EBRT, we must consider the maximum dose for organs containing normal tissue, critical organs which will absorb radiation from both the administered dose and the surrounding organs.

In addition to the considerations already mentioned, the type of decay process plays a large part in calculating internal radiation

TABLE 13.4 Decay processes/radiation weighting factors and organ/tissue weighting factors.

Decay Process	Radiation weighting factor (W_R)	Organ	Tissue weighting factor (W_T)
alpha particles	20	Bone marrow, colon, lung, stomach, breast, remainder tissues	0.12 (each organ)
beta particles	1	Gonads	0.08
gamma rays	1	Bladder, oesophagus, liver, thyroid	0.04
photons (all energies)	1	Bone surface, brain, salivary glands, skin	0.01
protons >2 MeV	2	Total	1.00
slow neutrons	3		

TABLE 13.5 Factors that must be considered in molecular radiotherapy (MRT) dosimetry.

Factors	
Metabolism	Varies with each individual patient
Critical Organs	Charted maximum values for each organ
Absorbed Dose	energy imparted per unit mass of tissue (Gy)
Dose Equivalent-H	Absorbed dose $\times W_R$ (Sv)
Effective Dose Equivalent	Dose Equivalent + the tissue weighting factor for each organ W_T (takes into account the radio sensitivity of each organ) (mSv/MBq)
Effective Half-life ($T_{1/2eff}$)	Related to biological half-life and radioactive half-life ($1/T_{1/2eff} = 1/T_{1/2bio} + 1/T_{1/2phys}$)

dosimetry; each type is assigned a radiation weighting factor Table 13.4.

The factors listed in Table 13.5 all play a part in determining the amount of dose administered.

The calculation of absorbed dose to patients from RPs is simplified somewhat by the Medical Internal Radiation Dose (MIRD) Committee. They calculate the organ weighting factors by assigning a standard geometry to the human body to allow approximations of individuals and apply a series of estimates,

averages, and guidelines to calculate the absorbed dose.

Often a 'tracer' dose is administered to the patient; a small diagnostic level dose that allows imaging. Since the administered dose in MBq is known, it is possible to use quantitation techniques to determine the tumour-absorbed and organ-absorbed doses that are obtained as a result. Normally the organ-absorbed dose will be expressed as a factor of the administered activity (mGy/MBq). This factor can then be utilised to calculate the dose required to deliver a specific absorbed dose to a specific organ or tissue. This works well if the radioisotope emits gamma radiation, however often the most applicable radioisotopes for therapeutic purposes are β emitters or occasionally α emitters, neither of which offer the opportunity to image with gamma cameras. In such cases 'surrogate' imaging can be undertaken using a gamma-emitting isotope to demonstrate the expected uptake (e.g. ^{111}In-DOTA-Octreotide/^{111}In-DOTA-Lanreotide), and α or β particles can be measured in blood and urine samples where appropriate and to assess the excretion rates from the body.

Dosimetry-based individualisation of treatment is more important than ever before. IR(ME)R 2017 were developed in response to European Directive 2013/59/Euratom which states that 'Exposures of target volumes shall be individually planned'. Definition within the legislation clearly states that this includes nuclear medicine for therapeutic purposes (article 56, definition 81). Individualisation is particularly significant because the maximum tolerated dose for organs can be lowered by cytotoxic chemotherapy.

The calculations of absorbed dose for MRT are therefore undertaken by a multidisciplinary team of clinicians, physicists, and therapeutic radiographers. The full explanation is beyond the remit of this chapter and readers with a further interest are directed to other texts [9].

References

1. Pichler, B., Wehrl, H.F., Kolb, A., and Judenhofer, M.S. (2008). PET/MRI: the next generation of multi-modality imaging? *Semin. Nucl. Med.* 38 (3): 199–208.
2. Musafargani, S., Ghosh, K.K., Mishra, S. et al. (2018). PET/MRI: a frontier in era of complementary hybrid imaging. *Eur. J. Hybrid Imaging* 2: 12.
3. Hutton, B., Occhipinti, M., Kuehne, A. et al. (2018). Development of clinical simultaneous SPECT/MRI. *Br. J. Radiol.* 90: 20160690.
4. Lux, F., Sancey, L., Bianchi, A. et al. (2015). Gadolinium-based nanoparticles for theranostic MRI-radiosensitization. *Nanomed. Fut. Med.* 10 (11): 1801–1815.
5. Goldberg, D.M. (2002). Targeted therapy of cancer with radiolabeled antibodies. *J Nucl Med* 43: 693–713.
6. Her Majesty's Stationery Office (2017). *The Ionising Radiations Regulations.* London: HMSO.
7. Her Majesty's Stationery Office (2017). *The Ionising Radiation (Medical Exposure) Regulations.* London: HMSO.
8. ICRP (2004). ICRP Publication 94: release of nuclear medicine patients after therapy with unsealed sources. *Ann. ICRP* 34 (2): v–vi): 71–79.
9. Baechler, S., Hobbs, R.F., Prideaux, A.R. et al. (2008). Extension of the biological effective dose to the MIRD schema and possible implications in radionuclide therapy dosimetry. *Med. Phys.* 35 (3): 1123–1134.

CHAPTER 14

Brachytherapy Physics and Equipment

Gemma Burke

Aim

The aim of this chapter is to present the fundamental principles and practice of brachytherapy and its associated equipment.

14.1 Introduction

Brachytherapy involves the accurate placement of a sealed source of radiation very close to a tumour or tumour bed, with the term 'brachy' itself meaning short or close. The mechanism of delivery is dependent on the presence of a body cavity, e.g. cervix, vagina, or uterus, or the ability to gain sufficient access to the tumour site, e.g. prostate, breast, or head and neck. Historically brachytherapy has been part of the management plan of a variety of cancer sites for over eight decades, however in the last 20 years the increasing sophistication of modern afterloading systems, combined with significant developments in pre-treatment imaging and planning systems, has facilitated an increase in the use and reach of brachytherapy, with respect to both treatment site and access to services.

In line with these technological developments, the role of the therapeutic radiographer in the delivery of brachytherapy has also significantly increased and many high dose rate (HDR) brachytherapy departments operate as an integral part of an external beam radiotherapy service.

Although the principles of radiobiology are the same for external-beam radiotherapy and brachytherapy, the advantage with brachytherapy lies in its ability to exploit the inverse square law, resulting in a high deposit of dose close to the tumour and then a rapid fall-off of dose a short distance away from the source, thus limiting dose to the surrounding healthy tissue. It is important to remember that the dose received to organs at risk (OAR) is still given careful consideration both when brachytherapy is used alone and when it is used following a course of external-beam radiotherapy, as the OAR may have already received a measurable dose. In addition, the smaller fractionation schedule and use of fixed applicators reduces opportunities for inter- and intrafraction variability. Brachytherapy can be utilised as a monotherapy or adjuvantly as a way of escalating dose beyond what external-beam radiotherapy can safely achieve. Although this chapter does not cover in any depth the principles of radioactivity

Practical Radiotherapy: Physics and Equipment, Third Edition. Edited by Pam Cherry and Angela M. Duxbury.
© 2020 John Wiley & Sons Ltd. Published 2020 by John Wiley & Sons Ltd.

and radionuclides it is important to acknowledge as a minimum the 'ideal' characteristics that a clinically useful radionuclide needs to have. These are:

- a high specific activity (Bq kg^{-1}) (can use small quantities);
- nontoxic and stable (i.e. insoluble);
- available in clinically useful physical forms (i.e. not a liquid or a gas);
- encapsulated (ensure rigidity/prevents leakage);
- an optimum gamma ray energy;
- an appropriate half-life which is long enough so that decay during treatment is negligible (e.g. iridium 192 has a half-life 74 days).

This chapter reviews aspects of the use of sealed sources in brachytherapy, with particular attention given to the use of remote afterloading, and the systems available to deliver it. Consideration will be given to all dose rate bandings (low, pulse, and high) but practical application will primarily focus on high and pulse dose rate delivery to reflect current and emerging practice. Some of the treatment delivery systems currently available, together with associated quality assurance procedures and safety considerations, will also be covered. Application of principles to practice will be considered and where appropriate the role of the therapeutic radiographer. This account of remote, or machine, afterloading is not exhaustive; rather it provides an indication of the types of technique and equipment that are available. A good discussion of remote afterloading safety and quality assurance may be found in the American Association of Physicists in Medicine (AAPM) Report No 61 [1].

Some equipment and techniques have been designed to be site specific whereas others are more flexible in the way that they can be adapted for use in several body sites, and the technical and financial considerations of whether a particular afterloading machine or method is suitable in a particular institution depends, in part, on the anticipated number of applications and the case mix. A brief overview of some of the main body sites treated will be covered within this chapter, however a more in-depth discussion of individual body sites can be found in Hoskin and Coyle [2].

This chapter inevitably has to refer to trade names of sources and equipment, and also to the names of equipment suppliers. This should not be taken to imply any recommendation of the products of any individual company, but because it is difficult to describe some of the techniques and equipment in purely generic terms. The reader will appreciate that machines that are similar (but not identical) in their mode of operation are available from various manufacturers and suppliers.

14.2 The Journey from Live Loading to Remote Afterloading

Most brachytherapy in the period before the 1960s entailed inserting a radioactive source directly into the patient, exposing all the operating room staff, radiographers, and transport personnel to radiation from the sources, and particularly giving high doses of radiation to the hands of the radiation oncologist performing the insertion. In the early days of manual brachytherapy, from the 1930s to the early 1980s, large implants were performed using many radium needles which were inserted manually in the operating theatre, with the consequent radiation exposure of the clinicians and other staff, and there are both documented and anecdotal reports of radiation injury to the fingers of clinicians.

Manual afterloading provided some additional protection often through the insertion of empty applicators with non-radioactive markers for localization purposes but the

TABLE 14.1 Radiation protection advantages of afterloading.

Advantage to	Non-afterloaded (handling live sources)	Manual afterloading	Remote afterloading
Theatre staff	No	Yes	Yes
Medical staff	No	Yes	Yes
Radiographer	No	Yes	Yes
Technician	No	No	Yes
Nursing staff	No	No	Yes

radiation protection advantage was gained only in this early part of the procedure, and eventually the radioactive sources had to be inserted into the applicators by the operator and the patient had to be cared for by nursing and clinical staff, with radioactive sources in position, for the duration of the treatment.

The development of remote afterloading systems in the late 1960s resulted in significant changes in brachytherapy practice. Applicators are now inserted into the patient by the radiation oncologist or therapeutic radiographer depending on the site being treated, and once all localization and planning is complete only then is the source released from the treatment unit safe into the applicators inside the patient. At this point all personnel apart from the patient are outside of the treatment room in a controlled area, thus limiting the radiation only to the patient. Table 14.1 summarises the relative advantages of the different types of afterloading with regard to radiation protection.

In 1985 the International Commission of Radiation Units and Measurements (ICRU) published document 38, *Dose and volume specification for reporting intracavitary therapy in gynaecology* [3], and subsequently in 1997 the ICRU 58 guidelines [4] were published for interstitial brachytherapy. These reports provide an international common language for recording and reporting both intracavitary and interstitial brachytherapy treatments which had been previously lacking.

14.3 Brachytherapy Terminology

To develop an understanding of brachytherapy delivery it is important to be familiar with some of the terminology used. Some terms are equipment manufacturer dependent and will be addressed in the relevant section but some of the more universally acknowledged terms are outlined here:

Insertion Mechanisms: Applicator placement can be defined within a number of distinct categories depending on the body site being treated. Four of the most common ones are outlined here.

- **Intracavitary** – The placement of applicators into an already existing cavity in the body, e.g. cervix, uterus, vagina. Applicators will often include a rigid rectal retractor as part of the set which aids in reducing rectal dose and is better tolerated when the treatment times are relatively short. Applicators are now also CT (computed tomography)-MRI (magnetic resonance imaging) compatible to facilitate more accurate verification and conformal/adaptive planning.

- **Intraluminal** – The placement of applicators directly into a lumen, e.g. oesophagus, bronchus. Flexible applicators inserted under image guidance and or endoscopy have enabled more challenging areas such as the bile duct and bronchus to be successfully treated.

- **Interstitial** – The placement of applicators directly into tissue, e.g. prostate, breast, head and neck. Applicators used in HDR brachytherapy are very similar to those utilised in low dose rate (LDR) interstitial treatments and consist of rigid or flexible needles housed in a fixed template. These facilitate the accurate planning and verification of the applicator and source positioning prior to the commencement of treatment, and the flexible needles enable the use of multi- and hypofractionated treatments, particularly in the head and neck and breast region.

- **Surface** – The placement of applicators directly into the skin surface, e.g. scalp, dorsum of hand. These are often custom-made moulds, however there are also a number of manufactured moulds and applicator systems available.

14.4 The Impact of Dose Rate

The effectiveness of radiation to produce an effect on tissue depends, amongst other things, on the type of tissue and the rate at which the dose is administered. Within brachytherapy practice an agreed set of dose limits are used and are predefined in distinct categories: low dose rate (LDR), medium dose rate (MDR), high dose rate (HDR) and more recently, pulsed dose rate (PDR).

Although there is no general agreement about the boundaries of low, medium, and high or even how the relevant dose rates are defined in relation to the treated volume, ICRU recognises these three categories, and the conventionally accepted boundaries between each of the categories are defined by ICRU 38 and outlined in the Table 14.2.

In a practical context a typical LDR fraction could last in the region of 12–18 hours in comparison to an HDR fraction which lasts typically between 4 and 8 minutes, depending on treatment site and the source strength at the time of treatment.

TABLE 14.2	ICRU 38 definitions of Low dose rate (LDR), Medium dose rate (MDR), and High dose rate (HDR).
Low dose rate (LDR)	0.4–2 Gy/h
Medium dose rate (MDR)	2–12 Gy/h
High dose rate (HDR)	> 0.2 Gy/min (i.e. 12 Gy/h)

There is no formal definition of PDR brachytherapy. The principle of PDR is to replace continuous LDR brachytherapy by a series of 'pulses' of HDR treatment. Historically research has focused on the delivery of PDR treatment and its effectiveness compared to the LDR approach [5–7]. However, more recent research is focused more on the role of PDR brachytherapy in comparison to HDR delivery [8, 9].

14.5 Afterloading Equipment

There are a number of different manufacturers who produce afterloading equipment, but for the purposes of this chapter examples of Varian and Elekta equipment will be provided. The focus will be on HDR and PDR afterloading equipment, however it is worth noting that some LDR/MDR afterloading equipment may still be in clinical use although production of LDR afterloaders has long since ceased.

14.6 HDR Afterloaders

The use of an HDR afterloading device has many advantages over historical afterloading equipment. The first is the length of treatment time, which is in the region of minutes rather than hours. Treatments tend to be fractionated with a 'beam on' time typically between four and eight minutes depending on factors such as the strength of the source, taking into account its half-life, and also the treatment site and number of applicators. Depending on the treatment site, treatment can be delivered on an outpatient basis or with patients attending as a day case or for an overnight stay. This brings significant advantages both for patients and at a service delivery level because greater number of patients can potentially be treated and there can be more flexibility in the service to meet changing demands and developments in the evidence base.

It is important to recognise that although the fraction delivery times are much shorter for many tumour sites, a significant amount of time (often hours) needs to be accounted for the applicator insertion, verification, and planning of treatments, as discussed further in this chapter.

14.6.1 Modern, Stepping Source HDR Units

Iridium-192 may be produced with a high specific activity. It is possible to manufacture iridium-192 sources that are physically small but that contain typically an activity of 10–20 Ci (370–740 GBq). This has led to the development of 'stepping source' treatment machines, in which a single iridium-192 source on the end of a computer-controlled cable sequentially moves through a series of dwell positions in each treatment applicator in turn. This technique avoids the need for several sources or source trains to be present in the machine because one source can simulate a series of sources.

There are several machines of this type in clinical use worldwide:

- GammaMedplus™ iX HDR/PDR Brachytherapy Afterloader;
- Elekta Flexitron® Aferloading platform;

- The microSelectron-HDR (Nucletron BV);
- The Varisource (Varian, USA).

Although there are variations between each of these systems, they all abide by similar principles of delivery. They use a single source attached to a drive cable or similar mechanism and the sources are housed in a safe within the treatment machine itself. When treatment is initiated the source leaves the safe and travels down the transfer tube which is connected at one end to the head of the treatment unit (in the indexer ring) and at the other end to the applicator which has been inserted into the patient; each of these trains is called a channel. The source then stops at a series of points, often referred to as a 'dwell position', and it stops for varying amounts of time, often referred to as a 'dwell time', and this is done for each of the applicators. Once treatment is complete the source automatically retracts to the safe within the machine.

The number of channels used for treatment will usually match the number of applicators inside the patient. For example, an oesophageal cancer treatment will have only one channel as there is only capacity for one applicator to be inserted into the patient, whereas an interstitial prostate cancer treatment will have multiple channels/catheters implanted. Different manufacturers offer equipment with varying numbers of channels. For example, the Flexitron afterloader shown in Figures 14.1 and 14.2 can deliver up to 40 channels.

The radiation protection requirements for the safe delivery of HDR afterloading brachytherapy are outside of the remit of this chapter and are addressed in detail in other texts and reports [2, 10, 11]. However in order to provide a basic context, single stepping unit HDR afterloaders should be ideally housed in a dedicated treatment room which meets legislative specifications for radiation protection and ideally with theatre capabilities, but where this isn't feasible, they can be housed in a room separate to the theatre. Due to the high activity source being permanently housed in the afterloader, the room should not be used for any other purpose.

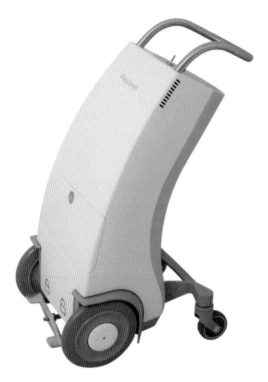

FIGURE 14.1 Showing the Elekta Flexitron Afterloading platform (Source: courtesy of Elekta).

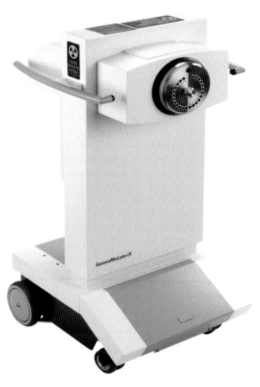

FIGURE 14.3 The GammaMedplus iX HDR/ PDR Brachytherapy Afterloader (Source: image courtesy of Varian Medical Systems, Inc. All rights reserved).

that unlike an external beam radiotherapy treatment room a designated HDR brachy-therapy room is always classed as a controlled area and will display the appropriate warning signs, including additional warnings to show that the source is out of its safe position. Safety mechanisms within the HDR unit itself and associated hardware and software will trigger an automatic source retraction should an entry barrier be broken during treatment delivery.

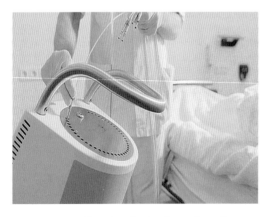

FIGURE 14.2 Showing the 40 channels and connection of transfer tube (Source: courtesy of Elekta).

14.6.2 Pulsed Dose Rate Systems

PDR afterloaders are very similar in appearance to HDR afterloaders, as shown in Figure 14.3. As previously highlighted, a HDR treatment fraction takes minutes where as a PDR fraction is in the region of hours or

Automatic entry warnings and systems that prevent persons entering the treatment room whilst the source is outside of the safe must be displayed. The appropriate designation of controlled and or supervised areas requires compliance with IRR (2017) regulation 17 [10]. It is important to recognise days which aligns more closely with LDR treatments. The radioactive source contains less radioactivity, typically having an activity of 0.5–1.0 Ci (37–18.5 GBq) of iridium-192. As a consequence, the source capsule is also physically smaller, having an active length of 0.5 mm and an overall length of 2.7 mm.

The operating software is also different, allowing the source movement to be programmed for the pulses as well as the intervals and overall treatment times. The pulsed nature of the treatments results in a delivery which is radiobiologically closer to LDR brachytherapy but because it is delivered by an afterloading device, there is the time for more accurate planning and dosimetry, as well as enabling the patient to have access to care from relevant healthcare professionals. Due to the mode of delivery, PDR units are housed in a dedicated ward side room which, as with the HDR rooms, requires appropriate and clear radiation protection warnings and signage in accordance with the legislation.

14.7 Brachytherapy Dosimetry

Inhomogeneous dose distributions are one of the well documented and recognised challenges within brachytherapy dosimetry and delivery. High dose gradients occur next to the source with a plateau of lower dose at a short distance away. Therefore, careful consideration has to be given to the spacing of the dwell positions and distribution in order to minimise this.

Prior to the development of more sophisticated computer systems and imaging modalities in the 1990's, brachytherapy dosimetry was calculated using a number of 'systems' which were developed to try and account for this inherent inhomogeneity. In very simple terms these systems were essentially a set of rules to which treatments could be safely and accurately calculated to ensure an accurate dose distribution and prescription [12].

The main systems utilised were the Manchester system for intracavitary brachytherapy and the Paris system for interstitial brachytherapy [13]. Although they could be adapted, it was important that their key principles were maintained to ensure plans could be compared and that accurate reporting and recording could be undertaken. However, one of their limitations was that the doses were prescribed and reported relative to a particular applicator set rather than to an individual patient's anatomy and tumour geometry. To facilitate safe treatment delivery 'standard' plans were generated from a preloaded library within the software of the afterloader with preconfigured dwell times and positions. For example, in the case of intracavitary cervical brachytherapy this data was provided for each set of differing size and angle of applicators.

Technological developments have resulted in a significant shift away from the use of these systems in routine HDR practice as the sophisticated nature of current planning systems in conjunction with CT and or MRI imaging enables dose optimization to be tailored to each patient's tumour and anatomy. However, the importance of the old systems should not be underestimated; they played a critical role in building the foundations on which modern brachytherapy treatments are delivered today, and they are still considered a reliable and well recognised starting point for brachytherapy dosimetry.

14.8 Transfer of Information to the Treatment Unit and Checking of Data

When not using a standard plan which is now more often the case, the requirements of the plan (treatment volume, prescribed dose, critical organ constraints, dose fractionation, etc.)

must be transmitted unambiguously to the staff delivering the treatment. Modern brachytherapy systems enable quick and accurate electronic transfer of data via DICOM links from the planning system to the delivery platform. In addition, paper prescription and planning data sheets may also be utilised for the treatment delivery staff; in the case of HDR treatments this is primarily therapeutic radiographers, to cross reference and perform data integrity checks prior to treatment commencing. In addition to these checks, physical checks must also be made on the patient as well as the actual applicators with respect to number, order, and where appropriate, relative coordinates.

14.9 Principles of Safe Treatment Delivery

14.9.1 Safety and Quality Assurance

Comprehensive quality assurance and safety systems must be in place resulting in a management programme which fully complies with current (inter)national and local legislation and protocol. This includes but is not exclusive to: room design; safe source storage and transportation; personal dose monitoring; quality assurance; designation of areas; and contingency planning. An overview of some of these components is provided below, although it is not possible to cover all of these in detail within this chapter. Readers should therefore refer to both Chapter 4 of Hoskin and Coyle [2] and Chapter 3 of Limbergen et al. [14] for a much more in-depth discussion.

A comprehensive quality assurance programme must be in place and consist of a series of specific tests, at defined repetition intervals, with appropriate record keeping. Typically, checks of the machine operation and selected safety features are performed on

a daily and three-monthly basis. In most institutions this is set up by the medical physics department and both therapeutic radiographers and physicists perform the checks. It is not appropriate here to define the details of these because they depend on factors such as the type of machine, local circumstances, frequency of use of the equipment. Quality assurance checks on the treatment planning system are beyond the scope of this chapter and readers are referred to the literature [15].

All remote afterloaders contain a 'check cable', which is essentially a dummy source on its own drive cable. The check cable is driven out through the transfer tubes and applicators before the source is transferred in order to check the correct connection of all the components and also for obstructions or tight curves. The check cable may also be used as a simulated source in some systems. The source and check cables are driven out and back by stepper motors with a positional accuracy of approximately ±1 mm.

14.9.2 Staff Training

As with any form of radiotherapy, safety is paramount. It is particularly so in brachytherapy because the treatment delivery is complex and often done under the pressure of having to work quickly in an operating theatre environment. It is vital that all staff groups are adequately trained and practised in the techniques, there are sufficient staffs to allow appropriate checking of machine programming, etc., and procedures are standardised wherever possible. In addition, robust quality assurance procedures for the equipment need to be in place.

Whereas LDR and PDR services tend to operate outside of the traditional radiotherapy department, often in a specialist room on a ward, HDR units are often an integral part of the external beam department either by locality and/or operational responsibility and so are primarily run by therapeutic radiographers as part of a multidisciplinary team which includes but is not exclusive to: clinicians; physicists; dosimetrists; anaesthetists; operating department practitioners; and theatre nurses. Depending on the level of service offered, therapeutic radiographers may be rotated on a full or part-time basis and may be in either rotational or fixed permanent roles. It is important that there is continuity of staffing to ensure that competency and confidence is maintained and the treatment delivery and care received by patients is of the highest standard. Due to the special application of brachytherapy and therefore often low patient numbers, this can be challenging. Refresher training, including local protocols, local rules, and regular 'walkthrough' of the safety procedures are imperative after a period of time away from the HDR department to ensure the safe operation of the unit.

14.9.3 Procedure in the Event of a Source Retraction Failure

Complex maintenance and quality assurance procedures should prevent this from occurring but in the event of the source failing to retract back into the safe and where all other equipment safety mechanisms have failed, a source retraction failure protocol has to be initiated, and this procedure should be an integral part of any brachytherapy department protocol. Clear roles and responsibilities under IR(ME)R [10] should be documented and part of the training to ensure the safety of all personal and patients. As stated earlier a regular 'walkthrough' of the procedure in the event of a retraction failure should be an intrinsic part of any training and competency. Although key principles and procedures should be adhered to, it may be necessary to adapt the protocol depending on the specific treatment technique being used and its complexity, e.g. outpatient endometrial cancer treatment or a prostate cancer implant under general anaesthetic. Where appropriate, sepa-

rate protocols should be developed for each of the techniques being delivered and staff should be fully informed of the procedure prior to the commencement of the treatment delivery. Accurate and timely documentation and reporting of any radiation incident must also be made to the local RPA (Radiation Protection Advisor) and RPS (Radiation Protection Supervisor).

14.10 Treatment Protocols in Brachytherapy

Brachytherapy facilities should have standard operating procedures to cover all of the sites being treated. The risk of an error occurring is reduced when treatments are given according to a documented protocol. Each treatment site and method of application should have its own protocol and include a description of localisation procedures and associated imaging equipment (including any radiographic markers, operating theatre procedure, treatment planning method, treatment delivery, and verification and recording procedures). It is important the protocols are reviewed regularly and where necessary updated to ensure their continued accuracy.

14.10.1 Treatment Prescription

The radiographer requires a signed treatment prescription, which should be clear, complete, and unambiguous, and specify exactly the treatment machine and technique to be used. Diagrams should be used routinely and particularly where this aids clarity. The type and size of applicators, radiation sources, prescribed radiation dose, and dose location should be clearly indicated. The prescription should be clearly signed and dated by the prescribing clinician. Any additional information on the prescription sheet, e.g. treatment planning information or data integrity checks of the dwell or treatment times, should be signed, and then checked and countersigned by a second suitably qualified person.

One of the difficulties with HDR treatments is that there is often only a short period of time available between the insertion of the applicators and the start of the treatment fraction. This is, of course, desirable from a clinical point of view because the patient may be intubated and anaesthetized whilst awaiting the start of the treatment. However, it does mean that the treatment parameters have to be determined and the treatment planned and checked in a timely manner with staff working under considerable pressure. Where permissible regional anaethesia e.g. spinal epidural are being increasingly used as an effective and safe alternative to general anaesthetic.

14.11 Clinical Examples

Although this chapter does not intend to cover in detail the clinical aspects of the provision of brachytherapy, it is important to be aware that the treatment regimens used in HDR and PDR brachytherapy are very different from those used for the equivalent LDR due to radiobiological considerations. The advantages of HDR brachytherapy are offset to some extent by the fact that, because of radiobiological considerations, the treatment has to be fractionated, so a patient will generally receive several of these albeit shorter treatment times within an overall course. Also, there may be a clinical disadvantage in that a patient may need several anaesthetics during the course of treatment, depending on the insertion or implantation procedure being performed.

What follows is a brief overview of some key aspects of clinical delivery for a selection of treatment sites and where applicable, examples of the applicators used are provided.

14.11.1 Uterine Tumours: Cervix, and Endometrium Brachytherapy

Intracavitary brachytherapy is an integral part of the management of both cervix and endometrial cancer and was one of the very first uses of brachytherapy. As already highlighted throughout the chapter, the treatment process for LDR/PDR and HDR brachytherapy can very different and so for the purpose of these examples, HDR brachytherapy only will be considered.

Vaginal Vault Brachytherapy for endometrial cancer is primarily given as an adjuvant treatment for post-hysterectomy patients who are at high risk of pelvic disease or developing local recurrence based on a number of predetermined criteria. Brachytherapy is delivered multifractionally either as adjuvant treatment following a course of external-beam radiotherapy to the pelvis or as a monotherapy following surgery to reduce the risk of local recurrence to the surgical scar site. Results from the PORTEC 2 trial [16] show that vaginal brachytherapy achieves comparable control for the prevention of vaginal recurrence to external beam radiotherapy in intermediate-risk patients and should be considered as the treatment of choice.

Applicators are generally inserted into the patient without the need for any anaesthetic or pain relief although it is available if required (see Figure 14.4). Patients are treated

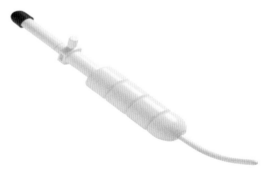

FIGURE 14.4 Example of vaginal applicator with option of a uterine tube (Source: courtesy of Elekta).

on an outpatient basis and treatments take in the region of 10 minutes. No specific patient preparation is required for the treatment and applicators are inserted and removed by the therapeutic radiographers responsible for delivering the treatment.

Cervix Brachytherapy is also delivered adjuvantly to patients who are at high risk of pelvic disease based on a number of predetermined criteria. Patients will not have had a hysterectomy and their primary treatment is concurrent radical chemo-radiotherapy to the pelvis followed by intracavitary brachytherapy.

Applicator insertion is undertaken in theatre either under general anaesthetic or spinal epidural. Ultrasound is more routinely being used in theatre to aid with accurate applicator placement and reduces the risk of adverse events occurring, e.g. uterine perforation.

There are a wide variety of applicator sets available and decisions are made locally based on service need as to the ones to be kept in stock. However, they are all designed with the same core principles. Most commonly applicator sets comprise a central uterine tube and then vaginal ring or ovoids to enable lateral dose to be delivered (see Figure 14.5). This ring/ovoid is designed to sit adjacent to the cervical OS. However, developments in applicator design have facilitated opportunities to deliver much more targeted and conformal doses with not only the addition of flexible needles (see Figure 14.6),

which means the dose distribution can be further tailored to the specific size and position of the tumour whilst still minimising the dose to critical structures, but also enable the treatment of any parametrium and/or vaginal disease.

Figure 14.7 shows the Advanced Gynaecological Applicator Venezia™ from Elekta which combines intracavitary and interstitial capabilities which can be used to treat all stages of disease from early to advanced.

Fixed rectal retractors are part of the applicator design which aids in dose reduction to the rectal wall. In addition, fixation of the applicators can be achieved either through vaginal gauze packing or the use of a fixating clamp, and this minimises movement of the applicator in the patient between insertion, localization, and the completion of treatment.

Following applicator insertion patients then undergo MRI and/or CT imaging as per local departmental protocol. The GEC-ESTRO working party published guidelines in 2006 [17] recommending minimum requirements for the transition from traditional to 3D imaging (MRI, CT) for 3D planning of cervical brachytherapy, with further guidelines in 2012 [18] with an emphasis on the use of MRI for adaptive image-based brachytherapy.

Once the images have been electronically transferred to the planning system, treatment plan can commence. During this time period it is imperative that the patient is waiting in

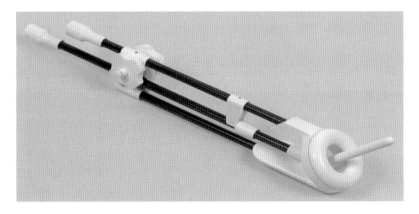

FIGURE 14.5   Ring CT/MR Applicator Set (Source: courtesy of Elekta).

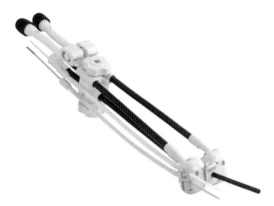

FIGURE 14.6 Utrecht Interstitial CT/MR applicator set (Source: courtesy of Elekta).

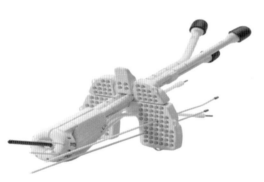

FIGURE 14.7 Advanced Gynaecological Applicator Venezia (Source: courtesy of Elekta).

an appropriate clinical area such as a ward, day case room, or dedicated theatre recovery bay and is monitored at all times. Following the completion and checking of the treatment plan and its associated data by the appropriately trained staff (physicists, clinicians, dosimetrists, therapeutic radiographers) the patient is then transported to the treatment room where treatment can commence. Upon completion of the treatment fraction or full treatment schedule the applicators are immediately removed and patients can be administered with pain relief for this. Applicator removal in some departments is routinely undertaken by therapeutic radiographers who have undergone a period of supervised practice competence. This development in skill set results in potentially less waiting time and

therefore a better experience for the patient and also a smoother workflow as the clinician can be undertaking other tasks. As stated earlier, as well as robust delivery protocols a comprehensive source retraction failure protocol must be in place for this technique.

14.11.2 Prostate Brachytherapy

For many patients with prostate cancer, radical brachytherapy is an integral part of their management plan. Prostate brachytherapy can be delivered in two different ways. This is either via the implantation of permanent LDR radioactive seeds, iodine- 125 or palladium -103, or through the use of an HDR afterloader. For both techniques the implantation procedure is very similar, the differences being in the permanent and/or temporary insertion of the radioactive source. Indications for which option should be used lie in the patients' risk status – low, intermediate, or high – which is determined by combining specific criteria such as the PSA (prostate-specific antigen) score, Gleason score, and stage of disease. Brachytherapy may be used as a monotherapy or as an adjuvant treatment either through the use of LDR seeds prior to external beam radiotherapy or using HDR brachytherapy as a boost following external beam radiotherapy [19].

Research is continually being undertaken to determine the most appropriate applications of LDR brachytherapy. ASENDE-RT [20] was a two-arm randomised controlled trial which compared two methods of dose escalation for intermediate- and high-risk prostate cancer patients, one of the arms being the use of a LDR brachytherapy boost following external beam radiotherapy and androgen deprivation. The study reported positive findings citing that compared to the external beam boost arm those randomised to the LDR boost 'were twice as likely to be free of biochemical failure at a median follow-up of 6.5 years' as those who had received external beam radiotherapy.

For both LDR and HDR methods the treatment is undertaken with the patient under a general anaesthetic and positioned in the lithotomy position for ease of access (Figure 14.8). Access is obtained through the perineum using trans-rectal ultrasound guidance to ensure accurate positioning of the needles.

For LDR seeds the planning and dosimetry is undertaken using ultrasound whilst the patient is under anaesthetic. The radioactive seeds are preloaded and inserted into the rigid applicators. Post-implant imaging is undertaken to ensure that none of the seeds have been misplaced during the procedure. Patients have a minimum one-night stay in hospital post-procedure and are required to have their urine output monitored through the use of a sieve in case any seeds have moved into the bladder and/or urethra.

For HDR afterloading, planning can be undertaken using the trans-rectal ultrasound (Figure 14.9) or alternatively through the use of MRI or CT imaging. There are pros and cons to each of these methods. The advantage of the single-step process using ultrasound is that the patient does not need to be moved to a different locality for the imaging to take place and this is more advantageous if the clinical department has a dual-use theatre/treatment room and the patient does not have to move for treatment delivery.

Following the completion and checking of the treatment plan and its associated data by the appropriately trained staff (physicists, clinicians, dosimetrists, therapeutic radiographers) treatment can commence. Applicator removal is either undertaken by the clinician or more routinely it is being undertaken by therapeutic radiographers who have undergone a period of supervised practice competence. This development in skill sets results in potentially less waiting time and therefore a better experience for the patients together with a smoother workflow as the clinician can be undertaking other tasks. As stated earlier, there must be robust delivery protocols and a comprehensive source retraction failure protocol in place for this technique.

14.11.3 Breast Brachytherapy

Surgery, external beam radiotherapy, and chemotherapy form the standard management for patients with breast cancer. However, for some specific indications, brachytherapy is considered an option, with the advantage of being able to deliver a high dose to the tumour/tumour bed whilst

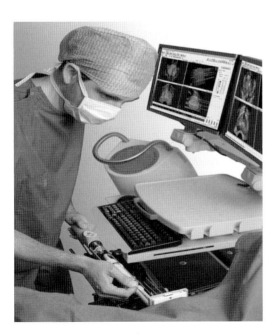

FIGURE 14.8 Showing the treatment setup (Source: courtesy of Elekta).

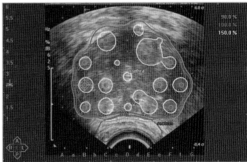

FIGURE 14.9 Ultrasound demonstrating needle positions (Source: image courtesy of Elekta).

sparing OAR which in this case would be primarily the skin, lungs, heart, and ribs, whilst also potentially offering better cosmesis. Brachytherapy can be used for a number of different circumstances including as a boost following radical external beam radiotherapy (as an alternative to electrons), adjuvantly for the management of locally advanced tumours, again following external beam radiotherapy (and chemotherapy), or as a form of postoperative management of low-risk patients through the mechanism of accelerated partial breast irradiation (APBI).

APBI delivered using brachytherapy can be undertaken via the insertion of multiple interstitial catheters or an intracavity balloon implant. Multi-catheter interstitial implants use either flexible or rigid interstitial needles which are implanted under operative conditions, but these are often complex and technically challenging procedures to undertake and so the development of intracavitary single channel applicators, for example, the Mammosite® balloon catheters, have made this a more accessible and less challenging procedure. The catheter is inserted into the tumour bed within the breast and then the balloon is expanded to fill the space. HDR afterloading can then be delivered multifractionally and twice daily with a six-hour gap. Follow-up data reported for the use of interstitial brachytherapy for APBI shows excellent cosmetic results as well as evidence of tumour control and survival [21]. The American Brachytherapy Society in 2018 [22] published consensus statements on the use of APBI and recognised within it the high value of both interstitial and single-catheter brachytherapy for specific categories of patients.

14.11.4 Head and Neck Brachytherapy

Brachytherapy as a treatment modality in the management of head and neck cancer is less common than some of the previously discussed treatment sites and as with all brachytherapy it relies heavily on there being the appropriate expertise within the clinical centre, and therefore in this instance it is often not utilised as a management option. The advantages for its use lie in the potential to preserve function and cosmetic effect compared to other modalities as well as being able to achieve excellent tumour control.

In 2017 the GEC-ESTRO [23] head and neck working group published recommendations for the use of brachytherapy in the treatment of squamous cell carcinomas for the following sites: lip; oral cavity; oropharynx; nasopharynx; and superficial cancers. Consideration is given within the recommendations to its use either alone or adjuvantly with external beam radiotherapy and its potential role as a salvage treatment for loco-regional recurrences including lymph nodes. The dose is primarily achieved through the use of interstitial flexible or rigid needles and delivered through multifractional bi-daily schedules. Figure 14.10a–c shows a clinical example of salvage interstitial brachytherapy for a patient with a neck recurrence which had occurred following radical external beam radiotherapy a number of years previously. A surgical neck dissection was carried out and the flexible interstitial catheters were placed in situ during the surgical procedure. Following a recovery period of a number of weeks, HDR brachytherapy commenced using a multifractional bi-daily regime. The applicators were incredibly well tolerated by the patient and steps were taken to reduce the risk of infection at the entry and exit points of the applicators. The applicators were removed after the last fraction in the treatment room with minimal preparation or pain relief required. Acute side effects were minimal and there was no superficial skin erythema.

14.12 Conclusion

In summary, brachytherapy plays a vital role in the management of many different cancer sites either as a sole therapy or adjuvantly as

(a)

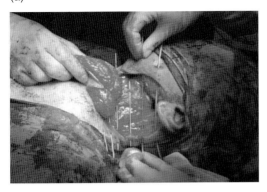

(b)

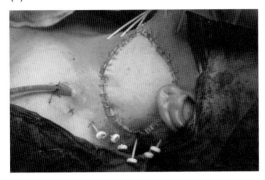

(c)

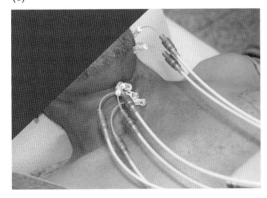

FIGURE 14.10 A clinical example of salvage interstitial brachytherapy for a patient with a neck recurrence.

part of a complex management plan. Its popularity as a treatment modality lies in the ability to be able to achieve a high dose to a localised area, whilst causing minimal critical structure dose; this in turn can create increased local control without an increase in long-term morbidity. This chapter has provided an overview of the key principles that underpin the safe delivery of brachytherapy as well as introducing key concepts, safety considerations, terminology, and examples of the equipment used. The clinical examples presented demonstrate the broad spectrum of applications brachytherapy has, including as a safe method of dose escalation when critical structure tolerances have been reached with external beam radiotherapy.

The delivery of HDR brachytherapy requires a multidisciplinary approach and therapeutic radiographers are critical to this team to ensure the safe operation of the HDR brachytherapy unit. All staff involved in the delivery of brachytherapy must be highly skilled/trained to ensure safe treatment delivery and high standards of patient care, however a lack of expertise and resources can be limiting factors in the availability and access of brachytherapy treatment. The role of the therapeutic radiographer has grown and expanded over the last two decades; the development of additional skills and competencies outside the boundaries of traditional roles are enabling both role extension and development in areas of advancing practice.

Some of the treatment techniques mentioned in this chapter are not commonplace in all brachytherapy departments. The future of brachytherapy remains exciting, as more research is published and the development of increasingly sophisticated equipment and planning solutions become available, offering realistic possibilities for the future for an increasing number of cancer sites.

References

1. Kubo, H., Glasgow, G., Pethel, T. et al. (1998). *American Association of Physicists in Medicine Report 61*: High dose-rate brachytherapy treatment delivery. *Med. Phys.* 25: 375–403.
2. Hoskin, P. and Coyle, C. (2011). *Radiotherapy in Practice: Brachytherapy*, 2e. Oxford University Press.

3. International Commission on Radiation Units and Measurements. *Dose and Volume Specification for Reporting Intracavitary Therapy in Gynaecology.* ICRU Report 38. Bethesda, MA: ICRU, 1985

4. International Commission on Radiation Units and Measurements. *Dose and Volume Specification for Reporting Interstitial Therapy.* ICRU Report 58. Bethesda, MA: ICRU, 1997

5. Swift, P.S., Fu, K.K., Phillips, T.L. et al. (1994). Pulsed low dose rate interstitial and intracavitary therapy. In: *Brachytherapy from Radium to Optimisation. Veenendaal* (eds. R.F. Mould, J.J. Batterman, A.A. Martinez and B.L. Speiser), 254–259. The Netherlands: Nucletron BV.

6. Bachtiary, B., Dewitt, A., Pintilie, M. et al. (2005). Comparison of late toxicity between continuous low-dose-rate and pulsed-dose-rate brachytherapy in cervical cancer patients. *Int. J. Radiat. Oncol. Biol. Phys.* 63: 1077–1082.

7. Harms, W., Krempien, R., Hensley, F.W. et al. (2002). 5-year results of pulsed dose rate brachytherapy applied as a boost after breast-conserving therapy in patients at high risk for local recurrence from breast cancer. *Strahlenther Onkol.* 178: 607–614.

8. Kumar, P., Sharma, N.D., Kumar, S. et al. (2016). Pulsed-dose-rate vs. high-dose-rate intracavitary radiotherapy for locally advanced carcinoma of cervix: a prospective randomized study. *Brachytherapy* 15 (3): 327–332.

9. Hannoun-Lévi, J.M. and Peiffert, D. (2014). Dose rate in brachytherapy using after-loading machine: pulsed or high-dose rate? *Cancer/Radiothérapie* 18 (5–6): 437–440.

10. Ionising Radiation (Medical Exposure) Regulations 2017 (IRR17) Statutory instruments 2017 no 1075. Available at www.legislation.gov.uk.

11. HSE, Working with ionising radiation. Ionising Radiations (Medical Exposure) Regulations. 2017. Approved Code of Practice and guidance.

12. Rivard, M.J., Venselaar, J.L.M., and Beaulieu, L. (2009). The evolution of brachytherapy treatment planning. *Med. Phys.* 36: 2136–2153.

13. Josyn, C., Flynn, A., and Hall, E. (eds.). *Principles and Practice of Brachytherapy: Using Afterloading Systems.* London: Arnold.

14. Van Limbergen, E.V., Pötter, R., Hoskin, P., and Baltas, D. (2014). Radiation Protection in Brachytherapy: ESTRO Radiotherapy and Oncology. In: *The GEC-ESTRO Handbook of Brachytherapy.* Brussels: ESTRO.

15. Thomadsen, B. (1999). *Achieving Quality in Brachytherapy.* London: Taylor & Francis.

16. Nout, R.A., Smit, V.T.H.B.M., Putter, H. et al. (2010). Lutgens, and LCHW et al for the POR-TEC Study Group: Vaginal brachytherapy versus pelvic external beam radiotherapy for patients with endometrial cancer of high-intermediate risk (PORTEC-2): an open-label, non-inferiority, randomised trial. *The Lancet* 375: 816–823.

17. Pötter, R., Haie-Mederb, C., Van Limbergenc, E. et al. (2006). Recommendations from gynaecological (GYN) GEC ESTRO working group (II): Concepts and terms in 3D image-based treatment planning in cervix cancer brachytherapy—3D dose volume parameters and aspects of 3D image-based anatomy, radiation physics, radiobiology. *Radiother. Oncol.* 78: 67–77.

18. Dimopoulosa, C.A., Petrow, P., Tanderup, K. et al. (2012). Recommendations from Gynaecological (GYN) GEC-ESTRO Working Group (IV): Basic principles and parameters for MR imaging within the frame of image based adaptive cervix cancer brachytherapy. *Radiother. Oncol.* 103: 113–122.

19. Hoskin, P.J., Colombo, A., Niehoff, P. et al. (2013). GEC/ESTRO recommendations on high dose rate afterloading brachytherapy for localised prostate cancer: an update. *Radiother. Oncol.* 107 (3): 325–332.

20. Morris, W.J., Tyldesley, S., Rodda, S. et al. Androgen Suppression Combined with Elective Nodal and Dose Escalated Radiation Therapy (the ASCENDE-RT Trial): an analysis of survival endpoints for a randomized trial comparing a low-dose-rate brachytherapy boost to a dose-escalated external beam boost for high- and intermediate-risk prostate cancer. *Int. J. Radiat. Oncol. Biol. Phys.* 98 (2): 275–285.

21. Shah, C., Harris, E.E., Holmes, D., and Vicini, F.A. (2018). Partial breast irradiation: accelerated and intraoperative. In: *The Breast: Comprehensive Management of Benign and Malignant Diseases*, 5e (eds. K.I. Bland, E.M. Copeland and S. Klimberg). Philadelphia, PA: Elsevier.

22. Shah, C., Vicini, F., Shaitelman, S.F. et al. (2018). The American Brachytherapy Society consensus statement for accelerated partial-breast irradiation. *Brachytherapy* 17: 154–170.

23. Strnad, V., Major, T., Polgar, C. et al. (2018). ESTRO-ACROP guideline: interstitial multi-catheter breast brachytherapy as Accelerated Partial Breast Irradiation alone or as boost. GEC-ESTRO Breast Cancer Working Group practical recommendations. *Radiother. Oncol.* 128: 411–420.

Index

abdominal compression plate 126
absorbed dose 2, 35–6
absorption 47, 62
absorption edge 52
accelerated partial breast irradiation 302
access interlocks 260
acoustic impedance 97–8
action levels 227–8
active breathing control 125
active screens 69
adaptive radiotherapy 188, 215–17, 229
additional dose 229–30
air kerma 38
air-wall concept 37
ALARA (ALARP) 256
alarm systems 259
alpha decay 21
aluminium filters 152
amorphous silicon detector 167
ampere 15
amplitude 96
amplitude-based sorting 83
anal margin disease 137
anatomical landmarks 113
ankle stocks 128
annihilation energy 21
annihilation radiation 56
anode 25
anode heel effect 149
antibodies, radiolabelled 282
anti-nodes 159
aperture size 78, 92, 112–13
applicators 150–1
as low as reasonably achievable/practicable
    (ALARA/ALARP) 256
ASENDE-RT trial 300
atomic energy 20
atomic numbers 19
atomic particles 18–19
atomic structure 18–20
attenuation 47–8, 62, 97
attenuation coefficients 49
average intensity projection 84, 85
azimuthal varying field cyclotron 178

background radiation 22
backscatter 54, 152

backscatter factor 152
barriers 57, 250, 257–8
baseplate systems 118
basic units 13
beam dump 155
beam-flattening filter 163
beam weighting 207
beam's eye view 205–6
becquerel 269
belly board 129
bending magnets 161–2
beryllium 148
beta decay 21
binding energies 29
bins 82
bipolar tubes 147
bite blocks 120–1
bladder, treatment verification 236
blood oxygen level dependent (BOLD)
    MRI 91, 107
body moulds 129
bolus 58, 116–17
bowtie filter 167–8
brachytherapy 1, 289–305
    afterloading equipment 292–5
    breast 301–2
    cervix 299–300
    check cable 296
    dose rate 292
    dosimetry 295
    electronic transfer of data 295–6
    head and neck 302
    high dose rate afterloaders 292–4
    insertion mechanism 291–2
    interstitial 292
    intracavitary 291
    intraluminal 291
    manual loading 290–1
    prostate 300–1
    pulsed dose rate 292, 294–5
    quality assurance 296
    remote afterloading 291
    safety 296–7
    source retraction failure protocol 297
    staff training 296–7
    stepping source machines 293
    surface 292

brachytherapy (*cont'd*)
   terminology 291–2
   treatment planning 214–15
   treatment prescription 297–8
   treatment protocols 297
   vaginal vault 298–9
Bragg curve 181
Bragg–Gray cavity theory 39
Bragg ionisation effect 57
Bragg peak 181
breast
   board 122–3, 124
   brachytherapy 301–2
   immobilisation 122–5
   treatment verification 232–4
breastfeeding 283
breath-hold techniques 125–6
bremsstrahlung 29, 57
Brown–Roberts–Wells device 140
buildup region 54, 57, 203–4
bunching section 157

C-band linear accelerators 170
calorimetry 36, 40
carbon fibre 166
cathode 24–5
cathode cup 156
cavity chamber 37
ceramic insulators 148
cervix brachytherapy 299–300
chair-based treatment 136–7
characteristic line spectrum 30
characteristic radiation 29–30, 51
check cable 296
chest board 128
chest treatment verification 234–5
child immobilisation 139–40
Clarity® Autoscan TPUS (Elekta) 134
classified people 264
clinical audit 252–3
clinical governance 247–8
clinical incidents 250–2
clinical target volume 115
collimation 150–1, 164–5, 203
colourwash display 207
composite filters 151–2
Compton scattering 52–5, 62, 152
computed radiography 62, 68
computed tomography (CT) 4, 73–85
   aperture size 78
   axial cine scan 82
   cone beam (CBCT) 167–8, 224–5, 231
   couch 78–9
   dosimetry 45

   dynamic contrast enhanced 107
   evolution 73–5
   external laser positioning system 79
   field of view 78
   4DCT 80–5, 126–7, 212–14, 228
   helical scanners 74
   hybrid imaging 103–4, 277–8
   image display 76–8
   image formation 75–6
   image reconstruction 76
   intrafraction motion 228
   intravenous contrast 79–80
   lasers within scanner 79
   multi-slice 74–5
   patient model 199–201
   PET-CT 103–4, 277–8
   region of interest 78
   scanner components 73–4
   simulators 78–80
   slow helical scan 82
   SPECT-CT 277
   spiral scanners 74
   treatment verification 224–5
   window width and level 76–7
   windowing 76
computer-controlled delivery 237–8
concession 247
concrete 57
conduction 14, 149
cone beam CT (CBCT) 167–8, 224–5, 231
conformance statement 71, 72
conformity 203
conformity index 208
contouring 199–202
contrast 62–7
contrast administration 79–80
controlled areas 264
convection 14
convergence error 211
cooling systems 149–50, 160
copper anode 149
copper filters 151–2
couches 78–9, 92, 166–7
CT dose index 45
CT number 76
Curie 269
current 15
CyberKnife 174–5, 189, 229
cyclotrons 176–81
cylindrical chamber 37

D2% 198
D98% 198
daughter product 20

dead-time 273
decay constant 269
deep expiration breath-hold 126
deep inspiration breath-hold 4, 126
deep X-ray 146
Dees 177
deformable algorithms 106
deformation 106
density 62–7
depth dose 196–7
derived units 13
deterministic effects 256
DICOM conformance statement 71, 72
DICOM RT 71–2, 201
diffusion-weighted MRI 91
digital images 67
digital imaging and communication in medicine
    (DICOM) 71–2, 201
digital radiography 62
diode gun 157
direct action 2
direct digital radiography 62, 68
distortion 106
doping 41
Doppler ultrasound 99–100
dose calculation 204–5
dose length product 45
dose limits 264
dose mapping 197
dose per fraction 7
dose–volume histogram 208
dosimetric shaping 207
dosimetry and dosimeters 35–46
    brachytherapy 295
    computed tomography 45
    megavoltage photons 38–40
    molecular radiotherapy 285–7
    MRI LinAcs 45
    personal dose monitoring 260
    treatment verification 230–1
dot pitch 69
double focused 172
double stacked 172
double strand break 2
drift tube 161
dynamic contrast enhanced CT/MR 107
dynodes 273

echo effect 96
echo time 89
elastic algorithms 106
elastic scattering 49, 50
electric fields 15
electromagnetic induction 16

electromagnetic radiation 16–17
electromagnetic spectrum 17–18
electromagnetic waves 16–17
electron beams 3, 156–7, 168–70
    treatment planning 211–12
electron catcher 155
electron cloud 28
electron dosimetry 39
electron gun 156–7
electron ranges 56–7
electron return effect 173
electron-scattering foils 169
electron target 162
electronic portal imaging device 167
electrons 19
Elekta
    Clarity® Autoscan TPUS 134
    Gammaplan 214
    Unity system 172–3
ELIOT trial 185
emergency radiotherapy 135–6
endometrial brachytherapy 298–300
energy 13
envelope 26
excitation 47, 56, 61
exponential relationship 48
exponentials 10–11
exposure 36
external beam radiotherapy 1
external laser positioning system 79, 92, 114–15
extrinsic registration 104–5

^{18}F-fluorodeoxyglucose (^{18}F-FDG) PET 103,
    107, 279–80
facial masks 119–20
feature detection and matching 105
fidelity 73
fiducials 132–4, 224
field gradient 91
field size 11
filament 25
filters 32–3
    beam-flattening 163
    bowtie 167–8
    composite 151–2
    inherent 149
    Thoraeus 152
    warmup 152
    wedge 206
fixed SSD method 203
flight tube 161
fluorescence 60
focal spot 24, 25–6, 149
focusing cup 25, 148

four-dimensional CT (4DCT) 80–5, 126–7, 212–14, 228
fractional reduction 8
fractions 7
frameless stereotactic radiotherapy 189
Fraxion device 189
free-air ionisation chamber 36–7
functional MRI 91, 107
functional PET 107–8
FusionArc 187–8

gamma analysis 231
gamma camera 272–5, 279
gamma decay 21
gamma knife 182, 214
gamma rays 21
gastrointestinal radiotherapy, treatment verification 236
geometrical shaping 207
graphite calorimeter 40
gray 35
Grenz rays 146
gross tumor volume 115
gynaecological cancer
    brachytherapy 298–300
    treatment verification 236

hadron therapy 177
hadrons 18
Halcyon linear accelerator 174
half-life 8, 21–2, 269
half-value layer 31, 48–9
halo device 140
head and neck
    brachytherapy 302
    immobilisation 117–21
    superficial radiotherapy 134–5
    treatment verification 231–2
head ring 140
head supports 118
heat 13–15
helical scanners 74
helical tomotherapy 170–1
Hertz 94
hinge angles 166
HL7 71
homogeneity index 208
hospital information systems 72
hot spots 101
Hounsfield unit 76
hybrid imaging 103–4, 107, 108, 277–9, 280–1
HybridArc IMRT 187–8

ICRU reference point 198
image fusion 104–7

image-guided radiotherapy 4, 224 *see also* treatment verification
image registration 104–7
image storage 72–3
immobilisation 4, 111, 112
    anal margin disease 137
    breast 122–5
    emergency radiotherapy 135–6
    extremities 138–9
    head and neck 117–21
    internal 131
    paediatric patients 139–40
    palliative radiotherapy 135–6
    pelvis 128–34
    penis 138
    perineum disease 137
    prostate 130, 131–2
    proton beam therapy 121–2
    seated treatment 136–7
    shells 117
    stereotactic radiotherapy 140–1
    superficial radiotherapy 134–5
    surgical 129
    thorax 128
    total body irradiation 137
incandescence 28
indirect action 2
inelastic scattering *see* Compton scattering
inherent filtration 149
intensity 31–3, 47, 96–7
intensity-modulated proton therapy 180
intensity-modulated radiotherapy (IMRT)
    breast 124
    forward planning 209
    HybridArc 187–8
    inverse planning 209
    planning target volume 116
    point dose verification 230–1
    quality assurance 217
    treatment delivery and planning 3–4, 186–7, 207, 209–11
interaction space 155
interfraction variability 116, 130
interlocks 259–60
internal margin 116, 198, 222
International Commission on Radiation Units and Measurements (ICRU) 260–1
    treatment planning guidelines 198–9
International Commission on Radiological Protection (ICRP) 261
interplay effect 85
Intrabeam® (Zeiss) 183–4
intrafraction motion 228–9
intrafraction variability 116, 130
intraoperative radiotherapy 5, 182–6

intrapelvic prostheses 129
intravenous contrast 79–80
intrinsic registration 105
inverse square law 11–12, 153
iodine-131 272
ion pumps 160
ionisation 47, 56, 61
Ionising Radiation (Medical Exposure)
    Regulations 2017/2018 (IR(ME)R) 242, 249,
    250–1, 256, 260, 261–2, 282–3
Ionising Radiation Regulations 2017 (IRR) 242,
    249, 260, 263–4, 282–3
IPerfexion® 182
iridum-192 293
ISO 9000 245
isocentric method 203
isochronous cyclotron 178
isodose curves 197
isotopes 20

kerma 38
kilovoltage equipment 3, 145–53
    applicators 150–1
    beam characteristics 152
    beam quality 151
    collimation 150–1
    control console 147
    cooling system 149–50
    filtration 151–2
    generators 146–7
    inverse square law 153
    low energy beams 146
    medium energy beams 146
    orthovoltage beams 146
    purposes 23–4
    quality assurance 153
    superficial beams 146
    tube design 148–9
    tube mounting 147–8
    very low energy beams 145–6
kinetic energy 13
klystron 155

landmarks 105, 113
Larmor frequency 87
laser positioning 79, 92, 114–15
latent image 60
lead 57
lead cutouts 135, 151
leg stocks 128
leptons 18
Liac system 184, 185
ligands 281
limb immobilisation 138–9
line focus principle 26

linear accelerators (LinAcs) 3, 153–76
    accelerating structure 157–60
    beam-flattening filter 163
    bending magnets 161–2
    C-band 170
    collimators 164–5
    components 154
    cooling system 160
    couches 166–7
    CyberKnife 174–5, 189, 229
    electron beams 168–70
    electron gun 156–7
    electronic portal imaging device 167
    flattening filter free mode 163
    focusing coils 160–1
    Halcyon 174
    helical tomotherapy 170–1
    imaging systems 167–70
    intraoperative 184–5
    ionisation chamber 163
    klystron 155
    loads 160
    magnetron 154–5
    MRI 45, 171–3
    multi-energy units 154
    multimodal units 154
    onboard imager 167
    optical system 163–4
    patient support system 166–7
    quality assurance 175–6, 243
    radiofrequency generators 154–5
    S-band 170
    steering coils 161
    target 162–4
    treatment head 162–6
    vacuum pumps 160
    waveguide 155–6, 158–60
    wedges 165–6
    X-band 170
linear array probe 99
linear attenuation coefficient 49
liquid crystal displays 69
lithium fluoride 43–4
local rules 263
logarithms 10
look-up tables 68
Lorentz forces 160, 173

magnetic resonance imaging (MRI) 86–93
    aperture size 92
    couches 92
    diffusion-weighted 91
    dynamic contrast enhanced 107
    external laser positioning systems 92
    functional (BOLD) 91, 107

magnetic resonance imaging (MRI) (*cont'd*)
  intrafraction motion 228
  limitation of use 91–2
  linear accelerators 45, 171–3
  patient model 200–1
  PET-MRI 108, 278–9, 280–1
  physical principles 86–91
  safety 92, 93
  signal-to-noise ratio 92–3
  simulators 92–3
  SPECT-MRI 279
  T1 and T2 relaxation 88–9
  T1- and T2-weighted images 89–90
  treatment verification 226
magnetism 16
magnetron 154–5
magnification 12
Mammosite® balloon catheters 302
map 62
mass numbers 19
mathematical skills 7–12
maximum intensity projection 84–5
mechanical movement probe 99
megavoltage photons 38–40
metal-ceramic tubes 148
metastability 268
microshells 123
millimetres of lead equivalent 57
minimum intensity projection 84, 85
Mobetron system 184–5
modified scattering *see* Compton scattering
molecular imaging 281–2
molecular radiotherapy 281–2, 284–7
molybdenum/technetium generator 269–71
monoclonal antibodies 282
Monte Carlo algorithms 205
motorized wedges 165
MR spectroscopy 107
multi-leaf collimators 164–5, 203
multi-slice CT 74–5
mutual information 105
MV EPID 230
mycosis fungoides 137, 189–90

n-type detectors 41
nanoparticles 281
negatron 55
net spin 86
neuroendocrine tumours 281–2
neutrons 18, 19
no action level protocol 227
nodes 158
non-conformance 247
non-rigid transformation algorithms 106

non-synchronous precession 87
normal tissue complication probability 3, 111
normalisation 197
Novac7 system 184, 185
nuclear magnetic resonance 86
nuclear spin 86–7
nucleus 19
nuclides 20

obese patients 129
object-oriented programming 71
offline adaptive radiotherapy 188
offline correction 227
Ohm's law 15–16
omentoplasty 129
onboard imager 167
online adaptive radiotherapy 188
online correction 227
optically stimulated luminescence
    dosimetry 44–5
optimisation 205–6, 209–11
organs at risk 4, 199
oversampling 82

p-type semiconductors 41
paediatric patients 139–40
pair production 55–6
palliative treatment 1, 3, 135–6
pancake chamber 38
parallel plate chamber 38
parent nucleus 20
Pareto optimal plan 211
particle accelerators 177–9
passive scattering 179–80
passive screens 69
patient model 199–201
pelvis
    immobilisation 128–34
    treatment verification 236
pencil-beam algorithms 204–5
pencil-beam scanning 180
penetration 31, 60, 62–3
penis immobilisation 138
penumbra 164, 203
percentage depth dose 196–7
percentages 8–9
performance interlocks 260
performance tolerance definitions 243
perineum disease 137
personal dose monitoring 260
PET-CT 103–4, 277–8
PET-MRI 108, 278–9, 280–1
PETG plastic shells 119
phantoms 58

phase-based sorting 83
photocathode 273
photoelectric absorption 50–2
photoelectrons 50
photographic effect 60
photomultiplier tubes 273
photons 3, 62
photonuclear disintegration 49–50
photostimulable phosphor imaging plate 60
picture archiving and communication system
    (PACS) 69, 71, 72
piezoelectric crystals 96
pixellated 68
pixels 67, 68
plain radiography 67–73
Plan-Do-Study-Act (PDSA) cycle 245
plan-of-the-day approach 188, 216, 229
planning target volume 115–16
play therapy 140
pneumotachograph spirometry 125
point dose verification 230–1
polyethylene terephthalate glycol plastic
    shells 119
polyurethane foam moulds 129
positioning patients 111–12
    laser use 79, 92, 114–15
    see also immobilisation
positron 55
positron emission tomography (PET) 21,
    101–4, 275–7
    ^{18}F-FDG 103, 107, 279–80
    functional 107–8
    hot spots 101
    hybrid imaging 103–4, 108, 277–9, 280–1
    image reconstruction 102–3
    patient model 201
    PET-CT 103–4, 277–8
    PET-MRI 108, 278–9, 280–1
    physical principles 102–3
    radiopharmaceuticals 103, 107–8, 279–80
potential difference 28
potential energy 13
precesses 86
precessional frequency 86–7
prefixes 13
pregnancy 283, 284
pressure-sensitive abdominal belts 81
pre-treatment imaging 59–110
primary barrier 257
primary collimator 164
primary dataset 106
primary standard 35
proactive risk assessment 249
probes 96, 98–9

prone positioning 112
proportionality 8
prostate
    brachytherapy 300–1
    fiducials 133–4
    immobilisation 130, 131–2
    spacers 131–2
    treatment verification 235–6
    ultrasound 134
proton beam therapy 3, 5, 176–81
    accuracy 180
    immobilisation 121–2
    intensity-modulated 180
    particle accelerators 177–9
    pencil-beam (spot) scanning 180
    radiation protection 257
    rationale 181
    shielding 179
    treatment planning 212
    treatment room and gantry 179–80
protons 18, 19
pulse-echo technique 97
pulse height analyser 274–5
pulse sequence 89–90

quality assurance 106–7, 153, 175–6, 217,
    242–4, 296
Quality Assurance in Radiotherapy report 244
quality control 217, 242–4
quality management 241–54
quality management systems (QMS) 244,
    245, 246–7
quantitation 275
quarks 18

radiation detection and measurement 35–46
    see also dosimetry and dosimeters
radiation of heat 14–15
radiation protection 57, 255–65, 282–3
Radiation Protection Advisor (RPA) 263
Radiation Protection Supervisor (RPS) 263–4
radical treatment 1, 3
radioactive decay 20–1, 268–9
radioactive family 20
radioactivity 20–2
radiofrequency pulse 87
radioimmunotherapy 282
radioisotopes 20, 268
radiology information systems 72
radionuclides 267–87
    generator systems 269–72
    imaging equipment 272–5
    imaging use 268
    therapeutic use 268

radiopharmaceuticals 103, 107–8, 267, 279–81
radiotherapy error 251
random error 222
RapidArc® 187
ratios 8
ray sum 76
reactive risk assessment 249–50
real-time position management system 126
receptor imaging 281–2
record and verify systems 208, 237–8
rectal balloon catheter 131
rectal spacers 131–2
reference dataset 106
reference points 113
reflection target 162
reflective surface markers 80–1
region of interest 78
relative biological effectiveness 181
relativistic change in mass 157
repetition time 89
reporting and learning systems 252
resistance 15–16
resolution 67, 69
respiratory correlated CT *see* four-dimensional CT
respiratory movements 125–7
retrospective data processing 82
rigid transformation algorithms 105–6
risk assessment 249–50
risk management 248–9
risk reduction 250
root cause analysis 249–50
rounding 9

S-band linear accelerators 170
safety issues 2, 92, 93, 100–1, 296–7
saturation recovery sequence 89
scatter maximum ratio 197
scattering 47
screen resolution 69
seated treatment 136–7
secondary barrier 257
secondary collimator 164
secondary dataset 106
secondary scatter grids 67
secondary standards 35
segmentation 105
semiconductor detectors 41–3, 230
semi-logarithmic scale 10
semipermanent skin marks 113–14
seromas 233
service class provider 71
service class user 71
service classes 71
service object pair 71

setup margin 116, 198, 222
shadow image 62
Sievert integral tables 214
signal-to-noise ratio 92–3
significant figures 9
silicon 41
similar triangles 11
similarity metrics 105
simulators 78–80, 92–3
single photon emission computed tomography
    (SPECT) 275, 279
  SPECT-CT 277
  SPECT-MRI 279
single strand break 2
skin-sparing effect 57, 203–4
SOP classes 71
source bushing assembly 182
source retraction failure protocol 297
space charge 28
space charge wheel 155
SPECT 275, 279
SPECT-CT 277
SPECT-MRI 279
spin-echo sequence 89
spin magnet 87
spiral scanners 74
spirometry 81–2, 125
spot scanning proton therapy 180
stand-in 153
stand-off 153
standard form 10
standing waveguide 158–60
stepping source machines 293
stereotactic ablative radiotherapy 5, 188
stereotactic body radiotherapy 5, 188
stereotactic bodyframe 141
stereotactic head frame 140
stereotactic radiosurgery 140, 188–9, 214
stereotactic radiotherapy 5, 140–1, 188–9
stochastic effects 256
sulphur hexafluoride 156
Sun Nuclear Daily QA™3 175
superficial radiotherapy 134–5
supervised area 264
supine positioning 112
support bras 124
surface-guided radiotherapy 226, 228
surface tracking 81, 126–7
surgical immobilisation 129
systematic error 222

T1 88
T1 relaxation 88–9
T1-weighted images 89

T2 88
T2 relaxation 88–9
T2-weighted images 89–90
target 24, 25–6
  angle 149
  definition 115–16
  interaction 28–30
TARGIT-A trial 185–6
tattoos 4, 113–14
technetium-99m 268, 279
temperature 13–15
tenth-value layer 49, 258
tertiary standards 35
theranostics 281
thermionic emission 25, 27–8, 148, 155
thermions 28
thermoluminescent dosimeters 43–4, 230
thermoplastic shells 119, 120
thimble chamber 37
Thoraeus filter 152
thorax immobilisation 128
three-dimensional (3D) conformal
    radiotherapy 124, 186, 230
three-dimensional (3D) printed bolus 117
time trend error 223
tin filters 151
tissue compensation 207
tissue equivalent material 58, 116
tissue interaction 2–3, 62
tissue maximum ratio 196–7
TomoDirect 171
tomotherapy 170–1
total body irradiation 137, 191–2
total mass attenuation coefficient 49
total skin electron beam therapy (total body
    electrons) 137–8, 189–91
Towards Safer Radiotherapy 246, 251, 253
transducer probes 96, 98–9
transformation model 105
transit dosimetry 230
transmission 97
transmission penumbra 164, 203
transmission target 162
travelling wave waveguide 158
treatment accuracy 4, 111–43
treatment delivery 3–4, 186–92, 228, 229,
    238–9, 296–7
treatment planning 3–4, 195–219
  adaptive radiotherapy 215–17
  beam setup 202–4
  beam weighting 207
  brachytherapy 214–15
  contouring 199–202
  dose calculation 204–5

electron beam 211–12
4DCT 212–14
ICRU guidelines 198–9
intensity-modulated radiotherapy 209–11
intensity modulators 207
objectives 199
optimisation 205–6, 209–11
plan evaluation 207–8
plan export 208–9
principles 196–7
process 199–209
proton beam 212
quality assurance 217
stereotactic radiosurgery 214
systems 4, 208
tissue compensation 207
treatment rooms 259
treatment verification 221–40
  action levels 227–8
  adaptive radiotherapy 229
  additional dose 229–30
  breast 232–4
  chest 234–5
  dosimetry 230–1
  geometric uncertainty 222–3
  head and neck 231–2
  imaging frequency 227
  imaging modality 223–6
  intrafraction motion management 228–9
  method of error correction 226–7
  pelvis 236
  prostate 235–6
  protocols 223
  site-specific uncertainties 231–6
triode gun 157
tumour control probability 3, 111
tumour (molecular) imaging 281–2
tungsten 25, 148
two-dimensional (2D) imaging 61–7

ultrasound (US) 93–101
  colour Doppler 99–100
  coupling medium 98
  Doppler imaging 99–100
  equipment 94–5
  image production 94, 96, 98
  intrafraction motion 228
  linear array probes 99
  mechanical movement probe 99
  physical principles 94–9
  safety 100–1
  spectral Doppler 100
  transducer probes 96, 98–9
  treatment verification 134, 225

unipolar tubes 147
units of measurement 13
Unity system (Elekta) 172–3
uterine brachytherapy 298–300

vacuum bag systems 128–9
vaginal vault brachytherapy 298–9
video-based patient motion tracking 126
ViewRay™ MRIdian system 171–2, 173
virtual wedges 165–6
voltage/volts 15
volume definitions 115–16
volumetric modulated arc therapy
    (VMAT) 3–4, 133, 187
voluntary reporting 252
voxel intensity 105
voxels 75–6

warmup filters 152
warning lights 259
warning signs 259

warping 106
wave–particle duality 17
waveguide 155–6, 158–60
wedge angle 166, 206
wedge filter 206
wedges 165–6, 206
windowing 76

X-band linear accelerators 170
X-ray
    beam quality 31–3, 62–3
    beam quantity 62
    interaction with matter 47–58
    output intensity 31–3
    production 3, 23–33, 62
    properties 59–61
    spectrum 30
    tube 24–7
Xoft Axxent (Xstrahl) 184

Zevalin 282